Aesthetic Surgery After Massive Weight Loss

Commissioning Editors: Sue Hodgson, Geoff Greenwood
Development Editor: Martin Mellor Publishing Services Ltd
Project Manager: Rory MacDonald
Design Manager: Andy Chapman
Illustration Manager: Bruce Hogarth
Illustrator: Paul Banville
Marketing Managers (UK/USA): John Canelon, Lisa Damico

Aesthetic Surgery After Massive Weight Loss

J. Peter Rubin MD

Director, Life After Weight Loss Program
Assistant Professor of Plastic Surgery
Department of Surgery
University of Pittsburgh
Pittsburgh, PA, USA

Alan Matarasso MD

Clinical Professor of Plastic Surgery
Albert Einstein College of Medicine
New York, NY, USA

SAUNDERS
ELSEVIER

SAUNDERS
ELSEVIER

An imprint of Elsevier Inc

ISBN-13: 978-1-4160-2952-6
ISBN-10: 1-4160-2952-4

British Library Cataloguing in Publication Data
A catalogue record for this book is available from the British Library

Library of Congress Cataloging in Publication Data
A catalog record for this book is available from the Library of Congress

Notice

Medical knowledge is constantly changing. Standard safety precautions must be followed, but as new research and clinical experience broaden our knowledge, changes in treatment and drug therapy may become necessary or appropriate. Readers are advised to check the most current product information provided by the manufacturer of each drug to be administered to verify the recommended dose, the method and duration of administration, and contraindications. It is the responsibility of the practitioner, relying on experience and knowledge of the patient, to determine dosages and the best treatment for each individual patient. Neither the Publisher nor the author assume any liability for any injury and/or damage to persons or property arising from this publication.
The Publisher

Printed in China
Last digit is the print number: 9 8 7 6 5 4 3 2 1

CONTENTS

CONTRIBUTORS

Siamak Agha-Mohammadi MD PhD
Clinical Assistant Professor of Surgery (Plastic)
Division of Plastic Surgery
University of Pittsburgh
Pittsburgh, PA, USA

Al S. Aly MD FACS
Plastic Surgeon
Iowa City Plastic Surgery
Coralville, IA, USA

Loren J. Borud MD
Plastic Surgeon
Beth Israel Deaconess Medical Center;
Harvard Medical School
Boston, MA, USA

Stacy A. Brethauer MD
Fellow, Advanced Laparoscopic and Bariatric Surgery
Cleveland Clinic
Cleveland, OH, USA

Joseph F. Capella MD
Plastic Surgeon
Surgical Weight Reduction and Body Contouring
Ramsey, NJ, USA

Robert F. Centeno MD
Plastic Surgeon
Body Aesthetic Plastic Surgery and Skincare Center
St Louis, MO, USA

Susan E. Downey MD FACS
Clinical Associate Professor of Plastic Surgery
Keck School of Medicine
University of Southern California
Los Angeles, CA, USA

Felmont F. Eaves III MD
Attending Surgeon
Charlotte Plastic Surgery
Charlotte, NC, USA

David T. Greenspun MD MSc
Plastic Surgeon
Private Practice
New York, NY, USA

Dennis J. Hurwitz MD FACS
Clinical Professor of Surgery (Plastic)
University of Pittsburgh Medical Center
Pittsburgh, PA, USA

Alan Matarasso MD
Clinical Professor of Plastic Surgery
Albert Einstein College of Medicine
New York, NY, USA

James P. O'Toole MD
Body Contouring Fellow
Division of Plastic Surgery
University of Pittsburgh Medical Center
Pittsburgh, PA, USA

Ivo Pitanguy MD
Head Professor
Department of Plastic Surgery
Pontifical Catholic University of Rio de Janeiro;
Carlos Chagas Post-Graduate Medical Institute;
Director
Clinica Ivo Pitanguy
Rio de Janeiro, Brazil

Henrique N. Radwanski MD
Assistant Professor of Plastic Surgery
Pontifical Catholic University of Rio de Janeiro;
Carlos Chagas Post-Graduate Medical Institute
Rio de Janeiro, Brazil

J. Peter Rubin MD
Director, Life After Weight Loss Program;
Assistant Professor of Plastic Surgery
Department of Surgery
University of Pittsburgh
Pittsburgh, PA, USA

Philip R. Schauer MD
Professor of Surgery
Cleveland Clinic Lerner School of Medicine;
Director, Advanced Laparoscopic and Bariatric Surgery
Bariatric and Metabolic Institute (BMI)
The Cleveland Clinic
Cleveland, OH, USA

Berish Strauch MD
Professor and Chair
Department of Plastic and Reconstructive Surgery
Albert Einstein College of Medicine and Montefiore Medical Center
Bronx, NY, USA

V. Leroy Young MD
Plastic Surgeon
BodyAesthetic Plastic Surgery and Skincare Center
St Louis, MO, USA

FOREWORD

The historian Arnold J. Toynbee explained the rise of civilization in terms of challenge and response. He could have been describing the history of plastic surgery. Our specialty began because of a need, perhaps the first being to rebuild the nose. Plastic surgery has continued, even flourished, because of its ability to recognize and respond successfully, although not always optimally, to the changing requirements of patients, as this well written, carefully edited and admirably illustrated book testifies.

That human beings have eating disorders, ranging from anorexia to obesity, is a fact and that the United States has an astonishing and disproportionate incidence of the enormously overweight is also a fact. Until recently, weight loss centers, psychotherapists, and questionably effective and frequently dangerous medications, were the usual recourse. Surgery for massive obesity was once considered farfetched, prohibitively dangerous, and even indulgent. Toward these patients our society has had, and to a lessor degree still has, a punitive attitude: "They should be able to work it out themselves through diet and restraint. Why should we devote our resources to their problem?" The reality is that their personal problem is our society's problem, now a healthcare crisis.

With the increasing numbers of the very obese, the realization of their compromised quality and length of life, with better education and more public understanding, as well as improvement in safety and success of bariatric surgery, operative treatment of this condition has not only been accepted by, but also welcomed by, the medical and surgical profession, and certainly by patients and their families.

As the editors, Dr Rubin and Dr Matarasso have so well documented in this book, *Aesthetic Surgery After Massive Weight Loss*, the combined best of our aesthetic as well as our reconstructive skills. The surgical demands are difficult, and not to be undertaken casually by someone inexperienced who has not seriously studied, and hopefully observed, surgeons who have learned how best to minimize complications and to secure results beyond merely satisfactory. For anyone contemplating doing these operations, whether plastic surgeon or general surgeon, and to anyone interested in this area of medicine, this book is important and essential. It is not just informative and helpful but honest, born of extensive experience on the part of the contributors, as well as the editors. They have been more than willing to share their mistakes in judgment, their errors of execution, and their ways of dealing with undesirable outcomes.

Bariatric surgery, in joining together with various specialties, including psychotherapy, internal medicine, general surgery, anesthesiology and plastic surgery, has been good for our specialty. It has returned us again to the mainstream where we belong and where we can interact and learn from colleagues in other fields who also can learn from us – all to the benefit of the patient who is and must always be our primary focus.

The bariatric surgeon now realizes, and certainly the patient has long known, that losing weight through an operation is not the end of the treatment. The long, painful journey for the patient is not over but the destination is in sight. That person still confronts physical deformity, emotional distress and additional operations because of excess tissue in numerous areas of the body. The patient, who has already endured so much, wants finally to look and be normal, a desire which is shared by most who seek plastic surgery.

My congratulations to the editors, the contributors, and the publishers for bringing this fine book to fruition.

Robert M. Goldwyn MD
Clinical Professor of Surgery
Harvard Medical School;
Editor Emeritus
Plastic and Reconstructive Surgery
Journal of the American Society of Plastic Surgeons

FOREWORD

Obesity is a rapidly growing disease that has spread widely in the western world and presents as an emerging issue in developing countries. The increase of the obese population has popularized the demand for bariatric surgery, and it is estimated that more than 70% of the patients who undergo such surgery state that, due to skin laxity and ptosis of certain anatomical areas, significant weight loss causes an unacceptable worsening of their body image. This becomes more relevant in our beauty-centered global society, where life is fast-paced and people are rapidly judged with regards to their appearance. It has therefore become more common for the patient who has undergone a great amount of weight reduction to present to the plastic surgeon requesting the removal of excess skin, from one or, more typically, many regions of the body.

In this timely book, *Aesthetic Surgery After Massive Weight Loss*, the various body contour deformities are addressed. Several authors, from many different medical specialties, and some who are well known for their work in aesthetic plastic surgery, present their experience in the treatment of the patient following great weight loss. Under the careful and competent supervision of Drs. Rubin and Matarasso, the medical issues pertaining to these patients and the complexity of the different deformities are focused in separate chapters, but with a clear editorial guidance. The editors and authors are to be commended for their contribution to this fascinating subject that is proving to be a new specialty in medicine and, particularly, in aesthetic plastic surgery.

Ivo Pitanguy MD FACS FICS
Professor of the Post-Graduate Courses in Plastic Surgery of the Pontifical Catholic University of Rio de Janeiro and the Carlos Chagas Post-Graduate Medical Institute. Member of the Brazilian Society of Plastic Surgery, the Brazilian National Academy of Medicine, and the Brazilian Academy of Letters.

ACKNOWLEDGMENTS

Each decade has witnessed major advances in our specialty leading to the establishment of new arenas of plastic surgery. Bariatric plastic surgery represents the next dimension in the evolution of our specialty and holds with it the promise and hope of helping many patients.

The editors are extremely grateful to the many experts who contributed to this text. It was only through their commitment of valuable time and energy that such a comprehensive textbook could be produced around an evolving field of plastic surgery. These are skillful surgeons who have focused their creativity on helping the massive weight loss patient achieve their ultimate goals. We recognize the sacrifice that academic contributions entail and appreciate how generous each of the contributors has been in sharing their surgical expertise. Indeed, their diverse perspectives and approaches make this book a valuable resource for all plastic surgeons.

We also wish to thank the editorial team at Elsevier. Their commitment to this project enabled us to invite the top experts in post-bariatric surgery as contributors, and allowed for the highest quality of production.

J. Peter Rubin MD
Alan Matarasso MD

DEDICATION

This book is dedicated to my wife Julie, whose partnership, patience, and constant support of my academic interests have enabled me to pursue this project. To my children, Eliana and Liviya, who inspire me to be more curious every day. And to the memory of my father, Leonard R. Rubin MD, who never stopped searching for new ideas.

J. Peter Rubin MD

Dedicated to:
Daniel MATARASSO ben
Hamaskil Albert MATARASSO

Alan Matarasso MD

WEIGHT LOSS SURGERY: STATE OF THE ART

1

Philip R. Schauer and Stacy A. Brethauer

Key Points

- Patients with a BMI of 40 kg/m^2, or 35 kg/m^2 with severe comorbidities of obesity, qualify for weight loss surgery.
- The type of weight loss procedure performed can have differential effects on weight loss and on long-term nutritional status.
- Most medical comorbidities associated with obesity improve after surgically induced weight loss.
- The most commonly performed procedure is Roux-en-Y gastric bypass.
- Laparoscopic approaches are becoming increasingly common.

OBESITY

Obesity is defined as the accumulation of excess body fat that leads to pathology. This disease can lead to an extensive list of comorbid conditions, the most serious of which are:

- hypertension,
- diabetes,
- heart disease,
- stroke,
- obstructive sleep apnea, and
- degenerative joint disease.

Body mass index (BMI = weight (kg)/height (m)^2) is the primary measurement used to categorize obese patients. In 1991, the National Institutes of Health (NIH) defined morbid obesity as a BMI of 35 kg/m^2 or greater with severe obesity-related comorbidity, or a BMI of 40 kg/m^2 or greater without comorbidity.[1] Patients with a BMI of 50 kg/m^2 or greater are often referred to as superobese or massively obese.

There has been increasing interest in obesity and major advances in bariatric surgery over the past 15 years as the problems associated with morbid obesity and the benefits of surgical treatment for this disease have become more clearly defined.

Epidemiology and risk factors

Obesity is a major public health problem in the USA that has significantly worsened over the past four decades and has now reached epidemic proportions. The National Center for Health Statistics has conducted periodic National Health and Nutrition Examination Surveys (NHANES) since 1960 to determine the prevalence of obesity.[2] According to this continuous study, 65% of US adults are overweight (BMI > 25 kg/m^2) or obese (BMI > 30 kg/m^2). These studies have shown an increase in the prevalence of obesity from 15% in 1980 to 30% in 2002. Additionally, 5% of Americans 20 years of age or older currently have a BMI > 40 kg/m^2. Children and older Americans are increasingly becoming obese as well. Thirty-one percent of children aged 6–19 are at risk for overweight (BMI for age > 85th percentile) or overweight (BMI for age > 95th percentile), and 16% are overweight. Thirty-three percent of Americans over the age of 60 are obese. These increases have occurred despite expenditures of over $45 billion annually on weight loss products.[3]

Obesity and morbid obesity affect women and minorities (particularly middle-aged black and Mexican American women) more than white males. However, in almost every age and ethnic group examined by NHANES, the prevalence of overweight or obesity exceeds 50%.[2]

Etiology

The etiology of obesity is not as straightforward as once thought. It is not simply an excess of caloric intake in relation to caloric expenditure, but a complex interaction of excessive intake, inefficient calorie utilization, reduced metabolic activity, a reduction in the thermogenic response to meals, and an abnormally high set-point for body weight. Genetic, environmental, and psychosocial factors all contribute to this problem. Children of obese parents have an 80–90% chance of developing obesity by adulthood, while only 10% of children of normal-weight parents will become obese. The high-fat and high-calorie American diet in conjunction with a sedentary lifestyle contributes significantly to this problem.

OVERVIEW OF BARIATRIC SURGERY

This section provides an overview of the different weight loss procedures and their physiologic effects.

Goals of surgery and mechanism of action

The goal of bariatric surgery is to improve the health of morbidly obese patients by reducing or eliminating their comorbid conditions. This is achieved by long-term weight loss that involves a significant reduction in caloric intake or absorption.

Bariatric operations that are currently performed involve:

- gastric restriction (vertical banded gastroplasty, VBG) (Fig. 1.1) or laparoscopic adjustable gastric banding (LAGB) (Fig. 1.2),
- malabsorption (biliopancreatic diversion, BPD) or biliopancreatic diversion with duodenal switch (BPD-DS) (Fig. 1.3), or
- a combination of restriction and malabsorption (Roux-en-Y gastric bypass, RYGB) (Fig. 1.4).

Between 1998 and 2003, the number of bariatric operations performed in the USA increased from 13 000 to 103 000 per year.[4] During that period, the percentage of gastroplasty procedures performed declined from 25% to 7%. Gastric bypass procedures comprise over 80% of bariatric procedures currently performed in the USA and 65% of bariatric procedures performed worldwide (Table 1.1).[5]

The choice of operation depends largely on patient preference. There are currently no data available to preoperatively predict which operation a specific patient should undergo. In surveys from the USA and Australia, safety and invasiveness had the greatest impact on patient choice for bariatric operations.[6] Most patients in the USA are currently seeking either gastric bypass or adjustable gastric-banding procedures, and the relative risks and benefits of each must be carefully explained.

- Gastric bypass generally provides more weight loss in a shorter time than LAGB does, but it is more invasive and has a higher mortality rate than LAGB.
- Adjustable gastric banding has the lowest mortality rate of any procedure currently used, but it generally results in less weight loss than with RYGB and involves a permanent foreign body in the abdomen.

Follow-up requirements must be considered preoperatively as well. Gastric bypass requires lifelong vitamin supplementation that can be a cost burden for some patients, while LAGB requires more frequent follow-up visits for band adjustments in

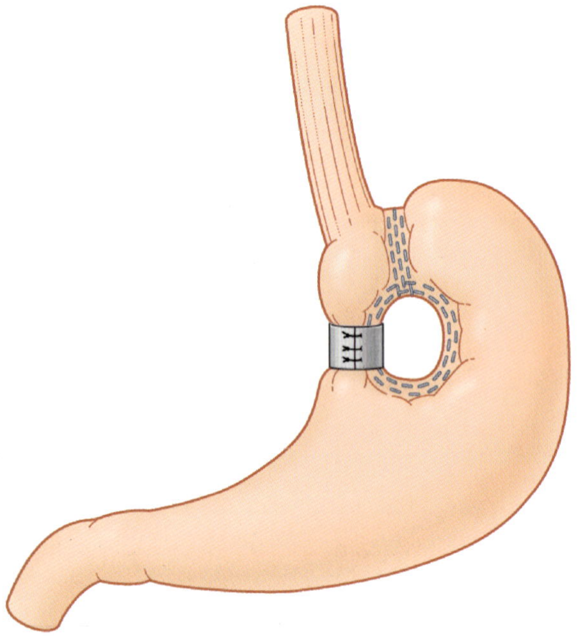

Figure 1.1 Vertical banded gastroplasty (VBS).

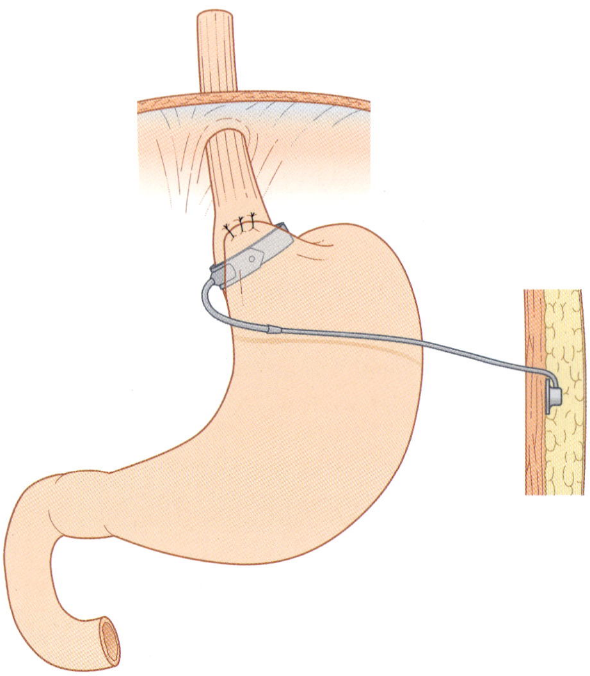

Figure 1.2 Adjustable gastric band (LAGB).

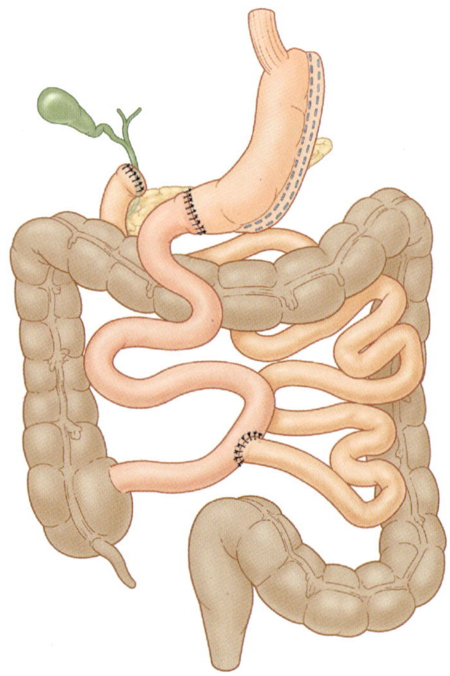

Figure 1.3 Biliopancreatic diversion with duodenal switch (BPD with or without DS).

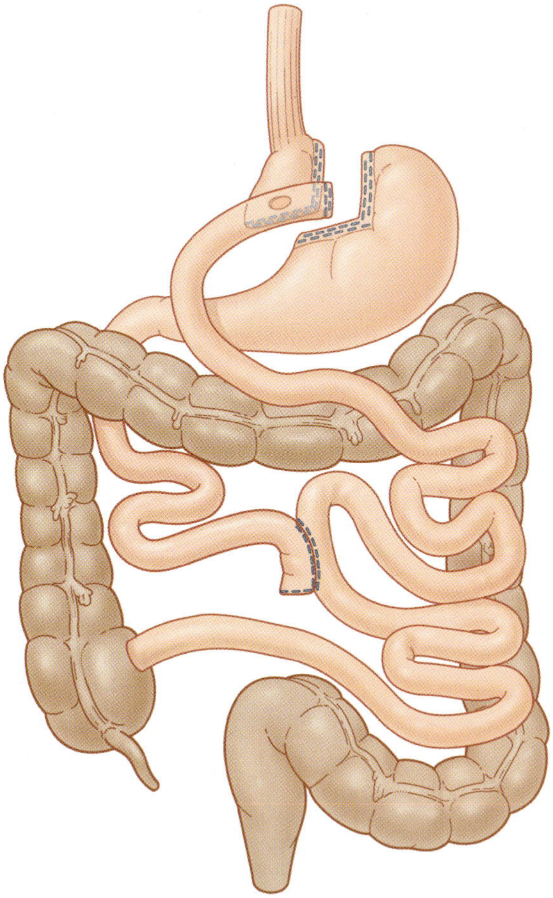

Figure 1.4 Roux-en-Y gastric bypass (RYGB).

Table 1.1 Types of bariatric procedure performed

Procedure	USA (%)	Worldwide (including USA) (%)
Gastric bypass	80	65
Laparoscopic adjustable gastric band	5–10	25
Vertical banded gastroplasty	<5	5
Biliopancreatic diversion/duodenal switch	5–10	5

(Adapted from Buchwald and Williams 2004,[5] with permission.)

the first year after surgery. BPD and duodenal switch procedures are performed at a few specialized centers and are more likely to be performed in superobese patients or patients specifically seeking these operations.

Restrictive procedures work by reducing the quantity of food that can be consumed at one time. In the case of LAGB, the degree of restriction can be increased or decreased based on the patient's weight loss. Malabsorptive procedures ensure that ingested food and digestive enzymes remain separated for a substantial bowel length to limit caloric absorption. RYGB provides a combination of restriction and decreased absorption. The restrictive component of the operation consists of the creation of a small (15–30 mL) gastric pouch. The standard Roux limb is 75 cm in length and results in mild, and probably transient, malabsorption. The long-limb (150 cm) RYGB used for superobese patients results in a greater degree of malabsorption.

The rapid reduction of comorbidities such as diabetes and the long-term weight loss achieved by RYGB and BPD cannot be explained exclusively by restriction or malabsorption. Other mechanisms of weight loss and glucose control following bariatric surgery are being investigated.

- Ghrelin, a peptide hormone produced by the stomach and duodenum, is normally released prior to meals and acts on the hypothalamus to increase appetite. Alterations in ghrelin production may play a role in the decreased appetite and sustained weight loss seen after certain bariatric procedures.
- Other gut hormones, such as peptide YY, glucagon-like peptide-1, and glucose-dependent insulinotropic peptide, may also contribute to the early satiety and rapid reduction of insulin resistance seen after bariatric surgery.
- Obesity is associated with a proinflammatory and prothrombotic state. Increased adipocyte activity, and the associated increase in circulating inflammatory cytokines, may be related to many of the cardiovascular risk factors seen with obesity. Preliminary studies have demonstrated improvement in these detrimental cytokines and adipokines after surgical weight loss.

Evolution of bariatric surgery

The initial operations to treat morbid obesity were performed in the 1950s and were malabsorptive procedures. The jejunocolic and jejunoileal bypass procedures resulted in electrolyte disturbances and liver failure. In 1967, Mason and Ito developed the gastric bypass procedure by creating a 50- to 100-mL proximal gastric pouch that emptied into a loop gastrojejunostomy.[7] Modifications to this procedure over the past 35 years have been directed towards minimizing the complications of bile reflux, anastomotic ulcers, and gastrogastric fistulas, and have resulted in the current Roux-en-Y divided gastric bypass. In the late 1970s, Scopinaro developed the BPD procedure.[8] In this procedure, the small bowel is divided 250 cm proximal to the ileocecal valve, and the alimentary limb is anastomosed to the gastric pouch. The duodenal switch (BPD-DS) is a modification of BPD in which the pylorus is left intact to prevent marginal ulceration and improve gastric emptying.

Gastric banding was also developed in the late 1970s, and the initial use of fixed banding material to create a proximal gastric pouch has evolved into the laparoscopic placement of an adjustable gastric band.

Indications

- Patients with a BMI > 35 kg/m^2 with obesity-related comorbidities, and those with a BMI > 40 kg/m^2 with or without comorbidities, are eligible for bariatric surgery.

- Patients must have attempted medical weight loss programs and should be highly motivated to change their lifestyle after surgery.
- The majority of patients undergoing bariatric surgery are between ages 18 and 60. There was insufficient evidence at the time of the 1991 NIH consensus to make recommendations about surgery at the extremes of age. There is a growing body of evidence, however, that supports bariatric surgery in carefully selected adolescents and in the elderly (> 60 years). The current indications for bariatric surgery may broaden as long-term safety and efficacy studies in these patient groups become available.

Contraindications

- Patients who cannot tolerate general anesthesia due to cardiac, pulmonary, or hepatic insufficiency are not candidates for surgery.
- Additionally, patients must be able to understand the consequences of the surgery and comply with the extensive preoperative evaluation and the postoperative lifestyle changes, diet, vitamin supplementation, and follow-up program.
- Patients who have ongoing substance abuse or unstable psychiatric illness are poor candidates for bariatric surgery.

Preparation for surgery

Surgical candidates must complete a thorough medical evaluation, a psychologic evaluation, and have preoperative testing appropriate for their comorbid conditions. There are over 30 comorbidities associated with obesity, and many of these predispose bariatric surgical patients to increased perioperative risk (Table 1.2). Because morbidly obese patients are at higher risk for having hypertension, diabetes, coronary artery disease, left ventricular hypertrophy, congestive heart failure, and pulmonary hypertension, an electrocardiogram should be performed on every patient, and a preoperative cardiology evaluation should be performed when there is evidence of cardiovascular disease.

Obstructive sleep apnea is frequently occult in this patient population until a thorough history prompts a preoperative evaluation. Patients with symptoms of loud snoring or daytime hypersomnolence should undergo polysomnography and, if positive, be treated with nasal continuous positive airway pressure (CPAP). Because these patients are at risk for upper airway obstruction, close monitoring and nasal CPAP should continue postoperatively. Asthma and obesity hypoventilation syndrome (chronic hypoxemia, hypercarbia, pulmonary hypertension, and polycythemia) are also severe pulmonary complications of obesity and should be evaluated by a pulmonologist preoperatively.

Upper gastrointestinal barium studies and endoscopy should be performed for patients with severe gastroesophageal reflux symptoms. Because the incidence of gallstones is high in this population, preoperative abdominal sonography is routinely performed in many centers.

Table 1.2 Comorbidities associated with obesity

System	Comorbidities
Cardiovascular	Hyperlipidemia Heart failure Myocardial infarction Hypertension Stroke Left ventricular hypertrophy Venous stasis ulcers/thrombophlebitis
Pulmonary	Asthma Obstructive sleep apnea Obesity hypoventilation syndrome Pulmonary hypertension
Endocrine	Insulin resistance Type 2 diabetes Polycystic ovarian syndrome
Hematopoetic	Deep venous thrombosis Pulmonary embolism
Gastrointestinal	Gallstones Gastroesophageal reflux disease Abdominal hernia
Genitourinary	Stress urinary incontinence Urinary tract infections
Obstetric/gynecologic	Infertility Miscarriage Fetal abnormalities and infant mortality
Musculoskeletal	Degenerative joint disease Gout Plantar fasciitis Carpal tunnel syndrome
Neurologic/psychiatric	Intracranial hypertension Depression Anxiety

All bariatric patients should undergo thorough nutritional evaluation and counseling preoperatively. Patients must understand how their diet will change after surgery, and what supplements are necessary to prevent specific nutritional deficiencies. The dietitian plays a key role in determining whether a patient understands the significant changes in diet that will occur after bariatric surgery.

Psychologic testing is performed preoperatively to assess patients' expectations and to ensure that there are no active psychiatric issues that would put the patient at risk for failure or poor compliance postoperatively.

Surgical techniques

Worldwide, two-thirds of bariatric procedures are performed laparoscopically.[5] Adjustable gastric banding is performed exclusively with the laparoscopic approach. Gastric bypass is performed open or laparoscopically, and the approach is primarily determined by the surgeon's training and advanced laparoscopic skills. Some bariatric surgeons perform open RYGB exclusively; others selectively choose the open approach for patients with very high BMIs or multiple prior abdominal operations. Previous abdominal surgery is not a contraindication to the laparoscopic approach, though, and revisional bariatric surgery (conversion of a failed VBG to a RYGB) can be accomplished laparoscopically. Some surgeons advocate performing all gastric bypass procedures with the open technique due to shorter operating times and lower costs, but the introduction of laparoscopy into bariatric surgery has increased the public's demand for this minimally invasive approach and attracted surgeons who are interested in advanced laparoscopic procedures. As experience is gained with the laparoscopic RYGB, operative times decrease and are comparable with those of open surgery. Because of the complexity of the procedures, BPD and BPD-DS have primarily been performed open. There are, however, small series that demonstrate the feasibility of performing these malabsorptive procedures laparoscopically.[9]

There are many well-documented advantages to the laparoscopic approach. The smaller incisions significantly reduce recovery time and postoperative pain compared with a laparotomy. Other benefits include:

- less surgical trauma in the wound and to the viscera;
- improved postoperative pulmonary function; and
- decreased incidence of wound-related complications such as hematomas, seromas, infections, hernias, and dehiscence.[10]

Assessment of results

Outcomes measurement in bariatric surgery is of paramount importance. The NIH consensus conference recommended statistical reporting in bariatric surgery, and it is imperative that surgeons maintain quality outcomes databases in order to track their results, to educate patients, and to demonstrate success to professional societies and insurance companies.

Follow-up

Bariatric surgery patients require lifetime follow-up. Early postoperative visits focus on complications and the dramatic changes in dietary habits. Diet is progressively advanced from liquid to solid food over the first month in consultation with the dietitian. Later follow-up visits focus on psychologic support, nutritional assessment and vitamin supplementation, and exercise programs. At the Cleveland Clinic, patient visits are at 1 week, 1 month, 3 months, 6 months, 9 months, 1 year, and annually thereafter.

Efficacy

Bariatric surgery is one of the few therapies in medicine that result in the simultaneous treatment of multiple diseases. Nonsurgical weight loss programs utilizing diet, exercise, medication, and behavioral modification can induce modest short-term weight loss, but there is currently no diet or medical therapy that results in sustained weight loss to adequately treat morbid obesity and its comorbidities.

There are two randomized controlled trials comparing surgical weight loss and non-surgical weight loss.[11,12] Both of these demonstrated the superiority of surgery over medical therapy in achieving long-term weight loss. The procedures used in these two trials have been replaced with the more effective and less morbid procedures used today.

The Swedish Obese Subjects Study Scientific Group is a prospective, controlled, matched-pair cohort study comparing surgery with non-surgical treatment for obesity. The procedures used were VBG, gastric banding, and gastric bypass.

- After 2 years, the control group's weight increased by 0.1%, and the surgery group had a 23.4% decrease from their preoperative weight.
- Ten-year follow-up of 1268 patients in this study revealed a weight increase of 1.6% in the control group and a weight decrease of 16.1% in the surgery group compared with preoperative weight.
- Only 3.8% of control patients achieved a 20% weight loss over the 10-year period, whereas 73.5% of the gastric bypass group, 35.2% of the VBG group, and 27.6% of the gastric-banding group achieved this level of long-term weight loss.
- Rates of recovery from hypertension, diabetes, hypertriglyceridemia, low high-density lipoprotein cholesterol, and hyperuricemia favored the surgical group at 2 and 10 years.
- The incidence of hypertension and hypercholesterolemia did not differ between groups at 10 years.

This study is ongoing with respect to analyzing mortality and the incidence of cancer, myocardial infarction, and stroke.[13]

A metaanalysis by Buchwald et al. analyzing 22 094 patients in 136 studies found that for all bariatric procedures, the average amount of excess weight loss (EWL = the amount of weight above ideal body weight that is lost, and is assumed to be adipose tissue in most patients) was 61.2%.

- BPD or duodenal switch procedures had the highest overall EWL (70%), followed by gastroplasty (68%), gastric bypass (61%), and gastric banding (47%).
- Overall, diabetes improved or resolved in 86% of patients, hyperlipidemia improved in 70%, hypertension improved or resolved in 78.5%, and obstructive sleep apnea improved or resolved in 83.6% of patients.
- Diabetes outcomes varied with operative procedure. Ninety-nine percent of BPD-DS patients, 84% of gastric bypass patients, 72% of gastroplasty patients, and 48% of gastric-banding patients had complete resolution of their diabetes.
- BPD and gastric bypass patients had the most improvements in hyperlipidemia postoperatively (99% and 97% resolution, respectively), but the reduction of blood pressure was independent of the surgical procedure performed.[14]

The Australian Safety and Efficacy Register of New Interventional Procedures—Surgical (ASERNIP-S) analyzed international data regarding LAGB and 55 papers evaluating VBG and RYGB.[15] The reported 56% EWL at 4-year follow-up after LAGB was comparable with the long-term weight loss achieved with RYGB.

In an observational cohort study, Christou and associates evaluated long-term morbidity and mortality in morbidly obese patients. They compared 1035 patients who underwent RYGB to 5746 age- and gender-matched morbidly obese controls who had non-surgical management of their weight.

- The surgery group had a mean EWL of 67% at 5-year follow-up; > 60% EWL at 16 years (72% follow-up); and significantly reduced risk of developing cardiovascular disease, cancer, infectious diseases, and endocrinologic, musculoskeletal, and respiratory disorders.
- Five-year mortality in the bariatric surgery group was 0.68%, compared with 6.17% in the control group (89% relative risk reduction).[16]

Complications

The risks of bariatric surgery have decreased with increasing experience and technical refinements. The operative mortality for restrictive procedures, gastric bypass, and BPD are 0.1%, 0.5%, and 1.1%, respectively. In the ASERNIP-S review, LAGB had an early mortality of 0.05%. Mortality after bariatric surgery is primarily due to pulmonary embolism and anastomotic leak. Early postoperative complications, particularly septic complications, are less common after restrictive procedures such as VBG and LAGB.

Vertical banded gastroplasty has largely been abandoned due to poor long-term weight loss and the late complications of gastroesophageal reflux, stomal stenosis, staple line dehiscence, and intractable vomiting. Patients with these complications frequently require conversion to a RYGB.

Biliopancreatic diversion and duodenal switch procedures have excellent results in terms of short- and long-term weight loss and resolution of comorbidities, but these procedures have a higher mortality rate than other bariatric procedures and a higher incidence of metabolic and nutritional problems. Operative mortality for BPD ranges from 0.5 to 1.3%. Early postoperative complications include intraperitoneal bleeding, wound dehiscence, wound infection, anastomotic leak, and gastric perforation. Nutritional deficiencies can occur after bariatric procedures that bypass segments of the small bowel (BPD, duodenal switch, and RYGB). Table 1.3 summarizes the data from a review of nutritional deficiencies after bariatric procedures.[17]

Protein malnutrition is characterized clinically by hypoalbuminemia (< 3.5 g/dL), anemia, edema, and alopecia, and occurs 3–18% of the time after BPD or BPD-DS. These patients may require total parenteral nutrition, and 6% will have a revision to lengthen their common channel. Protein malnutrition is seen less frequently after standard RYGB (0–1.4%), but long-limb (> 150 cm) RYGB for superobese patients can result in protein deficiency 3–13% of the time and typically occurs within 2 years of surgery. Iron is absorbed in the duodenum and proximal jejunum, and iron deficiency after

Table 1.3 Nutritional deficiencies after bariatric surgery

Deficiency	Procedure	Incidence (%)	Range of follow-up (months)
Protein malnutrition	BPD, BPD-DS	0–18	24–79
	RYGB	0–13	12–43
Iron	BPD, BPD-DS	23–44	28–48
	RYGB	6–52	20–60
Vitamin B12	BPD, BPD-DS	22	48
	RYGB	8–37	12–48
Folate	–	22–63	12–24
Calcium	Distal RYGB	10	24
	BPD, BPD-DS	25–48	9–48
Vitamin D	Distal RYGB	51	24
	BPD, BPD-DS	17–63	9–48
Thiamine	–	< 1	3–5
Vitamin A	Distal RYGB	10	48
	BPD, BPD-DS	5–69	12–96
Vitamin E	BPD, BPD/DS	5	28–48
Vitamin K	BPD, BPD-DS	50–68[a]	23–48
Zinc	BPD, BPD,DS	10–50	48
Magnesium	BPD, BPD-DS	5	28

BPD, biliopancreatic diversion; BPD-DS, biliopancreatic diversion with duodenal switch; RYGB, Roux-en-Y gastric bypass.
[a]No increased clinical bleeding.
(After Bloomberg et al. 2005,[17] with permission.)

bariatric surgery is seen most commonly after BPD and BPD-DS (23–44%) and RYGB (6–52%). Vitamin B_{12} is absorbed in the terminal ileum, and deficiencies are seen after BPD (22%) and RYGB (8–37%). Calcium absorption (duodenum and jejunum) and vitamin D absorption (jejunum and ileum) are impaired after BPD and RYGB as well, and these deficiencies can lead to secondary hyperparathyroidism and increased bone resorption. Calcium deficiency occurs 10–48% of the time and vitamin D deficiency occurs 17–63% of the time in published studies of malabsorptive procedures.[17] The absorption of fat-soluble vitamins is impaired after BPD due to the relatively short common channel.

Routine vitamin and mineral supplementation and careful attention to protein intake following bariatric surgery are necessary. Serious complications of these deficiencies can generally be avoided by early recognition and increased oral supplementation. Further studies are needed to better define these deficiencies and to determine guidelines for supplementation.

Hospital volume and surgeon experience are important factors in bariatric surgery outcomes. Nguyen and colleagues evaluated outcomes after RYGB according to hospital volume, and found higher morbidity and mortality rates for low-volume (< 50 cases/year) compared with high-volume (> 100 cases/year) centers (1.2% versus 0.3% mortality, respectively).[18] Bariatric surgery, particularly the laparoscopic approach, is technically challenging surgery that involves a learning curve, and complications such as anastomotic leaks and internal hernias are more common earlier in a surgeon's experience. Differences in complication rates between open and laparoscopic procedures are discussed later in this chapter.

BARIATRIC SURGICAL PROCEDURES

Vertical banded gastroplasty

Vertical banded gastroplasty is a purely restrictive procedure that limits the amount of solid food that can be consumed at one time. A proximal gastric pouch empties through a fixed, calibrated stoma that is reinforced with an external silastic band or ring of mesh (Fig. 1.1). The advantages of VBG include:

- improvement of comorbidities after weight loss,
- minimal nutritional deficiencies,
- the absence of any gastrointestinal anastomosis, and
- a lower morbidity and mortality rate than with RYGB.

It can be performed laparoscopically and is technically easier than RYGB. The disadvantages of this procedure include long-term weight loss that is inferior to that of RYGB, particularly in sweet eaters, and multiple long-term complications that frequently require reoperation.

Technique

1. A 32 French Ewald tube is passed into the stomach to size the pouch and stoma.
2. After the retrogastric dissection is completed from the gastrohepatic ligament to the angle of His, the anvil of an EEA circular stapler is placed behind the stomach and manually passed through both walls of the stomach 8–9 cm below the angle of His and adjacent to the Ewald tube.
3. The circular stapler is connected to the anvil and fired, creating a 2.5-cm window in the proximal stomach. Four rows of staples are then fired superiorly from the window to the angle of His to create a 50-mL pouch.
4. A 7 × 1.5 cm strip of polypropylene mesh is then sewn to itself around the outlet channel.

The laparoscopic approach has been used successfully for VBG. A linear-cutting stapler may be used to divide the vertical portion of the pouch or to excise a wedge of the fundus and eliminate the need for a circular stapler.

Efficacy

Vertical banded gastroplasty achieves acceptable early weight loss but has less favorable long-term weight loss than other procedures used today. Ashy and colleagues demonstrated a weight loss advantage of open VBG (87% EWL) over LAGB (50% EWL) at 6 months.[19] Some series have reported adequate long-term success with VBG, but EWL 3–5 years after VBG is typically 30–60%. Ten-year follow-up data show that only 26–40% of patients maintain acceptable weight loss (> 50% EWL), and one-third of patients in these series returned to or exceeded their preoperative weight.[20]

Complications

Early complications after VBG are infrequent, but late complications have resulted in a 17–30% reoperation rate. The most common late complications of VBG are:

- gastroesophageal reflux (16–38%),
- stomal stenosis (20%),
- staple line disruption (11–48%),
- incisional hernia (13%),
- band migration (1.5%), and
- intractable vomiting (30–50%).[21]

Because of the poor long-term weight loss and high late complication rate, VBG has largely been abandoned and is performed by less than 5% of bariatric surgeons in the USA.

Laparoscopic adjustable gastric banding

The LAGB is a restrictive procedure, and the device (Lap-Band; Inamed Corporation, Carpinteria, California) was approved for use in the USA in 2001, after having very good results in Europe and Australia. This silicone band with an inflatable inner collar is placed around the upper portion of the stomach to create a small gastric pouch. The band is connected to a port that is placed in the subcutaneous tissue of the abdominal wall. The inner diameter of the band can be adjusted by injecting saline through the port (Fig. 1.2).

- The adjustable nature of the LAGB is a major advantage that distinguishes it from VBG. Band adjustments are made according to weight loss.
- The LAGB is technically the simplest bariatric surgery to perform and requires less operating time than for other procedures.

- No anastomoses are created, and the morbidity and mortality are low.
- This procedure is reversible and, if patients fail to lose adequate weight after LAGB, it can be converted to a RYGB.

The disadvantages of the LAGB include:

- the need for frequent postoperative visits for band adjustments, and
- band slippage or gastric prolapse through the band (5–10%).

These mechanical complications require reoperation. Band erosion into the stomach, gastroesophageal reflux, esophageal dilatation, and dysmotility can also occur.

Technique

1. The patient is placed in steep reverse Trendelburg position, and six laparoscopic ports are placed.
2. The left lobe of the liver is retracted anteriorly, and a 15-mL balloon is placed transorally to calibrate the gastric pouch.
3. The pars flaccida technique is used to create a retrogastric tunnel from the base of the right crus of the diaphragm to the angle of His.
4. The band is passed through the retrogastric tunnel toward the angle of His and encircles the stomach approximately 1 cm below the gastroesophageal junction.
5. The tail of the band is passed through the buckle, and the band is locked in place around the gastric cardia.
6. A calibration tube is passed to assess the size of the stoma, and the anterior stomach is sutured over the band with interrupted sutures.
7. The tube attached to the band is brought out through a left-sided trocar site and attached to the port.
8. The port is then placed in a subcutaneous pocket and sutured to the anterior rectus sheath.

Patients remain in the hospital for 1 or 2 days, and a Gastrografin swallow is done prior to discharge to confirm band position and patency. Patients are kept on a liquid diet for 1 month postoperatively, at which time solid food can be introduced. Band adjustments can be made with or without fluoroscopic guidance. The first band adjustment is performed 4–8 weeks postoperatively, and patients are then observed monthly for the first year to assess weight loss and to make further adjustments if necessary.

Efficacy

Reports of weight loss after LAGB have been variable but generally fall in the 40–55% EWL range 3 years after the procedure. Weight loss after LAGB is more gradual than with RYGB, and most of the weight loss after LAGB takes place in the first 3 years after surgery. O'Brien reported results on 706 patients undergoing the LAGB in Australia, with a mean EWL of 57% at 72 months and major improvements in diabetes, asthma, gastroesophageal reflux, dyslipidemia, sleep apnea, depression, and quality of life.[22] The Italian Collaborative Study Group for the Lap-Band system reviewed 1863 patients undergoing LAGB. Six-year follow-up showed a steady decrease in BMI from a preoperative average of 43 kg/m^2 to a BMI of 32 kg/m^2 at 72 months.[23]

Initial results with the LAGB in the USA were not as favorable as those in Europe and Australia. EWL at 2-year follow-up was typically reported to be between 35 and 45%. Some recent US studies of LAGB have approached the success rates seen in international studies, though, including a report of 1014 Lap-Band procedures with 64% EWL at 4 years (> 85% follow-up). In this study, 75% of patients achieved satisfactory weight loss (> 50% EWL) at 4 years.[24]

Complications

Laparoscopic adjustable gastric banding has a low operative mortality (0.05%) and an 11% rate of perioperative and late complications.[15] Postoperative mortality was 0.53% in the Italian Collaborative Study, and the ASERNIP-S review reported three deaths in 5827 LAGB cases (0.05%). Intraoperative bleeding or injury to the stomach, esophagus, or spleen occurs less than 1% of the time.

- Early postoperative complications include bleeding (0.5%), wound infection (0–1%), and food intolerance (0–11%).
- Late complications include band slippage or gastric prolapse through the band (7–21%), band erosion (2–7%), tube-related problems (4%), persistent vomiting (13%), pouch dilatation (5%), and gastroesophageal reflux.

In a study of 1120 patients, O'Brien and Dixon reported a 1.5% early major complication rate.[25] These complications included 10 access port infections; four patients with delayed emptying through the band; and one case each of deep venous thrombosis, hepatotoxicity, and bile leak from the liver. The most common late complication requiring reoperation after LAGB is gastric prolapse or slippage. As experience was gained, the rate of this complication decreased from 25% to 4.7%. Erosion of the band into the stomach occurred in 3% of patients early in the authors' experience, and problems with the access port occurred in 5.4% of their patients. Although esophageal dilatation was common after prolapse or aggressive band adjustments, no persistent esophageal dilatation or dysmotility was found after appropriate treatment of the prolapse or decreased band restriction.

Roux-en-Y gastric bypass

Roux-en-Y gastric bypass combines a restrictive and a malabsorptive procedure, and is the most commonly performed bariatric procedure in the USA (80%). A small 15- to 30-mL gastric pouch is created to restrict food intake, and a Roux-en-Y gastrojejunostomy provides the malabsorptive component (Fig. 1.4).

The advantages of RYGB include:

- superior weight loss when compared with VBG,
- excellent long-term reduction in EWL, and
- resolution or elimination of comorbidities.

Early and late complication rates are reasonably low, and operative mortality ranges from 0 to 0.5%. Dumping syndrome may occur after RYGB, and this may discourage patients from eating sweets.

Disadvantages of RYGB include:

- the potential for anastomotic leaks and strictures,
- severe dumping syndrome symptoms, and
- procedure-specific complications including distension of the excluded stomach and internal hernias.

The RYGB is technically more challenging to perform than the restrictive procedures, particularly using the laparoscopic approach.

Open RYGB technique

1. The abdomen is entered through an upper midline incision, and a thorough exploration is completed.
2. The anterior and lateral phrenoesophageal ligament is opened to the angle of His.
3. The distal esophagus is mobilized and encircled with a Penrose drain, and the gastrohepatic ligament is opened over the caudate lobe.
4. The mesentery between the second and third branches of the left gastric artery is divided, and a retrogastric space is developed from the lesser curvature to the angle of His.
5. The pouch can be formed using a series of firings with a linear-cutting stapler to create a vertically oriented pouch, or a red rubber tube placed in the retrogastric space can be used to guide 90-mm linear staplers behind the stomach to create a 15- to 30-mL pouch.
6. The ligament of Treitz is identified, and the jejunum is divided with a linear stapler 15–45 cm distal to the ligament.
7. A standard length (75 cm) or long-limb length (150 cm for BMI > 50 kg/m^2) Roux limb is measured, and the jejunojejunostomy is created with the linear stapler.
8. The mesenteric defect at the jejunojejunostomy is closed with suture.
9. The Roux limb can be brought up to the gastric pouch retrocolic and retrogastric, retrocolic and antegastric, or antecolic and antegastric, depending on the surgeon's preference and tension on the Roux limb. If the Roux limb is brought through the transverse mesocolon, the space between the jejunal and transverse colon mesenteries is closed (Peterson's space) to prevent internal herniation of small bowel.
10. A 1- to 1.5-cm gastrojejunostomy is either hand-sewn over a 30-F dilator or created with a circular stapler.
11. The anastomosis is tested with air insufflation or injection of methylene blue through a carefully guided nasogastric tube or with intraoperative endoscopy.

Laparoscopic RYGB technique

1. After pneumoperitoneum is established, five or six access ports are placed.
2. The sequential firings of a linear cutting stapler are used to create a vertically oriented gastric pouch measuring 15–30 mL.
3. The ligament of Treitz is identified, and the jejunum is divided 10–12 cm distally with a linear stapler.
4. A 75- to 150-cm Roux limb is measured, and a side-to-side jejunojejunostomy is created with a linear stapler. Several techniques can be used to create the gastrojejunal anastomosis.
   If a circular stapler is used, the anvil can be pulled into the pouch transorally using endoscopy and placement of a loop wire percutaneously into the gastric pouch.
   In the transgastric method, the anvil is placed in the stomach through a distal gastrotomy prior to pouch formation. The anvil is then positioned in the upper stomach and included in the pouch that is created with a linear stapler.
   The current method favored by the authors is placement of continuous layer of sutures to approximate the Roux limb and pouch, followed by the creation of a side-to-side anastomosis with a linear stapler.
5. The anastomosis is completed with two layers of running suture anteriorly over a flexible endoscope. The anastomosis can also be completely hand-sewn in two layers.
6. The anastomosis is tested for integrity and hemostasis with the flexible endoscope. The conversion rate to open RYGB is < 5%.

Efficacy

The RYGB results in mean EWL ranging from 65 to 80% in studies with follow-up of 2 years or less. There is no significant difference in weight loss between the open and laparoscopic approach, and weight loss typically reaches a nadir 18–24 months after surgery. In a study by Schauer and colleagues, the mean EWL was 83% at 1 year and 77% at 30 months.[26] Longer follow-up after RYGB reveals some weight regain, with 60–70% EWL at 5 years. The Swedish Obese Subjects Study demonstrated 10-year weight loss (as a percentage of initial body weight) of 25% for RYGB.[13]

Nguyen and colleagues compared laparoscopic ($n = 79$) to open ($n = 76$) RYGB and found a longer operative time but shorter hospital stay (3 versus 4 days) in the laparoscopic group. Weight loss at 1 year was similar between groups, but the laparoscopic group had fewer wound complications and a more rapid return to daily activities.[27]

The RYGB results in significant improvement or resolution of many major obesity-related comorbidities (Table 1.4). Degenerative joint disease, hyperlipidemia, gastroesophageal reflux, hypertension, obstructive sleep apnea, depression, stress urinary incontinence, asthma, migraine headaches, venous insufficiency, congestive heart failure, and diabetes improve or resolve in the majority of patients after surgery. Type 2 diabetes resolves in over 80% of patients after RYGB.

Complications

Overall, the incidence of major early postoperative complications is similar between open and laparoscopic RYGB (10–15%). Notable exceptions to this, though, are the higher

Table 1.4 Changes in comorbidities after laparoscopic Roux-en-Y gastric bypass[13]

Comorbidity	Aggravated (%)	Unchanged (%)	Improved (%)	Resolved (%)
Diabetes	0	0	100	82
Sleep apnea	2	5	93	74
Gastroesophageal reflux disease	0	4	96	72
Gout	0	14	86	72
Hypertension	0	12	88	70
Hypercholesterolemia	0	4	96	63
Hypertriglyceridemia	0	14	86	57
Migraine headaches	0	14	86	57
Urinary incontinence	0	11	89	44
Degenerative joint disease/osteoarthritis	2	10	88	41
Peripheral edema	0	4	96	41
Anxiety	0	50	50	33
Asthma	6	12	82	13
Depression	8	37	55	8

(After Schauer et al. 2000,[26] with permission.)

rate of anastomotic leak rate (1–5%) and internal hernias with the laparoscopic approach. Anastomotic leak rates decrease as a surgeon gains experience with the laparoscopic technique. The higher incidence of internal hernia may be due to a combination of technical factors, surgeon experience, and the formation of fewer intraabdominal adhesions following laparoscopic surgery. Pulmonary embolism occurs in 1–2% of patients after RYGB. Late complications after RYGB include anastomotic stricture (3–10%) and marginal ulcers (3–10%). Vitamin and nutritional deficiencies can be prevented or corrected with supplementation.

Complications after open RYGB ($n = 2771$, 8 series) and laparoscopic RYGB ($n = 3464$, 10 series) were reviewed by Podnos and colleagues.[28]

- There were five intraoperative spleen injuries requiring splenectomy in the open cases, and none in the laparoscopic reports.
- The anastomotic leak rate was 1.68% for open RYGB and 2.05% for laparoscopic RYGB (not significant).
- Gastrointestinal tract hemorrhage was higher in the laparoscopic group (1.93% versus 0.60%, $P = 0.008$), but wound infections and death occurred more frequently after open RYGB than after laparoscopic RYGB (6.63% versus 2.98%, $P < 0.001$, and 0.87% versus 0.23%, $P = 0.001$, respectively).
- There was no significant difference in rates of postoperative pneumonia (0.33%, open; 0.14%, laparoscopic).
- Late complications for open and laparoscopic RYGB included bowel obstruction (2.11% versus 3.15%, $P = 0.02$), incisional hernia (8.58% versus 0.47%, $P < 0.001$), and stomal stenosis (0.67% versus 4.73%, $P < 0.001$).

There is clearly a higher wound complication rate with open RYGB, and this was demonstrated in Nguyen's randomized, controlled trial of laparoscopic versus open RYGB as well, with a wound infection rate and hernia rate of 7.9% each in the open group. This study also showed less pulmonary impairment during the first 3 postoperative days for the laparoscopic group.[27]

Biliopancreatic diversion

Biliopancreatic diversion is a malabsorptive procedure developed by Scopinaro. The procedure consists of a distal gastrectomy and the creation of a long Roux-en-Y limb and an enteroenterostomy 50–100 cm from the ileocecal valve to form the common channel. A modification of BPD with a duodenal switch (BPD-DS) consists of a sleeve gastrectomy and duodenoileostomy with a long alimentary limb and a common channel measuring 50–100 cm (Fig. 1.3). The BPD-DS was developed to reduce the incidence of marginal ulceration, diarrhea, dumping syndrome, and protein calorie malnutrition seen with BPD. These procedures are primarily designed to limit intestinal energy absorption. Initial weight loss relies on decreased stomach capacity and rapid delivery of nutrients to the hindgut to limit appetite. Patients eventually regain their appetite and eating capacity, though, and the long-term success of BPD and BPD-DS relies on malabsorption, which is determined by the length of the common channel.

The advantages of BPD include:

- substantial, durable weight loss (> 70% beyond 10 years); and
- resolution of many obesity-related comorbidities.

After the initial adaptation period, patients can eventually consume more calories than are expended and not regain weight. This procedure may be more effective than RYGB or restrictive procedures for superobese patients, and can be used as a secondary procedure in patients who have failed to lose weight with gastric bypass or restrictive procedures. BPD-DS can be performed laparoscopically.

Disadvantages include:

- a higher operative mortality rate (1.1%) than with other bariatric procedures; and
- metabolic complications including vitamin, mineral, and protein deficiencies that occasionally require reoperation to lengthen the common channel.

Liver disease and diarrhea occur with BPD and BPD-DS, although less frequently than was seen with jejunoileal bypass. After surgery, patients typically have four to six foul-smelling stools per day and flatulence as a result of fat malabsorption. Inability or unwillingness to comply with a strict nutritional supplementation regiment postoperatively is a contraindication to performing this procedure. BPD and BPD-DS, particularly if done laparoscopically, are technically challenging operations performed routinely only at specialized centers.

Technique

Biliopancreatic diversion

Biliopancreatic diversion consists of a subtotal gastrectomy leaving a proximal 200- or 400-mL pouch. The smaller pouch is used for superobese patients.

1. The small bowel is divided 250 cm from the ileocecal valve, and the distal end is anastomosed to the gastric pouch with a 2- to 3-cm stoma.
2. A common channel is formed by completing the Roux-en-Y enteroenterostomy 50–100 cm from the ileocecal valve.

If present, the gallbladder is routinely removed at the time of BPD due to the high incidence of postoperative cholelithiasis.

Duodenal switch

The duodenal switch consists of a greater curvature sleeve gastrectomy, leaving the antrum, the pylorus, and the first portion of the duodenum in continuity. The remaining gastric reservoir is 150–200 mL.

1. The proximal duodenum is divided, and a duodenoileostomy is created using a 250 cm long alimentary limb.
2. A Roux-en-Y anastomosis is then created to form a 100 cm long common channel.

Efficacy

Weight loss after BPD is excellent, and the results are durable. A recent metaanalysis demonstrated that BPD had a higher percentage of EWL (70%) than other bariatric procedures.[14] Scopinaro reported overall EWL of 74% at 8 years and 77% at 18 years. There was no difference in long-term EWL between morbidly obese and superobese (> 120% ideal body weight) subjects.[29] Ren and colleagues performed 40 laparoscopic BPD-DS procedures and reported EWL of 58% at 9 months. Operative time and perioperative morbidity were higher in patients with BMI > 65 kg/m^2.[9]

Complications

Postoperative complication rates for BPD are relatively high, and postoperative mortality ranges from 0.4 to 1.3%. Marginal ulceration can occur up to 10% of the time, but this can be reduced to 1–3% with the duodenal switch and acid suppression therapy. Other complications include:

- dumping syndrome;
- protein calorie malnutrition and anemia in up to 12% and 40% of patients, respectively;
- vitamin B_{12} deficiency;
- hypocalcemia;
- fat-soluble vitamin deficiency; and
- bone demineralization (6%).

Failure to screen for such problems can lead to an unfavorable wound healing after body-contouring surgery. The plastic surgeon reading this chapter should also be cognizant of the expected outcomes from these procedures in terms of magnitude of weight loss and effect on medical problems. A basic appreciation of how the specific procedures impact nutritional status is crucial.

In Scopinaro's series of over 1700 BPD patients, the overall rate of early major surgical complications (intraperitoneal bleeding, wound dehiscence, wound infection, anastomotic leak, and gastric perforation) decreased from 2.7% in his first 738 cases to 1.4% in his last 500 cases. Late complications of BPD included iron deficiency anemia, which was decreased to less than 5% with supplementation. Other late complications included stomal ulcer in 3% of patients, incisional hernia (8.7%), and protein malnutrition (7%). Four percent of patients required elongation of the common channel or reversal of BPD.

In Ren's laparoscopic series, there was one death (2.5%). Postoperative complications included anastomotic leak (2.5%), venous thrombosis (2.5%), subphrenic abscess (2.5%), and staple line hemorrhage (10%), with an overall major morbidity rate of 15%.

CONCLUSION

Obesity is a major public health problem in developed countries worldwide. Currently, the only treatment for this disease that provides long-term weight loss is surgery. Restrictive, malabsorptive, and combination procedures have been developed, and each has its merits and unique set of risks and complications. Weight loss after bariatric surgery is accompanied by improvement or resolution of obesity-related comorbidities and improved life expectancy.

Careful patient selection for bariatric surgery and selection of the appropriate procedure for each patient are keys to success when performing these operations. Close monitoring for nutritional deficiencies and short- and long-term complications is required to completely assess outcomes after these procedures.

REFERENCES

1. National Institutes of Health Conference. Gastrointestinal surgery for severe obesity. Ann Intern Med 1991; 115:956–961.
2. Hedley AA, Odgen CL, Johnson CL, et al. Overweight and obesity among US children, adolescents, and adults, 1999–2002. JAMA 2004; 291:2847–2850.

3. Wolf AM, Colditz GA. The costs of obesity: the US perspective. Pharmacoeconomics 1994; 5:34–37.
4. Santry HP, Gillen DL, Lauderdale DS. Trends in bariatric surgical procedures. JAMA 2005; 294(15):1909–1917.
5. Buchwald H, Williams SE. Bariatric surgery worldwide 2003. Obes Surg 2004; 14(9):1157–1164.
6. Ren CJ, Cabrera I, Rajaram K, et al. Factors influencing patient choice for bariatric operation. Obes Surg 2005; 15(2):202–206.
7. Mason EE, Ito C. Gastric bypass. Ann Surg 1969; 170:329–339.
8. Scopinaro N, Adami FG, Marinari GM, et al. Biliopancreatic diversion. World J Surg 1998; 22:936–946.
9. Ren CJ, Patterson E, Gagner M. Early results of laparoscopic biliopancreatic diversion with duodenal switch: a case series of 40 consecutive patients. Obes Surg 2000; 10(6):514–523; discussion 524.
10. Cottam DR, Mattar SG, Schauer PR. Laparoscopic era of operations for morbid obesity. Arch Surg 2003; 138(4):367–375.
11. [Anonymous]. Randomised trial of jejunoileal bypass versus medical treatment in morbid obesity. The Danish Obesity Project. Lancet 1979; 2:1255–1258.
12. Anderson T, Backer OG, Stokholm KH, et al. Randomized trial of diet and gastroplasty compared with diet alone in morbid obesity. N Engl J Med 1984; 310:352–356.
13. Sjostrom L, Lindroos AK, Peltonen M, et al. Lifestyle, diabetes, and cardiovascular risk factors 10 years after bariatric surgery. N Engl J Med 2004; 351(26):2683–2693.
14. Buchwald H, Avidor Y, Braunwald E, et al. Bariatric surgery. A systematic review and meta-analysis. JAMA 2004; 292(14):1727–1737.
15. Chapman A, Kiroff G, Game P, et al. Systematic review of laparoscopic adjustable gastric banding in the treatment of obesity (ASERNIP-S report no. 31). Adelaide: Australian Safety and Efficacy Register of New Interventional Procedures—Surgical; 2002:18–48.
16. Christou NV, Sampalis JS, Liberman M, et al. Surgery decreases long-term mortality, morbidity, and health care use in morbidly obese patients. Ann Surg 2004; 240(3):416–424.
17. Bloomberg RD, Fleishman A, Nalle JE, et al. Nutritional deficiencies following bariatric surgery: what have we learned? Obes Surg 2005; 15:145–154.
18. Nguyen NT, Paya M, Stevens M, et al. The relationship between hospital volume and outcome in bariatric surgery at academic medical centers. Ann Surg 2004; 240(4):586–594.
19. Ashy AR, Merdad AA. A prospective study comparing vertical banded gastroplasty versus laparoscopic adjustable gastric banding in the treatment of morbid and superobesity. Int Surg 1998; 83:108–110.
20. Ramsey-Stewart G. Vertical banded gastroplasty for morbid obesity: weight loss at short and long-term follow up. Aust N Z J Surg 1995; 65:4–7.
21. DeMaria EJ, Jamal MK. Surgical options for obesity. Gastroenterol Clin North Am 2005; 34:127–142.
22. O'Brien PE, Brown WA, Smith A, et al. Prospective study of a laparoscopically placed, adjustable gastric band in the treatment of morbid obesity. Br J Surg 1999; 86:113–118.
23. Angrisani L, Furbetta F, Doldi B, et al. Lap-Band adjustable gastric banding system: the Italian experience with 1863 patients operated on 6 years. Surg Endosc 2003; 17:409–412.
24. Ponce J, Dixon JB. 2004 ASBS Consensus Conference. Laparoscopic adjustable gastric banding. Surg Obes Relat Dis 2005; 1:310–316.
25. O'Brien PE, Dixon JB. Weight loss and early and late complications—the international experience. Am J Surg 2002; 184:42S–45S.
26. Schauer PR, Ikramuddin S, Gourash W, et al. Outcomes after laparoscopic Roux-en-Y gastric bypass for morbid obesity. Ann Surg 2000; 232(4):515–529.
27. Nguyen NT, Goldman C, Rosenquist J, et al. Laparoscopic versus open gastric bypass: a randomized study of outcomes, quality of life, and costs. Ann Surg 2001; 234(3):279–291.
28. Podnos YD, Jiminez JC, Wilson SF, et al. Complications after laparoscopic gastric bypass: a review of 3464 cases. Arch Surg 2003; 138:957–961.
29. Scopinaro N, Gianetta E, Adami GF, et al. Biliopancreatic diversion for obesity at eighteen years. Surgery 1996; 119:261–268.

EVALUATION OF THE MASSIVE WEIGHT LOSS PATIENT WHO PRESENTS FOR BODY-CONTOURING SURGERY

2

James P. O'Toole and J. Peter Rubin

Key Points

Proper evaluation of the weight loss patient includes the following key components.

- Calculating BMI at time of presentation and assessing stability of weight.
- Screening for residual medical problems associated with obesity and gastric bypass.
- Elucidating relevant psychosocial issues.
- Diagnosing the deformities that result from massive weight loss.
- Understanding the patient's goals and expectations.
- Formulating a safe treatment plan.

With the universal increase in morbid obesity and the concomitant development of advanced laparoscopic techniques, a large number of patients are opting for surgical therapy to reduce excess body weight and ameliorate the myriad of associated medical problems. The US Centers for Disease Control and Prevention estimate that in excess of 64% of the US population is either overweight or obese.[1] On a global scale, the International Obesity Task Force estimates that more than 1 billion individuals are overweight.[2] The American Society for Bariatric Surgery estimated that greater than 150 000 weight loss procedures would be performed in the USA alone in the year 2005.[3] As surgical techniques have evolved, and weight loss surgery has been performed with greater frequency, the tremendous health benefits have been noted in many studies.[4–13] However, the enormous benefits that the patients receive also come at the cost of redundant, loose, hanging rolls of skin and fat. Nearly every region of the body can be affected. This has fueled a rapid increase in the number of patients presenting to the plastic surgeon's office for body-contouring procedures. It is essential that the plastic surgeon approach these patients in a concise, well-thought-out fashion with safety as the primary concern.

PATIENT INTERVIEW

The individuals who seek the advice and expertise of a plastic surgeon regarding the removal of excess skin after massive weight loss have undergone a major life-altering event. While their overall body shape has changed dramatically, they retain a daily reminder of their obese state in the form of loose, hanging skin. It is important for the clinician to realize this, and to recognize that patients may still view themselves as 'fat' and 'different'. Despite successful weight loss, self-esteem may be low. These patients often state that they feel triply stigmatized:

- first for being morbidly obese,
- second for choosing surgical therapy to lose weight (the 'easy way out'), and
- third for being considered vain and seeking the help of a plastic surgeon.

Patients will be looking for a specialist who understands the emotional as well as the physical needs of the postbariatric patient, and their comfort with you will be influenced by your sensitivity to self-esteem issues. We often start the interview by congratulating patients on the progress they have made in the process of weight loss and for taking steps to reclaim their lives. Key historical components specific to the weight loss patient are described in detail below, and provide the basis for a thoughtful assessment. Figure 2.1 shows an office data collection sheet that we use in our center to summarize some of the important data points.

Weight loss history and nutritional assessment

While the initial interview is an excellent time to establish a rapport with your patients, it is also an opportunity to elicit a detailed history of their weight loss surgery and compliance with the nutritional regimen after weight loss. The surgeon should know what type of procedure the patient had, as different operations will have varying potential to cause nutritional deficits. Other important data points include:

- the timing of the weight loss surgery relative to the plastic surgery consult,
- Body Mass Index (BMI) prior to surgery,

Patient name: ______________________

Date of consult: __________ GBP Surgeon: ______________ GBP Complications: __________

Date of GBP: __________

Max weight: __________

Lowest post-GBP weight: __________ Referral source: __________

Goal weight: __________ Max BMI: __________

Current weight: __________ Current BMI: __________

Recent weight loss

Last month: __________ Previous body contouring: ______________ History of DVT/PE? (Circle one) Y N

Last 3 months: __________ Therapy: ______________

Nutritional status (circle one): Adequate protein Inadequate protein Significant nutritional risk

Patient's primary concern (circle one): Abdomen Arms Chest Buttock Thighs Face Neck Flank

Patient's order of priority/goals: ______________________________

Physician notes/surgical plan: ______________________________

Photos taken and date:

☐ Abdomen: __________ ☐ Breast: __________ ☐ Arms: __________

☐ Full body: __________ ☐ Thighs: __________ ☐ Face/neck: __________

Figure 2.1 Sample clinic data sheet for quick reference, evaluation of patient's goals, and surgical plans. GBP, gastric bypass procedure.

- lowest weight reached since bariatric surgery,
- current BMI,
- goal weight, and
- the last time the patient has met with his or her bariatric team.

We ask specifically about weight loss (or gain) in the 3 months prior to the plastic surgery consult to assess stability.

The plastic surgeon takes a nutritional history relevant to the weight loss surgery patient. Most weight loss patients will have adequate food intake for the unstressed state. Indeed, it is rare to see a weight loss surgery patient with overt signs of malnutrition. The plastic surgeon should determine if nutritional intake is adequate to meet the demands of a major surgical procedure. This begins by inquiring about any prolonged problems, such as nausea, which may preclude adequate protein intake to heal large surgical wounds. Beware of patients with persistent nausea at a year or more following gastric bypass; they may have a mechanical problem warranting treatment by the bariatric surgeon. The surgeon should inquire if the patient is taking all recommended supplements. Calcium, vitamin B_{12}, and iron are usually prescribed by the bariatric surgeon after Roux-en-Y gastric bypass to prevent micronutrient deficiencies.[14] It is valuable to get an assessment of the patient's daily protein intake. Three ounces of lean poultry or fish provides approximately 20 g of protein, 3 ounces of beef provides 25 g, 8 ounces of cottage cheese contains 28 g, 8 ounces of milk contains 8 g, and most hard cheeses contain about 7 g per ounce.[15]

Ask about any food aversions. Many patients will struggle with concentrated animal protein after gastric bypass and may have a difficult time maintaining a high protein intake.[16] In our center, we require patients to take at least 50–70 g of protein per day before elective body-contouring surgery. A referral for formal nutritional evaluation and counseling, followed by dietary modification and repeat assessment, would be recommended if protein intake is poor. Even patients with food aversions can find protein sources that they can tolerate well if they are coached through the process. It is essential for the surgeon to understand that a weight loss patient with a favorable BMI does not necessarily represent a good surgical candidate. Major surgery can increase the body's nutritional requirements by 25%, and many weight loss patients may have to adjust their oral intake.[17]

Screening for medical problems

The initial patient interview also provides the clinician with the first opportunity to appreciate any medical issues that may increase the risk of surgery. While body-contouring surgery after massive weight loss may make a patient look and feel better, it does not have the same level of overall health benefit as gastric bypass does.[18] The key focus is patient safety, and a history of significant medical problems, including hypertension, ischemic cardiac disease, sleep apnea, and diabetes, must be fully delineated and addressed before body-contouring surgery. While most medical comorbidities of obesity are significantly improved, if not resolved, following weight loss, the plastic surgeon must search for residual disease. Exercise tolerance is a useful indicator of surgical risk. Patients who routinely do 45 min of vigorous exercise without shortness of breath or other symptoms will likely tolerate the stress of surgery. However, beware of the inactive patient. These patients may have cardiac disease that will be unmasked by a major surgical procedure. We advise liberal use of medical consultants, as warranted, for preoperative evaluation and recommendations for managing chronic disease states. Patients who smoke are encouraged to take responsibility for stopping in order to decrease their perioperative risk.

Psychosocial and lifestyle issues

Permanent lifestyle modifications are essential to long-term weight loss success for patients after bariatric surgery. Do they have a definitive exercise regimen? Do they have an exercise 'buddy' or at least a source of encouragement from friends and family? Does the patient attend support group meetings? Delineate the follow-up routine the patient has with their bariatric surgeon. The majority of trained weight loss surgeons have well-developed postoperative routines and support groups. If your patient has gone to such a surgeon, and has not been faithful with the postoperative regimen, explore the reasons. Issues with compliance may be elucidated. These queries give a reasonable assessment of how invested the patient is in her or his own care. We find that the more motivated patient generally represents a better candidate for elective body-contouring surgery. We look for patients who understand that it is not just the gastric bypass surgery that made them lose weight, but rather their own personal commitment and responsibility to the process.

Weight loss can often be accompanied by major changes in interpersonal relationships. Relationships may be strengthened as family and friends rally behind the successful bariatric patient. However, the radical change in appearance and lifestyle of the patient also has the potential to evoke feelings of envy, jealousy, and abandonment in people close to them. Turmoil may ensue. While patients may be reluctant to discuss these issues, it is vital to understand the stability of their support network and the stressors that may be active before adding the additional burden of recovering from surgery. Our approach is to ask patients about their personal lives, their marriages, their living arrangements, their level of contentment with their lives personally and professionally, and their support network. Example questions include the following.

- 'Who lives at home with you, and are they able and willing to help?'
- 'Who are the other people available to help you in the first few days to weeks?'
- 'Who can drive you to post op visits?'

Observe the affect of the patient during the interview. Individuals who have triumphed over the problems associated with obesity can reasonably be expected to be proud of their accomplishments. Be cautious of the patient who gives elusive or vague answers to questions about their social situation. The withdrawn individual should prompt further questioning about symptoms of depression. While it is common to see patients treated with antidepressants after a gastric bypass procedure, simple depression is not a contraindication to surgery. Inquire about general mood and any depressive episodes during the past year. Patients with poorly treated (or untreated) depression should be referred for psychiatric clearance. Additionally, any patients with bipolar disorder or schizophrenia should also have formal psychiatric clearance.

PHYSICAL EXAMINATION

All aspects of a thorough physical examination should be included in the initial patient evaluation in order to fully appreciate the deformities and screen for residual medical problems. The massive weight loss patient will present with a wide range of physical anomalies. BMI, overall body type (truncal versus peripheral), remaining adipose tissue, and rolls and folds should be noted. Body fat distribution will vary greatly in this patient population and will influence surgical options. Attention should be given to the patient's skin tone and elasticity, as well as regional variations in skin elasticity. On the abdominal examination, make note of:

- thickness of the subcutaneous tissue,
- presence of any hernias,
- degree of diastasis, and
- overall laxity of the abdominal wall.

To facilitate analysis of deformities in each anatomical region of the body, a four-point rating scale can be applied. Table 2.1 shows the Pittsburgh Weight Loss Deformity Scale, which serves as a tool to delineate the severity of deformities.[19] During the examination, consideration may be given to the number of procedures required, the interactions of each procedure, and whether staging would be appropriate. Look for stigmata of nutritional depletion, including thin hair, brittle nails, and BMI < 23 kg/m^2 (it is rare for patients to reach this level). Be observant for any physical limitations that will make the recovery period too physically demanding or be aggravated by surgical trauma. For example, a patient with chronic shoulder pain that limits range of motion may have a difficult time recovering from a brachioplasty.

MANAGING PATIENT EXPECTATIONS

Our approach is to ask patients to list the regions of their bodies that they would like to correct in order of priority. We then discuss surgical options that would effect changes in these regions, including the location of the scars and the extent of recovery. We emphasize the concept of trading excess skin for scar, and assess the patient's willingness to accept these scars. We also emphasize the concept that, in general, body-contouring procedures are major surgical procedures. Having adequate time available to recover from the procedure is something that should be addressed before surgery; this will allow patients to make arrangements with their employer or, if necessary, delay surgery until a more suitable time. Patients are also informed that skin relaxation (relapse of skin laxity) is unpredictable and can be severe enough to lead to operative revision. We recommend advising patients about any office policies regarding fees associated with revision surgery.

We find it useful to stand patients in front of a mirror and review how areas of skin laxity might be improved on their body, including a demonstration of how the surgeon pulls on the skin to estimate the amount of resection and the resultant impact on contour. During this part of the examination, limitations of the procedures, given the patient's body type, are discussed. This often includes an explanation of which anatomical regions can be changed with a given procedure and, importantly, which adjacent regions will not be impacted. How existing scars will be handled, and the effect of the procedure on stretch marks inside and outside the area of planned resection, is explained. The quality of previous scars is noted and used as a guideline to predict how future scars may appear. To further emphasize the issue of surgical scars, a skin marker is often used to draw the location of the scars directly on the patient's body and photographs are taken. This also helps the patient review scar location with their spouses or significant others after the consultation.

Patients who comprehend these issues and whose priorities are addressed first are likely to be satisfied with the procedures performed. If the points outlined in this section are thoroughly conveyed by the surgeon, unrealistic expectations on the part of the patient will emerge during the discussion. If these expectations cannot be balanced, an unsatisfactory result is likely.

PATIENT SELECTION

Patient selection must be focused on maximizing safety. With that goal in mind, the following key principles should be applied.

- The patient should be weight-stable.
- BMI should be favorable.
- Nutrition must be adequate.
- Medical and psychosocial issues should be stable.
- The patient should have reasonable goals and expectations considering their age, health, and body habitus.

It is also desirable for the patient to be on a definitive exercise regimen. One may be lured into operating on a patient whose anatomical deformities are easy to correct. However, underappreciated nutritional, medical, and psychosocial issues may lead to an unfavorable outcome. Any issue that may influence the safety of the planned procedure must be remedied prior to operative intervention. If surgery is not to be offered at the initial consultation, remain the patient's advocate and encourage his or her continued progress. Inform patients that you respect all that they have accomplished. We emphasize that there is a correct time for elective surgery, and that this may not be the best time. While they may be disappointed, they will understand and appreciate that you are keeping their best interests in mind. It is a common practice in our center to have patients work on problematic nutritional or medical issues after the initial consultation and follow-up for another evaluation in 1–3 months. Figure 2.2 shows a checklist of the important components to consider.

All patients considered candidates for body-contouring surgery must be weight-stable for 3 months (this usually occurs between 12 and 18 months after a gastric bypass procedure). This is important for several reasons.

- For large surgical wounds, nutritional homeostasis and a positive nitrogen balance are necessary to facilitate the healing process.[20]
- A more predictable outcome can be achieved when the patient is not actively losing weight.
- A high BMI is associated with increased wound-healing complications.[21,22]

The BMI at presentation is an important factor. As the patient's BMI decreases, we are able to offer more safe surgical options and expect better aesthetic outcomes. The best candidates have a BMI of 28 kg/m^2 or less. We are more cautious in our level of aggressiveness with patients who have a BMI between 29 kg/m^2 and 32 kg/m^2. Patients whose BMI is between 32 and 35 kg/m^2 should be selected with great care, and procedures may be more limited than for patients with a lower BMI. If a patient in this BMI range desires significant contouring, we recommend delaying the operation until further weight loss can be achieved. The technical challenge and subsequent outcome are impacted by body fat distribution.

Table 2.1 Pittsburgh Weight Loss Deformity Scale

Area	Scale	Definition	Preferred procedure(s)
Arms	0	Normal	None
	1	Adiposity with good skin tone	UAL and/or SAL
	2	Loose, hanging skin without severe adiposity	Brachioplasty
	3	Loose, hanging skin with severe adiposity	Brachioplasty with UAL and/or SAL
Breasts	0	Normal	None
	1	Ptosis grade 1 or 2 or severe macromastia	Traditional mastopexy, reduction, or augmentation techniques
	2	Ptosis grade 3, or moderate volume loss, or constricted breast	Traditional mastopexy ± augmentation
	3	Severe lateral roll and/or severe volume loss with loose skin	Parenchymal reshaping techniques; consider autoaugmentation
Back	0	Normal	None
	1	Single fat roll or adiposity	UAL and/or SAL
	2	Multiple skin and fat rolls	Excisional lifting procedures versus liposuction
	3	Ptosis of rolls	Excisional lifting procedures
Abdomen	0	Normal	None
	1	Redundant skin with rhytids or moderate adiposity without overhang	Miniabdominoplasty, versus full abdominoplasty
	2	Overhanging pannus	Full abdominoplasty
	3	Multiple rolls or epigastric fullness	Modified abdominoplasty techniques, including fleur de lis and/or upper body lift
Flank	0	Normal	None
	1	Adiposity	UAL and/or SAL
	2	Rolls without ptosis	UAL and/or SAL
	3	Rolls with ptosis	Excisional lifting procedures
Buttocks	0	Normal	None
	1	Mild to moderate adiposity and/or mild to moderate cellulite	UAL and/or SAL
	2	Severe adiposity and/or severe cellulite	UAL and/or SAL ± excisional lifting procedure
	3	Skin folds	Excisional lifting procedure
Mons	0	Normal	None
	1	Excessive adiposity	UAL and/or SAL
	2	Ptosis	Monsplasty
	3	Significant overhang below symphysis	Monsplasty
Hips/lateral thighs	0	Normal	None
	1	Mild to moderate adiposity and/or mild to moderate cellulite	UAL and/or SAL ± excisional lifting procedure
	2	Severe adiposity and/or severe cellulite	UAL and/or SAL ± excisional lifting procedure
	3	Skin folds	Excisional lifting procedure
Medial thighs	0	Normal	None
	1	Excessive adiposity	UAL and/or SAL ± excisional lifting procedure
	2	Severe adiposity and/or severe cellulite	UAL and/or SAL ± excisional lifting procedure
	3	Skin folds	Excisional lifting procedure
Lower thighs/knees	0	Normal	None
	1	Adiposity	UAL and/or SAL
	2	Severe adiposity	UAL and/or SAL ± excisional lifting procedure
	3	Skin folds	Excisional lifting procedure

SAL, suction-assisted lipectomy; UAL, ultrasound-assisted lipoplasty.
(Adapted from Song et al 2005,[19])

Evaluation/screening checklist

- ☐ What is the current BMI?__________
- ☐ Has the patient's weight been stable for at least 3 months?
- ☐ Active nausea or vomiting? ☐ If yes, immediate referral to gastric bypass surgeon.
- ☐ Would the patient benefit from further weight loss? ☐ If yes, return in 2–3 months for weight check.
- ☐ Is the patient's nutrition adequate? ☐ If no, comprehensive nutritional evaluation.
- ☐ Is the psychosocial situation stable and adequate?
- ☐ Are there medical issues that preclude safe surgery and/or require further evaluation?
- ☐ Is the patient willing to accept visible scars?
- ☐ Does the patient understand the magnitude of the planned procedure?
- ☐ Does the patient appreciate the recovery involved and have an adequate support network?
- ☐ Are expectations reasonable?

Figure 2.2 Screening and evaluation checklist.

The patient should be counseled that additional weight loss allows for a safer operation with better aesthetic outcomes. Work on a weight loss plan with the patient and nutritionist, and schedule a 2- to 3-month follow-up appointment. This way, the patient will remain under your care and not feel abandoned; moreover, you are able to serve as a motivating source. Some patients in this BMI range may benefit from a first-stage breast reduction or simple panniculectomy if such a procedure would improve their ability to exercise and progress with further weight loss. For patients with a BMI greater than 35 kg/m^2, our practice is, in most cases, to avoid operations because of increased risk of complications and less potential for satisfying aesthetic results.[22,23] Patients in this BMI range would generally be offered only a truly functional panniculectomy, with strict indications of severe panniculitis or a profoundly disabling pannus.

The importance of the nutritional status of the postbariatric patient cannot be overstressed.[24–27] If patients have symptoms consistent with a physical impedance to eating, have them see their bariatric surgeon to rule out stricture. Because gastric bypass patients have altered gastrointestinal physiology, and subsequent dietary issues are to be expected, nutritional issues should be revisited in the postoperative period if any wound-healing complications arise.[28] As mentioned earlier, our practice is to require at least 50–70 g of protein intake per day before surgery will be offered. A patient who is incapable of 50 g per day does not represent a surgical candidate, and dietary modification is essential.

Medical and psychosocial issues must also be stable prior to any operation. Patients with significant medical comorbidities are routinely sent to an appropriate medical specialist for further evaluation and clearance. An adequate support network should be in place. Active smokers are encouraged to stop at least 1 month prior to surgery. If this is not possible, then the extent of the procedure performed, especially the amount of tissue undermining, is limited. Similar caution is exercised with diabetic patients and those treated with steroids.

The final component is a reasonable set of goals and expectations. Patients should be willing to accept extensive scars in exchange for loose skin, understand both the power and limitations of the intended procedures, and appreciate which areas of the body will not be affected by the planned surgery. This last point is important because improving one area of the body may highlight deformities in adjacent areas.

COMBINATION PROCEDURES, STAGING, AND DEALING WITH ABDOMINAL HERNIAS

Performing body-contouring procedures in two or more stages should be considered if the patient has goals of reshaping multiple regions. The advantages of staging are:

- less anesthetic time,
- less blood loss,
- less surgeon fatigue,
- avoidance of opposing vectors of pull on regions of skin, and
- the ability to have a second chance to correct any contour irregularities or skin relaxation seen after the first stage.

Disadvantages of staging include:

- multiple anesthetics,
- increased time off work, and
- increased expense for the patient.

While it may be feasible to do two or three procedures in a single stage, the surgeon should be guided by his or her level of experience, experience of the operating room team, and treatment setting. Individual procedures may be performed safely at a fully equipped surgery center, assuming that adequate personnel are available for recovery and that adequate arrangements are in place should extended recovery be necessary. Great caution should be exercised in the surgery center setting if combined procedures are considered. Multiple (more than two) procedures performed in a single anesthetic should take place in a hospital setting.

It is not uncommon for the plastic surgeon to encounter a massive weight loss patient with an incisional hernia. When approaching these patients, we first consider whether there has been sufficient weight loss to avoid excessive pressure on the repair exerted by a still obese intraabdominal compartment. It is reasonable to recommend further weight loss and use of an abdominal binder for comfort before performing surgery on a large asymptomatic hernia, if necessary. If the patient has reached an appropriate body weight for hernia repair, consideration is then given to the extent of the procedure. For small or moderate-sized hernias, we will combine the repair with major body-contouring procedures (e.g. lower body lift). Very large hernias may require extensive lysis of adhesions and/or separation of the abdominal wall components to achieve closure. When such an abdominal wall reconstruction is anticipated, we limit the body-contouring procedures to a concurrent panniculectomy and stage any other desired surgeries. We routinely bowel-prepare patients with hernias, and seek recommendation from the patient's bariatric surgeon regarding the preferred method. Bariatric surgeons may be dogmatic about which gastrointestinal medications are prescribed for their patients. Moreover, the referring weight loss surgeon may want to be involved with these cases in a team approach.

CONCLUSION

Body contouring is a wonderful adjunct to bariatric surgery and completes the weight loss process for many patients. Any plastic surgeon who evaluates patients after massive weight loss will see the full spectrum of patient subtypes. The majority of patients who present to the office for contouring surgery will be well adjusted and have undertaken great measures to reclaim their lives. However, there will be individuals who are not quite prepared for surgery. A thoughtful and organized approach to the massive weight loss patient will identify the individuals who represent good surgical candidates. Carefully devised operations for the appropriate patient at the right time have the potential to provide a tremendously rewarding experience for the patient and surgeon. As the surgeon, you have the capability to eradicate the last reminders of the obesity that these patients have labored so long to be rid of.

REFERENCES

1. National Center for Health Statistics. National Health and Nutrition Examination Survey. Online. Available: http://www.cdc.gov/nchs/nhanes.htm 2006.
2. International Obesity Task Force. About obesity. Online. Available: http://www.iotf.org 2006.
3. American Society for Bariatric Surgery. Online. Available: http://www.asbs.org/ 2006.
4. Dixon JB, O'Brien PE. Changes in co-morbidities and improvements in quality of life after LAP-BAND placement. Am J Surg 2002; 184:51S–54S.
5. Dhabuwala A, Cannan RJ, Stubbs RS. Improvement in co-morbidities following weight loss from gastric bypass. Obes Surg 2000; 10:428–435.
6. Choban PS, Onyejekwe J, Burge JC, et al. A health status assessment of the effect of weight loss following Roux-en-Y gastric bypass for clinical obesity. J Am Coll Surg 1999; 188:491–497.
7. Vidal J. Updated review on the benefits of weight loss. Int J Obes 2002; 26:25S.
8. Dietel M. How much weight loss is sufficient to overcome major co-morbidities? Obes Surg 2001; 11:659.
9. Goldstein DJ. Beneficial health effects of modest weight loss. Int J Obes 1991; 16:397.
10. Carson JL, Ruddy ME, Duff AE, et al. The effect of gastric bypass surgery on hypertension in morbidly obese patients. Arch Int Med 1994; 154:193–200.
11. Pories WJ, Swanson MS, MacDonald KG, et al. Who would have thought it? An operation proves to be the most effective therapy for adult-onset diabetes mellitus. Ann Surg 1995; 222:339–341.
12. Sugerman JH, Baron PL, Fairman RP, et al. Hemodynamic dysfunction in obesity hypoventilation syndrome and the effects of treatment with surgically induced weight loss. Ann Surg 1998; 207:603–605.
13. Frezza EE, Ikramuddin S, Gourash W, et al. Symptomatic improvement in gastroesophageal reflux disease (GERD) following laparoscopic Roux-en-Y gastric bypass. Surg Endosc 2002; 16:1027–1031.
14. Rubin JP, Nguyen V, Schwentker A. Perioperative management of the post–gastric-bypass patient presenting for body contour surgery. Clin Plast Surg 2004; 31(4):601–610.
15. US Department of Agriculture. USDA National Nutrient Database for Standard Reference, release 17. Washington: USDA; 2004.
16. Brown EK, Settle EA, Van Rij AM. Food intake patterns of gastric bypass patients. J Am Diabet Assoc 1982; 80(5):437–443.
17. Van Way CW. Nutritional support in the injured patient. Surg Clin North Am 1991; 71:537–548.
18. Gleysteen JJ, Barboriak JJ. Improvement in heart disease risk factors after gastric bypass. Arch Surg 1983; 118:681–682.
19. Song AY, Jean RD, Hurwitz DJ, et al. A classification of weight loss deformities: the Pittsburgh Rating Scale. Plast Reconstr Surg 2005; 116:1535–1554.
20. Halverson JD. Micronutrient deficiencies after gastric bypass for morbid obesity. Am Surg 1986; 52(11):594–598.
21. Matory WE, O'Sullivan J, Fudem G, et al. Abdominal surgery in patients with severe morbid obesity. Plast Reconstr Surg 1994; 94:976–987.
22. Vastine VL, Morgan RF, Williams GS. Wound complications of abdominoplasty in obese patients. Ann Plast Surg 1999; 42:33–35.
23. Choban PS, Flancbaum L. The impact of obesity on surgical outcomes: a review. J Am Coll Surg 1997; 185:592–593.

24. Charles P. Calcium absorption and calcium bioavailability. J Int Med 1992; 231(2):161–168.
25. Rhode BM, Arseneau P, Cooper BA, et al. Vitamin B-12 deficiency after gastric surgery for obesity. Am J Clin Nutr 1996; 63(1):103–109.
26. Lash A, Saleem A. Iron metabolism: a comprehensive review. Ann Clin Lab Sci 1995; 25(1):20–30.
27. Kushner R. Managing the obese patient after bariatric surgery: a case report of severe malnutrition and review of the literature. JPEN: J Parenter Enteral Nutr 2000; 24(2):126–132.
28. Halverson JD. Metabolic risk of obesity surgery and long-term follow-up. Am J Clin Nutr 1992; 55(2 suppl):602S–605S.

APPROACH TO THE FACE AND NECK AFTER WEIGHT LOSS

3

Ivo Pitanguy, Henrique N. Radwanski and Alan Matarasso

Key Points

- Description of the round-lifting technique.
- Avoiding dislocation of anatomical landmarks.
- Addressing the forehead.
- Description of main ancillary procedures.
- Overview of complications.
- Short scar facelift in the MWL patient.

In the past few decades, facial aesthetic surgery has undergone enormous progress, with a greater understanding of anatomy and the development of newer technology and products that complement the operation. In our beauty-centered global society, where life is fast-paced, people are rapidly judged with regards to their appearance. The face is frequently the main focus of anxiety, especially in individuals who have attained a certain stage in their lives. Job competition, interpersonal relationships, and physical well-being are reasons that many times motivate the patient to come to the plastic surgeon seeking a more youthful look. On the other hand, bariatric surgery has permitted significant loss of weight in the morbidly obese. It has therefore become more common for the patient who has undergone a great amount of weight reduction to present to the plastic surgeon requesting the removal of excess skin from one or, more typically, many regions of the body. When there is redundant facial skin, this causes social embarrassment and needs to be addressed by a surgical procedure.

The surgeon must be knowledgeable in details of different surgical approaches and variations thereof to attain the best result for each individual case. The round-lifting technique, as described by the senior author, is very well indicated for the treatment of excess facial skin, as the vectors of traction allow for the repositioning of tissues without causing anatomical distortion, such as dislocation of the hairline and visible signs of skin traction. Ancillary procedures present the surgeon with a vast array of surgical and non-surgical techniques that should be used in an individualized manner, as each patient presents differences not only in anatomy but also regarding regional complaints.

In this chapter, the surgical treatment of the aging face in the patient with massive weight loss will be presented, giving emphasis to the correct traction applied to the facial flaps (the round-lifting technique) and the forehead (the 'block' lifting), assuring that all anatomical landmarks are precisely preserved. The reader should note the importance of planning incisions for facial aesthetic surgery in this population, so that redundant skin can be removed without distorting key landmarks.

SURGICAL TECHNIQUE

A satisfactory outcome of an aesthetic facial procedure is obtained when signs of an operation are undetectable and anatomy has been preserved. Visible scars and dislocation of the hairline are among the most common complaints, and everything should be done to avoid these stigmas. The round-lifting technique evolved with these concerns as its principal guidelines.

Rhytidoplasty is one of the most frequently performed surgeries in the practice of the plastic surgeon. In the senior author's private clinic, a total of 7927 personal consecutive cases have been analyzed to date (see Fig. 3.1). More recently, a noticeable increase in male patients has been noted. In the 1970s, men represented 6% of face-lifting procedures; in the eighties, approximately 15%; currently, 20% of patients who seek aesthetic facial surgery are men (see Fig. 3.2).

After appropriate intravenous sedation and preparation, local anesthetic infiltration is performed. The standard incision is demarcated, beginning in the temporal scalp, and proceeds in the preauricular area in such a way as to respect the anatomical curvature of this region. The incision then follows around the earlobe and, in a curving fashion, finishes in the cervical scalp (Fig. 3.3). (This S-shaped incision creates an advancement flap that prevents a step-off in the hairline, allowing patients to wear their hair up without revealing the scar.)

Variations of this incision are chosen depending on each case. The choice of which incision is most appropriate should have the following goals in mind:

- the treatment of specific regions for optimal distribution of skin flaps,

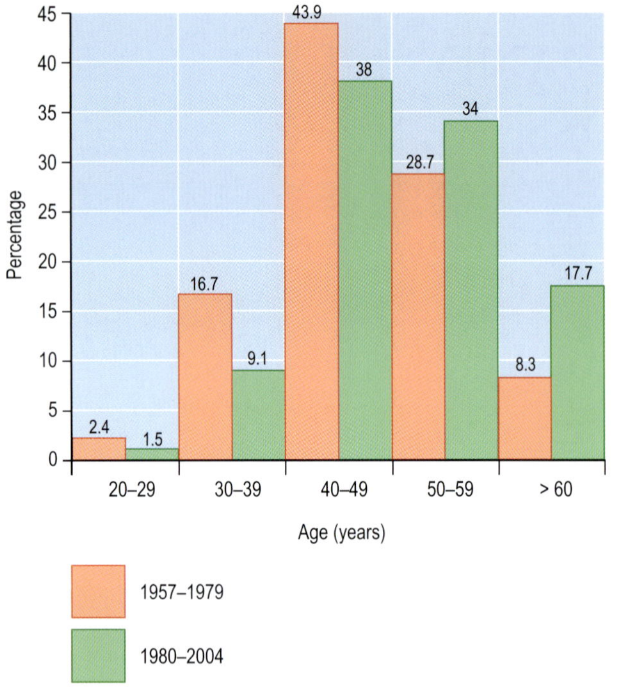

Figure 3.1 Collated data for facial rejuvenation surgery, by age group, from the senior author's personal clinic. Number of cases for 1957–1979, 2934; for 1980–2004, 4993. (Total number: 7927 cases.)

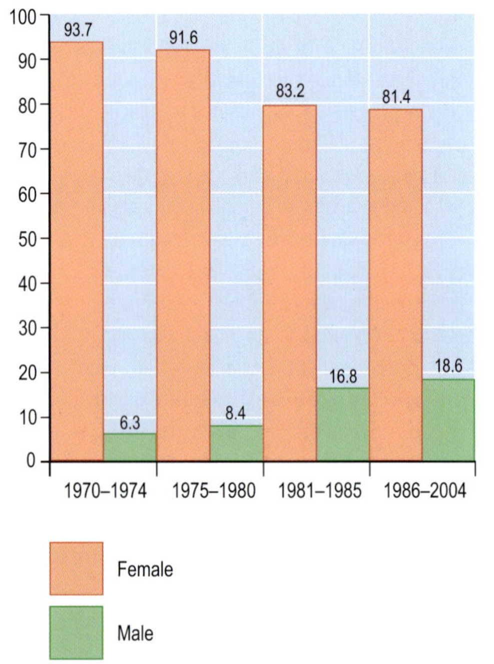

Figure 3.2 Grouping by gender for facial rejuvenation surgery. (Total number: 7927 cases.)

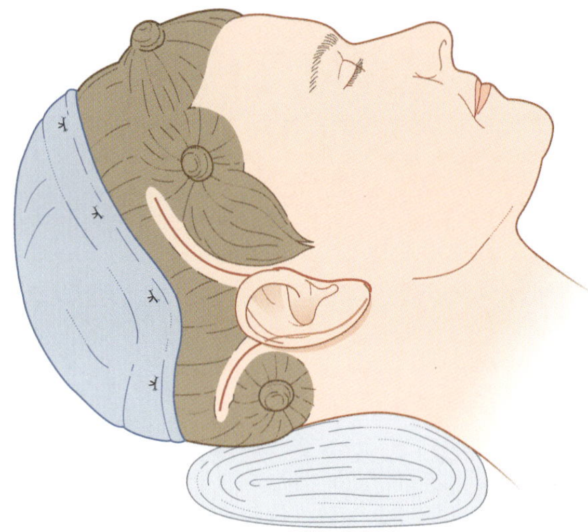

Figure 3.3 The classic incision, as described for the round-lifting.

- the resection of previous scars in secondary rhytidoplasty, and
- the maintenance of anatomical landmarks.

Secondary face-lifts especially present elements that require different incisions, and the versatile surgeon will establish the indications and advantages of each different incision often by using a sideburn incision to avoid excess hairline elevation.

Undermining of the facial and cervical flaps is performed in a subcutaneous plane, the extension of which is variable and individualized for each case. A danger area lies beneath the non–hair-bearing skin over the temples, which we have called 'no man's land', where most of the temporofrontal branches of the facial nerve are more frequently found. Dissection over no man's land should be superficial, and hemostasis carefully performed, if at all. Larger vessels should be tied.

The patient who has undergone a significant loss of weight will usually complain of the very heavy, fatty neck. Treatment of this area requires that the dissection proceed all the way to the other side under the mandible. With the advent of suction-assisted lipectomy, submental lipodystrophy is mostly addressed by liposuction, in a crisscross fashion (Fig. 3.4). On the other hand, direct lipectomy using specially designed scissors may still be useful to defat the submental region, as has been described historically. Following this, treatment of medial platysmal bands is carried out under direct vision. Approximation of diastasis is done with interrupted sutures, plicating down to the level of the hyoid bone.

Undermining of the facial flaps is extended over the zygomatic prominence to free the retaining ligaments of the cheek. Dissection of the deeper elements of the face has evolved over the past 20 years. Almost no treatment was advocated before the publications that first described the submuscular aponeurotic system (SMAS). The approach to this structure has been a topic of much discussion. Currently, we determine whether to dissect or simply plicate the SMAS only after subcutaneous dissection has been completed. Pulling of the SMAS is done, noting the effects on the skin.

Although extensive undermining of the SMAS was performed in an earlier period, it has been noted that plication of this structure in the same direction as the skin flaps, with repositioning of the malar fat pad, has given satisfactory and natural results. The durability of this maneuver is relative to the individual aging process. Tension on the musculoaponeurotic system allows support of the subcutaneous layers, corrects the sagging cheek, and reduces tension on the skin flap.

Techniques that treat the pronounced nasolabial fold include traction of skin flaps, and traction on the SMAS or the fascial fatty layer, with variable results. Filling with different substances may also be done at the end of surgery, either with fat grafting or other material. Direct excision of the nasolabial fold is reserved for the older male patient as a secondary procedure. In very selected cases, this technique gives a definite solution to the nasolabial fold, with a barely noticeable scar that mimics the nasolabial fold itself.

The direction of traction of the skin flaps is a fundamental aspect of the round-lifting technique. In this manner, the undermined flaps are rotated rather than simply pulled, acting in a direction opposite to that of aging, and assuring a repositioning of tissues with preservation of anatomical landmarks. A second advantage in establishing a precise vector of rotation is that the opposite side is repositioned in the exact manner.

This vector of traction connects the tragus to Darwin's tubercle for the facial—or anterior—flap. A Pitanguy flap demarcator (Padgett Instruments, Kansas City, Missouri) is placed at the root of the helix to mark point A on the skin flap (Fig. 3.5). The edge of the flap is then incised along a curved line crossing the supraauricular hairline so that bald skin, not pilose, is resected. A key suture is located here.

Likewise, the cervical flap should also be pulled in an equally precise manner, in a superior and slightly anterior vector of traction, to avoid a step-off of the hairline. Key stitches are placed to anchor the flap along the pilose scalp at point B so that there is no tension on the thin skin at the peak of the retroauricular incision.

Only when the temporary sutures have been placed will excess facial skin be resected. Skin is accommodated and demarcated along the natural curves of the ear, with no tension whatsoever (Fig. 3.6). Final scars are thus not displaced or widened. The tragus is preserved in its anatomical position, and the skin of the flap is trimmed so as to perfectly match the fine skin of this region.

When performing a brow lift, placing these key sutures at points A and B is mandatory before any traction is applied to the forehead flap, essentially blocking the facial flaps.

Forehead lifting

Aging in the upper face becomes evident with a descent in the level of the eyebrow and the appearance of wrinkles and furrows, sometimes from an early age. These are a direct consequence of muscle dynamics, responsible for the multitude of expressions so characteristic of humans, and also due to loss of skin tone. The use of botulinum toxin has been a valuable adjunct to temporarily correct these lines of expression and

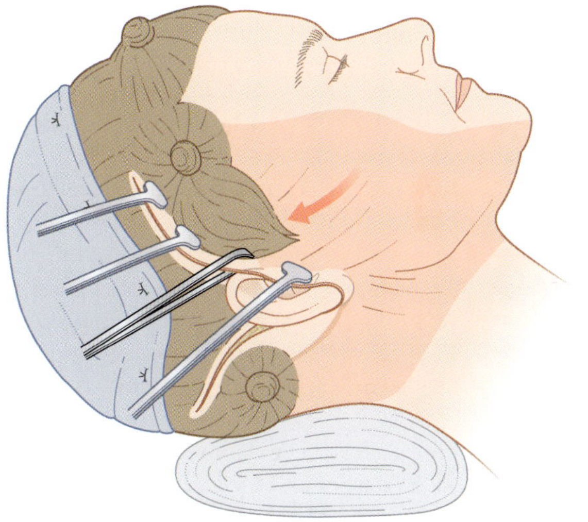

Figure 3.5 The direction of traction of the anterior or facial flap follows a vector that connects the tragus to Darwin's tubercle. Excess tissue is marked with a Pitanguy flap demarcator.

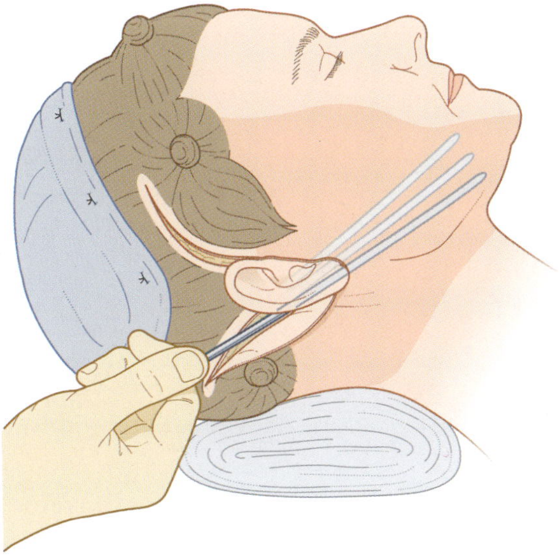

Figure 3.4 Liposuction has been useful to complement a face-lift.

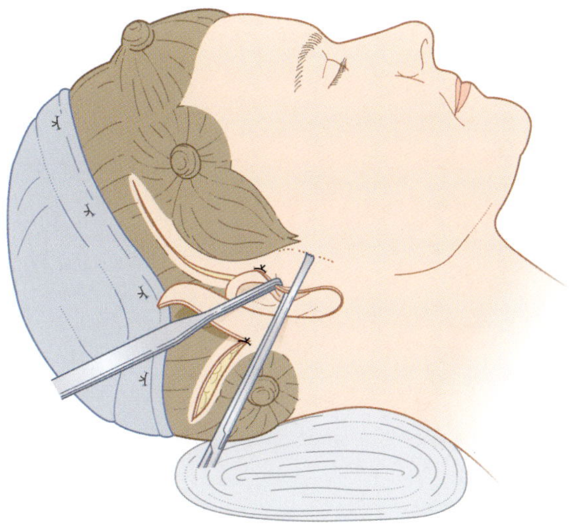

Figure 3.6 The posterior flap has been rotated and fixed at point B. Excess facial skin is demarcated with no tension on the flap.

has been widely indicated as a non-surgical application, either by itself or as a complement to surgery.

Elements of the upper face that must be considered preoperatively for any procedure are:

- the length of the forehead and the elasticity of the skin,
- muscle force and wrinkles,
- the position of the anterior hairline, and
- the quality and quantity of hair.

An important decision to be made regarding a brow lift is the placement of incisions. There are basically two classic approaches: the bicoronal incision and the limited prepilose or juxtapilose incision. The first allows for treatment of all elements that determine the aging forehead, while hiding the final scar within the hairline. Certain situations, however, rule out this incision. Patients with a very long forehead or those who have already been submitted to previous surgery should not be considered for this incision, because they will have an excessively recessed hairline if the forehead is further pulled back. The final aspect will be displeasing, giving the patient a permanent look of surprise.

Having blocked the facial flaps at points A and B, as described above, the forehead may be pulled in any direction, either straight backward or more laterally (Fig. 3.7). The amount of scalp flap to be resected is determined by the length of the forehead and the effect that traction causes on the level of the eyebrow. The midline is positioned, demarcated, incised, and blocked with a temporary suture. Sometimes no traction is necessary and no scalp is removed in the midline. Two symmetric flaps are created, and lateral resection can now be performed, allowing the eyebrow to be raised as necessary (Fig. 3.8).

The second approach is the juxtapilose incision, performed when the patient presents with ptosis of lateral eyebrow and scant lines of expression of the forehead. The short distance required to reach the eyebrow region is easily performed by subperiosteal blunt dissection (Fig. 3.9).

Endoscopic instrumentation has permitted treatment of the brow through minimal access, and has proved useful in selected cases.

Optimizing outcomes

The effects of the round-lifting technique have been studied by analyzing the mechanical forces applied and the displacements produced. The method of finite elements was employed and, by means of computers, the relevant equations were defined. Human skin was modeled as a pseudoelastic, isotropic, noncompressible, and homogeneous membrane, and a computational study of the fields of displacement and the forces applied to the flaps during a rhytidoplasty demonstrated that the

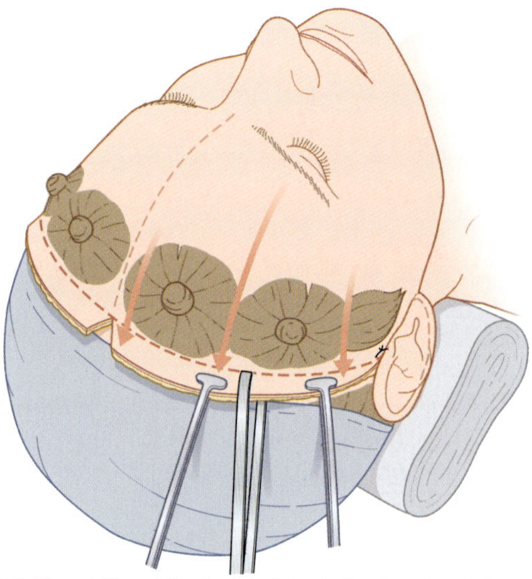

Figure 3.8 The midline of the forehead flap is fixed, and each lateral flap is tractioned according to the amount of correction required.

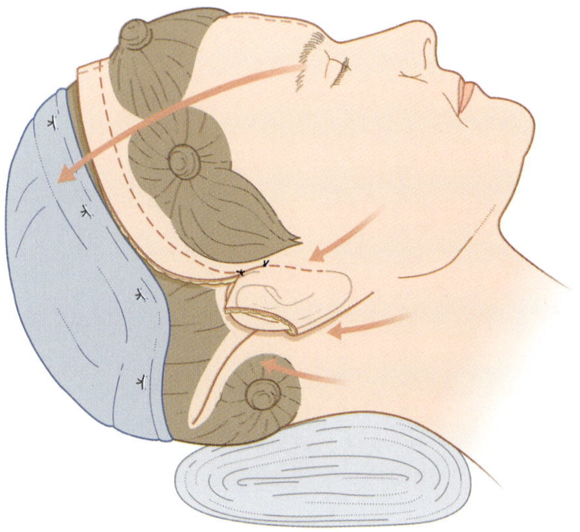

Figure 3.7 Positioning of the forehead flap is done only after the facial flaps have been rotated and 'blocked'. This avoids excessive elevation of the facial tissues and alteration of the hairline.

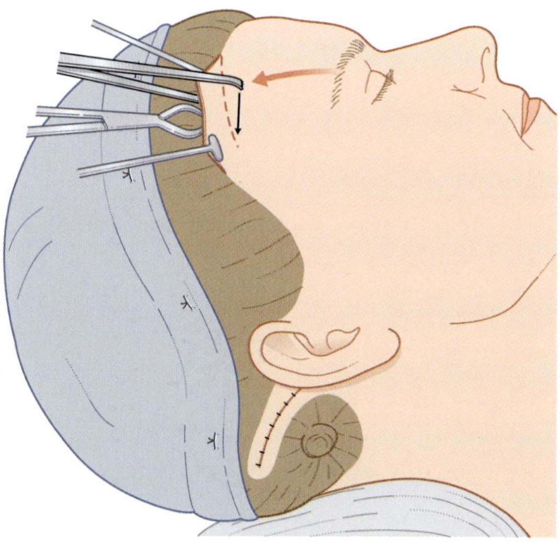

Figure 3.9 Correction of the level of the brow to a more elevated position may be done by the juxtapilose incision, with a subperiosteal blunt dissection.

direction of traction creates areas of tension that can be either negative or positive. These forces ultimately result in the correction of signs of aging.

Interestingly, the vectors described in the round-lifting technique address both the main features that suffer distortion with aging as well as maintaining anatomical parameters. Although there were limits due to the variety of factors involved because of the complexities of human skin (basic properties and individual variations), the study holds a close parallel to a real surgical procedure.

ANCILLARY PROCEDURES

Several surgical techniques are part of the armamentarium that a surgeon should have to enhance the result of a rhytidoplasty. These procedures may be complementary to the face-lift or may be indicated by themselves. Two of the more frequently performed procedures are blepharoplasty and treatment of the aging lip. In general these areas are treated as they might be in a non massive weight loss patient. Occasionally massive weight loss patients can be observed to have persistence of periorbital lower eyelid fat after their weight loss—not associated with generalized facial aging.

The short scar face-lift in the massive weight loss patient. Technique by Dr Alan Matarasso

The short scar face-lift with or without fibrin sealant is the preferred method of treatment in all aging and massive weight loss patients.

The characteristics of patients faces following massive weight loss are similar to the changes seen in the aging face. However, in certain massive weight loss patients, there may be a greater absence of subcutaneous fat, more loss of fixed points at areas of osteodermocutaneous ligaments, more damage in dermal elements and "better" scar formation.

The face-lift technique is a result of a continuous evolution from the traditional open face-lift incision (Fig. 3.10), into the modified open technique (Fig. 3.11) and finally into the short scar face-lift (Fig. 3.12). All of the patients who have had this short scar face-lift also had concomitant suction-assisted lipoplasty, and most (76%) underwent a submentalplasty with a platysmaplasty. The short scar approach provides

- a shorter more appealing, and well-hidden scar,
- essentially no hair abnormalities or changes in hair position or density,
- potentially shorter operative time, and
- greater patient acceptance at the expense of a slightly narrower operative field with limited access to the orbicularis oculi muscle and temporalis muscle.

The short scar incision begins in the horizontal aspect of the sideburn 'sideburn incision', extends to the preauricular region (either pre- or posttragal), curves around the ear lobe posteriorly up to the postauricular notch, and ends in the sulcus approximately 2–3 cm above the lobule. It spares incisions in the temporal and mastoid areas (see Fig. 3.12).

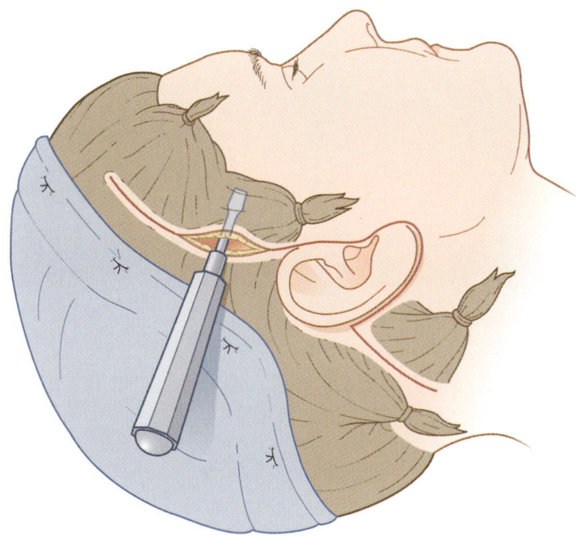

Figure 3.10 Traditional open face-lift approach, which allows wider access (i.e. the temporalis muscle). Modified from Matarasso A, Rizk SS, Markowitz J. Short scar face-lift with the use of fibrin sealant. Dermatol Clin 2005; 23:495–504.

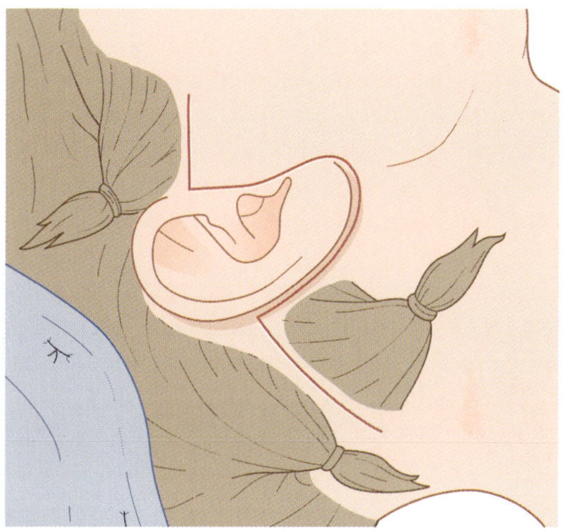

Figure 3.11 Modified open face-lift approach. In the course of evolving to a short scar lift this was useful. Modified from Matarasso A, Rizk SS, Markowitz J. Short scar face-lift with the use of fibrin sealant. Dermatol Clin 2005; 23:495–504.

The short scar face-lift may require additional midline platysmal work, accounting for the higher rate of submentalplasty than is done with the traditional face-lift (76% versus 10.6%). The face-lift procedure begins with liposuction of the neck through a submental incision. A subcutaneous neck dissection is performed and jowl liposuction through a preauricular stab wound. The midline platysma is then isolated. A wide strip wedge platysmaectomy is performed to shorten redundant platysma muscle and deepen the cervicomental angle. When fat excision is indicated, the exposed fat deep to the platysma muscle is excised under direct vision and eletrocoagulated to further reduce it. The medial (anterior) borders of the platysma muscle are then identified, and a back cut is performed at the

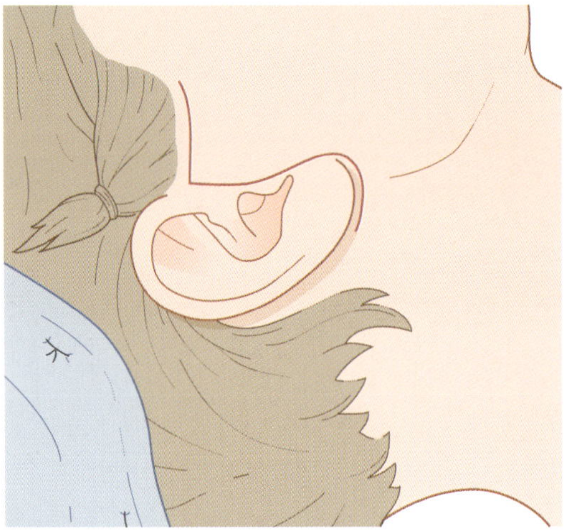

Figure 3.12 5-STAR incision. Note incision inside sideburn hairline, extending preauricularly (either pretragal or posttragal) and for a short distance postauricularly (short scar transauricular rhytidectomy). Modified from Matarasso A, Rizk SS, Markowitz J. Short scar face-lift with the use of fibrin sealant. Dermatol Clin 2005; 23:495–504.

level of the hyoid if indicated. The medial borders of the platysma are then sutured in the midline with nonabsorbable sutures. This medial vector pull on the platysma is important for defining the cervicomental angle and for the redraping of excess skin into the submental hollow that occurs with the short scar face-lift following the concept Pythagorium Theorem. It is not necessary or desirable to have excess lateral vector pull on the platysma.

The authors have found that 'fatty necks' after being aggressively defatted often have a surprising degree of tissue elasticity and retraction and that less skin excision than expected is required accounting for the dramatic result that can be achieved in the short scar face-lift in 'large' necks. In contrast, thin necks in older patients with 'chicken skin' lack elasticity and have poor collagen structure in addition to the diminished number of pilosebaceous units normally found in neck skin. Consequently, no amount of excessive pulling or tightening ultimately overcomes these characteristics. Indeed, attempting to compensate in these situations by excessive pulling by any surgical approach is a futile exercise that does not benefit poor-quality skin.

Next, the face and neck skin on the right side is undermined widely beyond the sternocleidomastoid muscle and then across the cheek and along the jowl, freeing any retaining ligaments. The superficial musculoaponeurotic system (SMAS) in the face is addressed with a SMAS resection, SMAS plication, or anterior imbrication as indicated. The lateral platysma is tightened and secured to the mastoid fascia. Final subcutaneous contouring is done with a ball tip cautery. The skin flaps on one side are redraped obliquely and vertically, so that the mandible no longer represents a border to the advancement of the neck skin (Fig. 3.13). This is done while adjusting the flap position to minimize bunching at the proximal (anterior end of sideburn) and distal (posterior lodule) incisions. The addition of the Tisseel glue provides a significant draping advantage in the neck and postauricular region and may result in not using drains which also enhances flap redraping though drains are liberally used and can be used with tissue glue.

After the SMAS is tightened and the skin flaps rotated, positioned, and trimmed they are tacked at the apex with an absorbable suture and at the tragus with a 5-0 nylon suture. The tissue glue is sprayed in an even, thin layer (<1 mL per side) on the undersurface of the flap and on the raw dissected surfaces through the sideburn, preauricular, and postlobule incisions (Fig. 3.14). The preauricular incision is then closed with 5-0 nylon suture. The Tisseel glue is sprayed in 60 seconds or less,

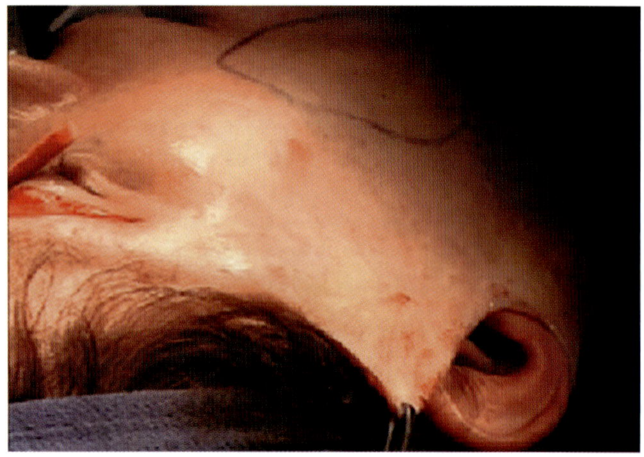

Figure 3.13 Flap redraping in an oblique and vertical vector before sealant application. Note the circle depicting the area of the jowl that was liposuctioned. With permission from Matarasso A, Rizk SS, Markowitz J. Short scar face-lift with the use of fibrin sealant. Dermatol Clin 2005; 23:495–504.

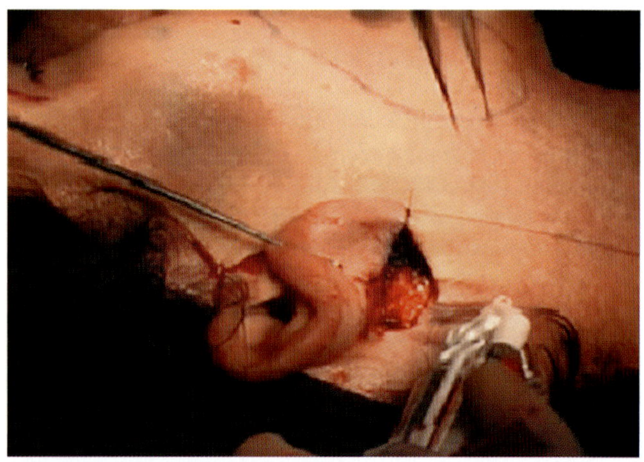

Figure 3.14 Intraoperative fibrin sealant application with dual-injection device before closing. Key sutures at the helical rim and tragus. The preauricular suture begins at the lobule and is then used in a running fashion up to the helical rim. Note the redundant postauricular skin that redrapes and flattens. This is aided by the fibrin sealant and 'walking out' the excess tissue while closing with staples. With permission from Matarasso A, Rizk SS, Markowitz J. Short scar face-lift with the use of fibrin sealant. Dermatol Clin 2005; 23:495–504.

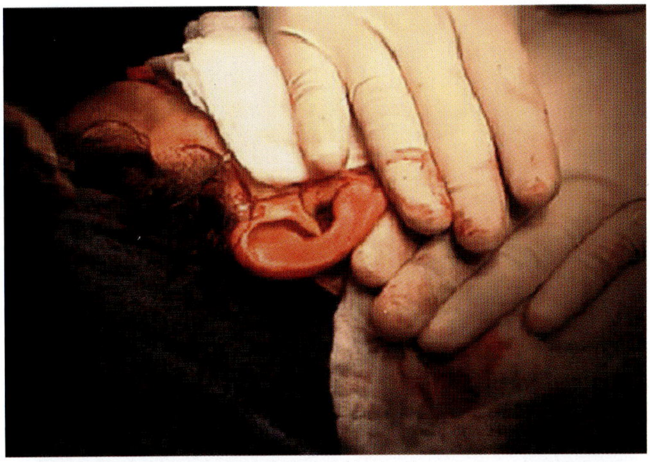

Figure 3.15 Fibrin sealant is applied within 1 minute and manual pressure for 3 minutes after application. During this time, wounds are closed. With permission from Matarasso A, Rizk SS, Markowitz J. Short scar face-lift with the use of fibrin sealant. Dermatol Clin 2005; 23:495–504.

and then external gentle pressure must be applied to the flaps with moist gauze for 3 minutes while avoiding shearing (Fig. 3.15). The postauricular sulcus incision is closed with staples carefully walking out the excess skin to avoid pleating. The transverse sideburn incision is closed from lateral to medial, similarly adjusting the bulge at the lateral end that can occur. At the completion of one side, the patient is turned and surgery continues on the opposite side. Finally, final hemostasis is obtained and sealant is sprayed at the submental incision, and while pressure is applied, the wound is closed with a 5-0 nylon suture. Three layers of gauze are applied and covered with a surginet dressing (examples; Figs 3.16–3.18). No unique postoperative care is necessary.

Facelifting in massive weight loss patients – timing and results

Facial rejuvenation is a part of a comprehensive, staged approach to the patient. The results are very satisfying (following similar principles as in the typical indications seen in an aging patient) as this often completes the long journey of weight loss, facial scars are well hidden and heal demonstrably better than other anatomic sites. Facelift surgery can be combined with other facial or body contour procedures. Safety of combining procedures is determined by the patients medical history, overall operative time required, a coordinated team approach and the patient desires. The goals of surgery are improved contour and rejuvenation with the least conspicuous incision.

Blepharoplasty

Although changes around the eyes generally accompany the aging process of the face, it is not uncommon to observe younger patients who complain of excess skin and baggy lower lids. In the massive weight loss patient, herniated fat compartments persist even after weight loss. There are several important points that should be emphasized regarding surgical technique. Final scars should be well hidden, lying in the supratarsal fold in the upper lids, and along the ciliary margin in the lower lids, when an external incision is made. If possible, the incision should not extend beyond the orbital rim because of the difference in thickness between these two regions. Since the advent of laser resurfacing, there has been an increase in the transconjunctival access for removal of fat pads of the lower lids.

When associated with a face-lift and/or forehead lift, as is generally the case, treatment of the periorbital region is done only after the face and the brow have been blocked, as traction of the flaps may alter the amount of excess skin that needs to be removed. The shape of the incision is tailored to each patient, matching the individual's anatomical features and correcting for asymmetry when this is present. Both sides are demarcated before any infiltration is performed.

COMPLICATIONS AND THEIR MANAGEMENT

Complications in rhytidoplasty are infrequent yet can bring great distress to the patient and to the surgeon.

- It is essential to eliminate from surgery patients who continue to smoke, as the risk for skin slough is greatly increased. Smoking must be stopped completely at least 2 weeks in advance.
- In the immediate postoperative period, blood pressure must be constantly monitored by the nursing staff to prevent hypertension and consequently hematoma formation.
- If an expansive hematoma is diagnosed, the surgeon may initially attempt to drain the collection at the bedside. Early identification and treatment of large hematomas is essential to prevent sequelae.
- Nerve injuries, dehiscence, and other complications are infrequent and should be treated conservatively.

CLINICAL CASES

See Figures 3.19–3.23 for descriptions of clinical cases.

CONCLUSION

With the advent of bariatric surgery, the obese and morbidly obese person can significantly improve his or her quality of life. Nevertheless, these patients will present with excess skin covering in several different body areas, which requires the attention of the plastic surgeon. It has currently become more frequent for the plastic surgeon to be requested to improve the signs of facial aging in the patient who has undergone significant weight loss. Myriad variations of established techniques are available, allowing for the correction of loose facial skin without leaving visible signs that a surgical procedure was performed. When well understood and executed, the round-lifting technique has proven to be reliable in consistently improving the different aspects of the aging face. The short scar facelift variation has been demonstrated to be a feasable alternative in the massive weight loss population.

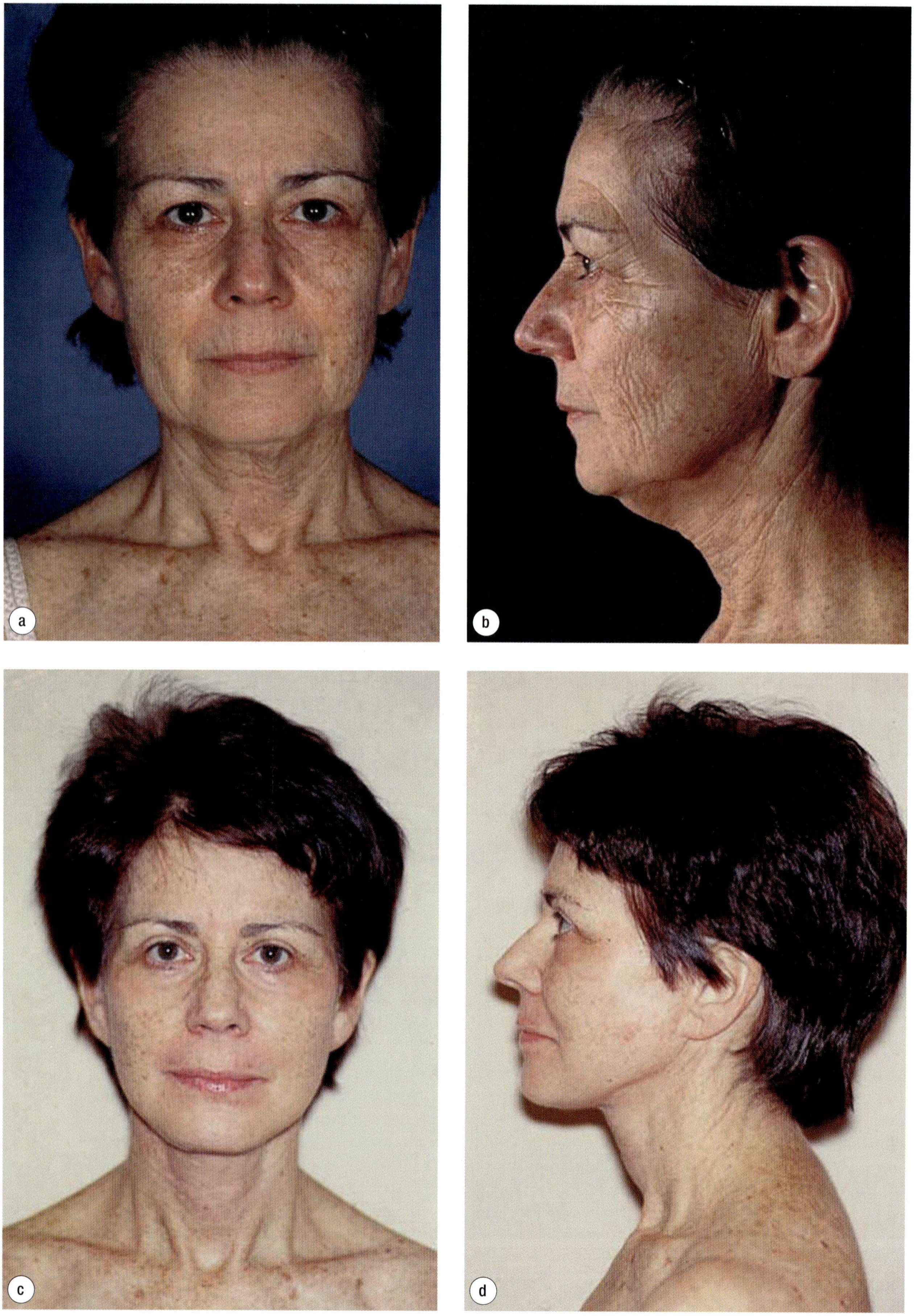

Figure 3.16 (**a** and **b**) This 60-year-old woman underwent short scar face-lift, submentalplasty, upper and lower blepharoplasty, and periocular and perioral erbium laser skin resurfacing. (**c** and **d**) Postoperative views shown at 1 month. Note the dramatic improvement in neck contour with the short scar face-lift. With permission from Matarasso A, Rizk SS, Markowitz J. Short scar face-lift with the use of fibrin sealant. Dermatol Clin 2005; 23:495–504.

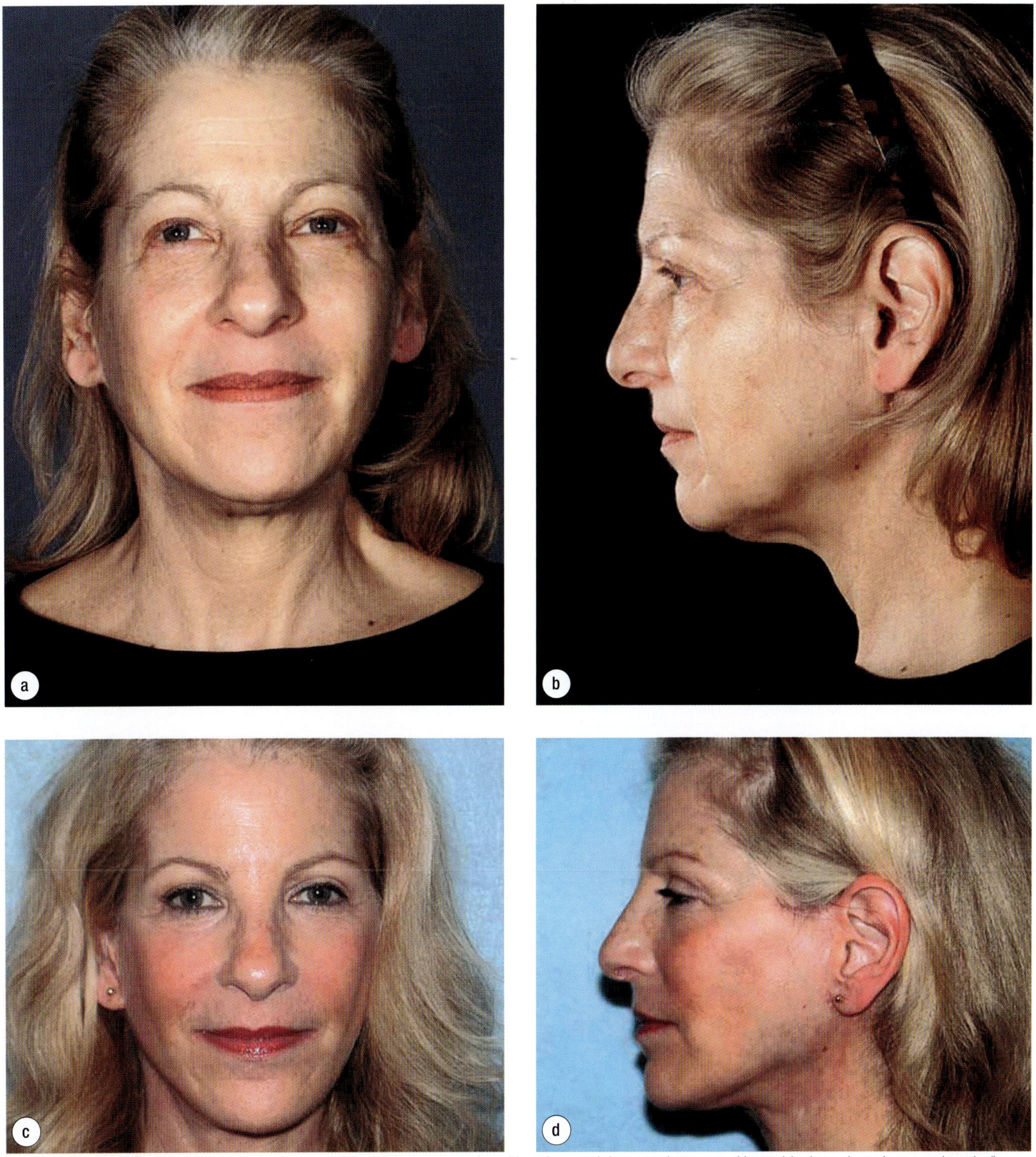

Figure 3.17 (**a** and **b**) This 64-year-old woman underwent a short scar face-lift, submentalplasty, and upper and lower blepharoplasty (transconjunctival). (**c** and **d**) Postoperative views shown at 2 months. With permission from Matarasso A, Rizk SS, Markowitz J. Short scar face-lift with the use of fibrin sealant. Dermatol Clin 2005; 23:495–504.

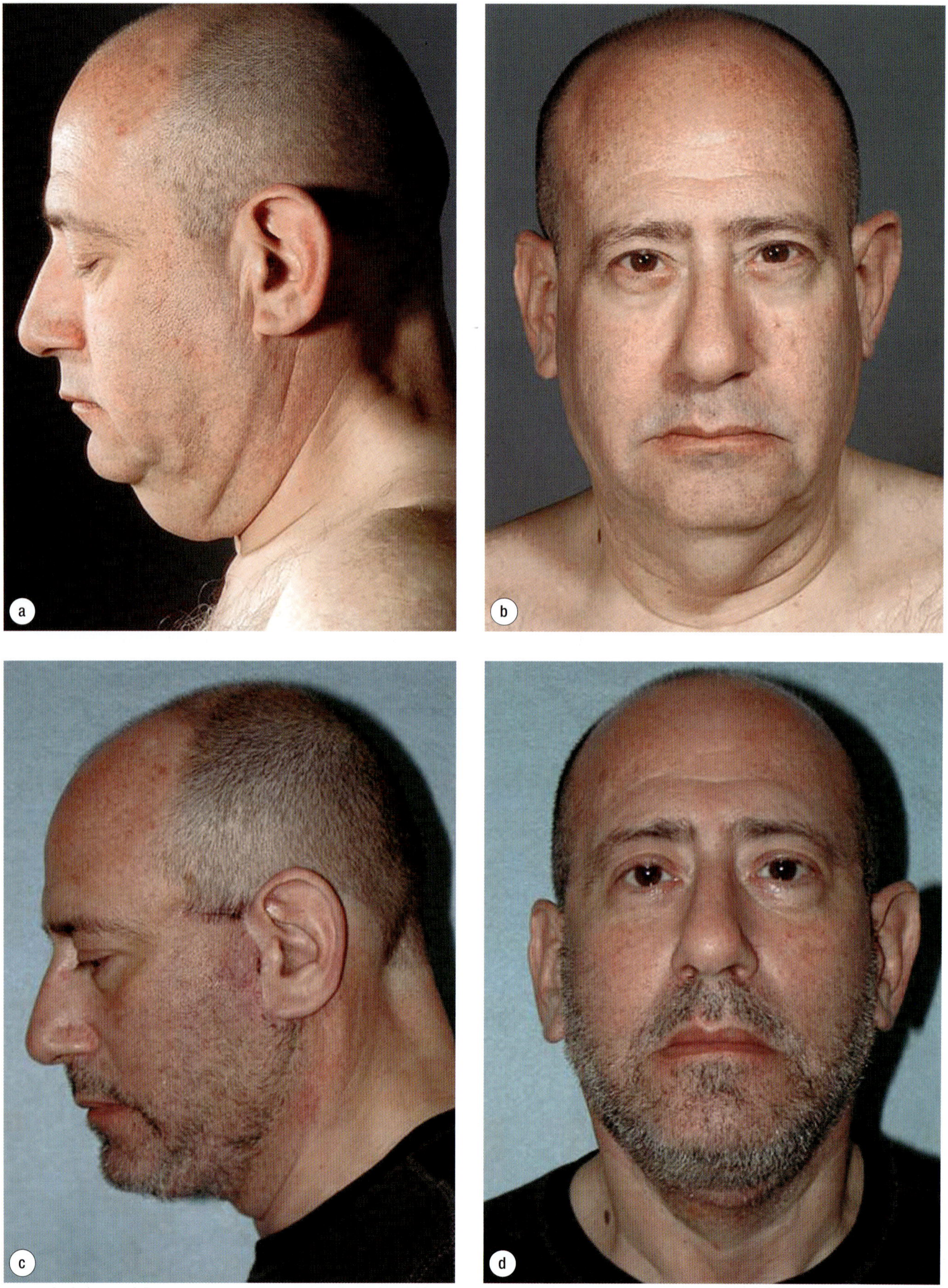

Figure 3.18 (**a** and **b**) This 55-year-old diabetic man underwent a short scar face-lift and submentalplasty after a 100 lb (45 kg) weight loss. (**c** and **d**) Postoperative views shown at 2 weeks. With permission from Matarasso A, Rizk SS, Markowitz J. Short scar face-lift with the use of fibrin sealant. Dermatol Clin 2005; 23:495–504.

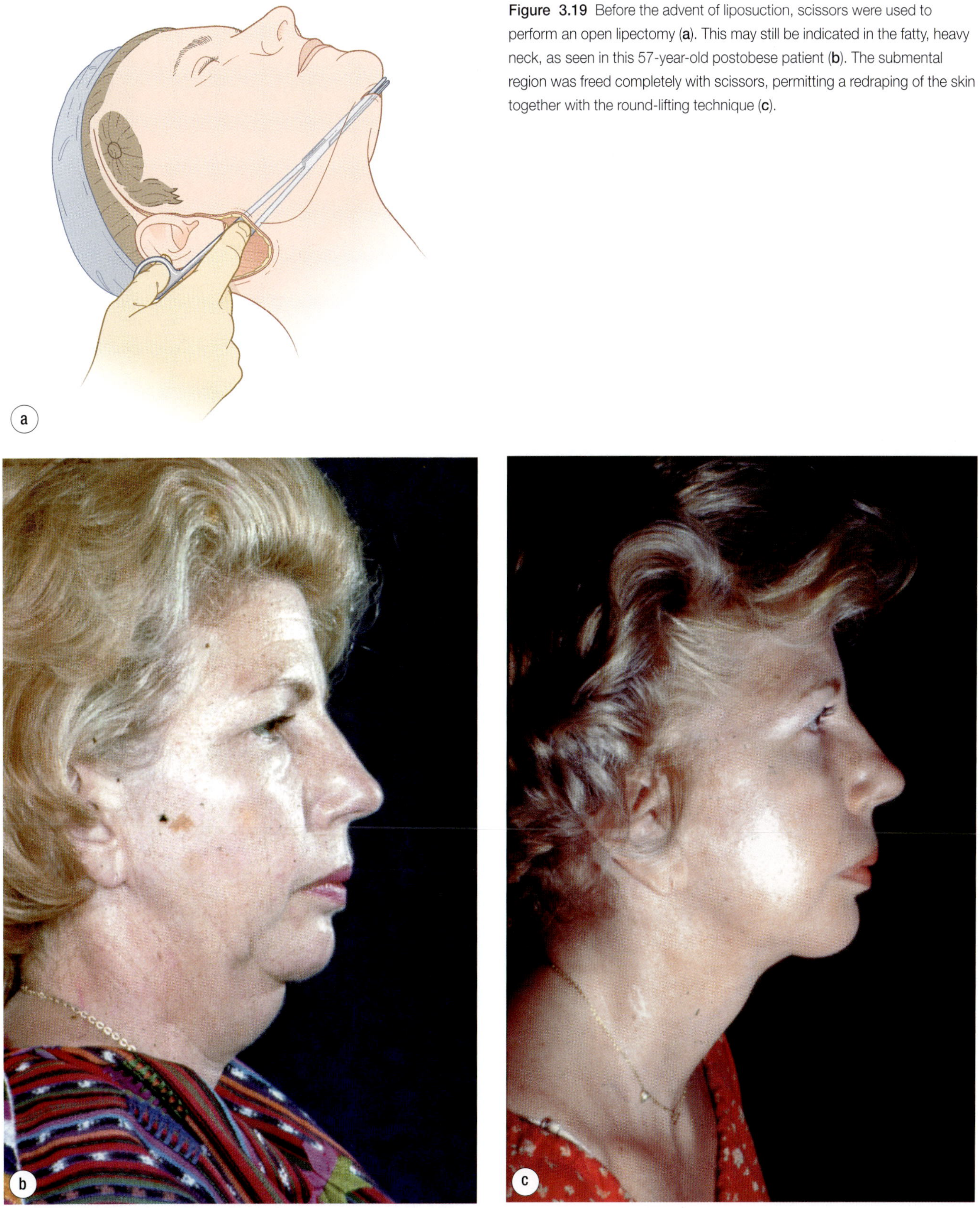

Figure 3.19 Before the advent of liposuction, scissors were used to perform an open lipectomy (**a**). This may still be indicated in the fatty, heavy neck, as seen in this 57-year-old postobese patient (**b**). The submental region was freed completely with scissors, permitting a redraping of the skin together with the round-lifting technique (**c**).

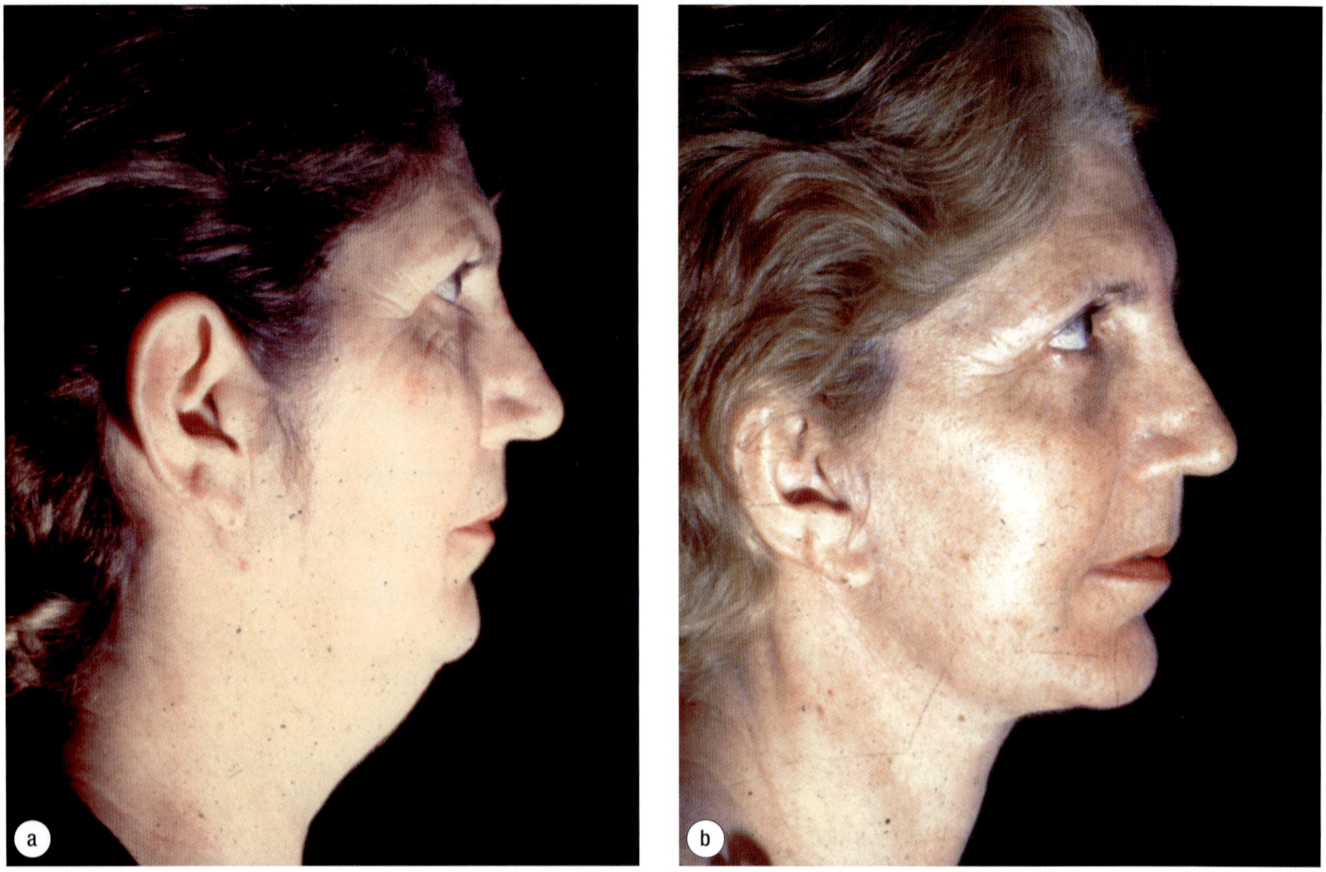

Figure 3.20 A main complaint of the postobese patient is flaccidity of the submental region. Following ample liposuction of the submental area, the round-lifting technique allows for a repositioning of undermined facial and cervical flaps without causing dislocation of anatomical landmarks, as seen in this 49-year-old female patient (**a**, before; **b**, after).

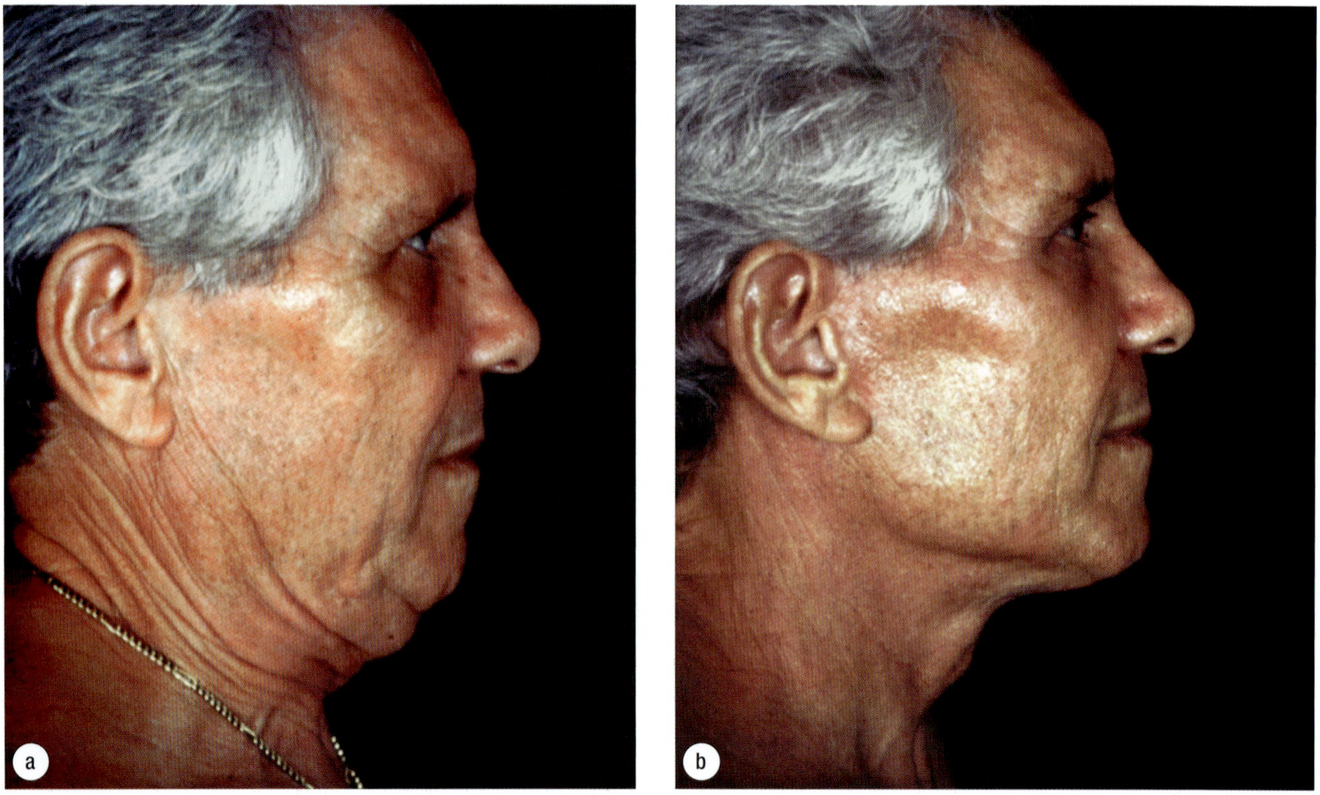

Figure 3.21 Men requesting a facial rejuvenation are seen more frequently than they were previously. Currently, weight reduction is strong motivation for a rhytidoplasty, as in this 61-year-old man (**a**, before; **b**, after).

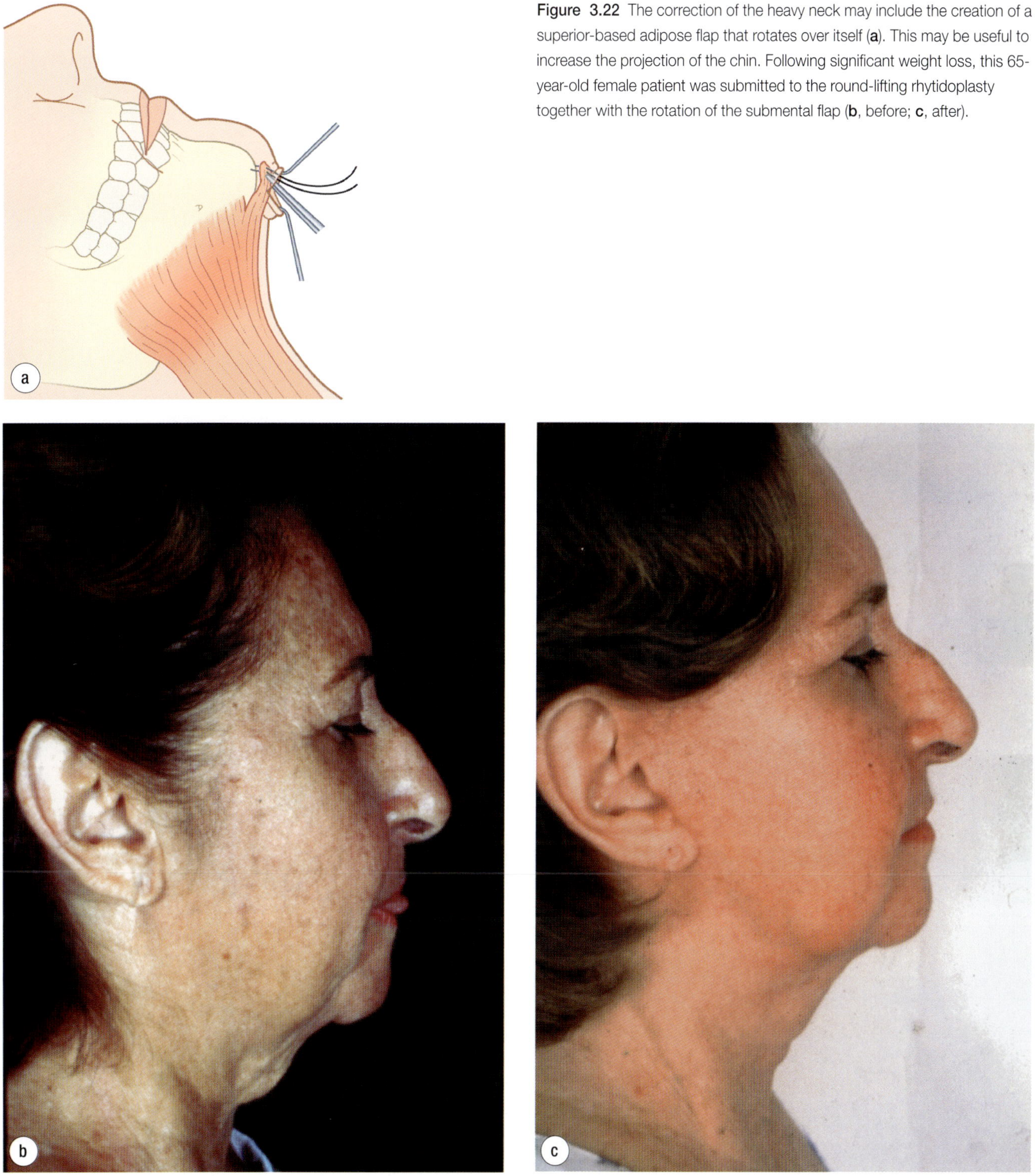

Figure 3.22 The correction of the heavy neck may include the creation of a superior-based adipose flap that rotates over itself (**a**). This may be useful to increase the projection of the chin. Following significant weight loss, this 65-year-old female patient was submitted to the round-lifting rhytidoplasty together with the rotation of the submental flap (**b**, before; **c**, after).

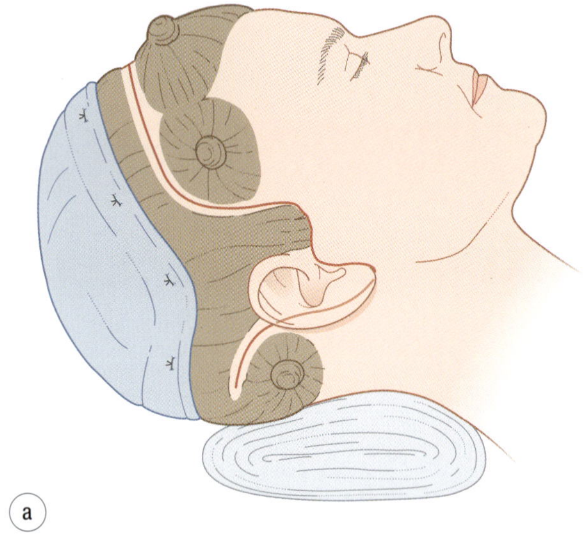

Figure 3.23 An atypical approach to the heavy neck and face may be indicated, as in this secondary face-lift. The incision becomes prepilose over the temporal hairline and then meets the opposite coronal incision, allowing for treatment of the forehead without dislocation of the hairline (**a**). This alternative incision was chosen in this 58-year-old female patient after weight loss (**b**, before; **c**, after).

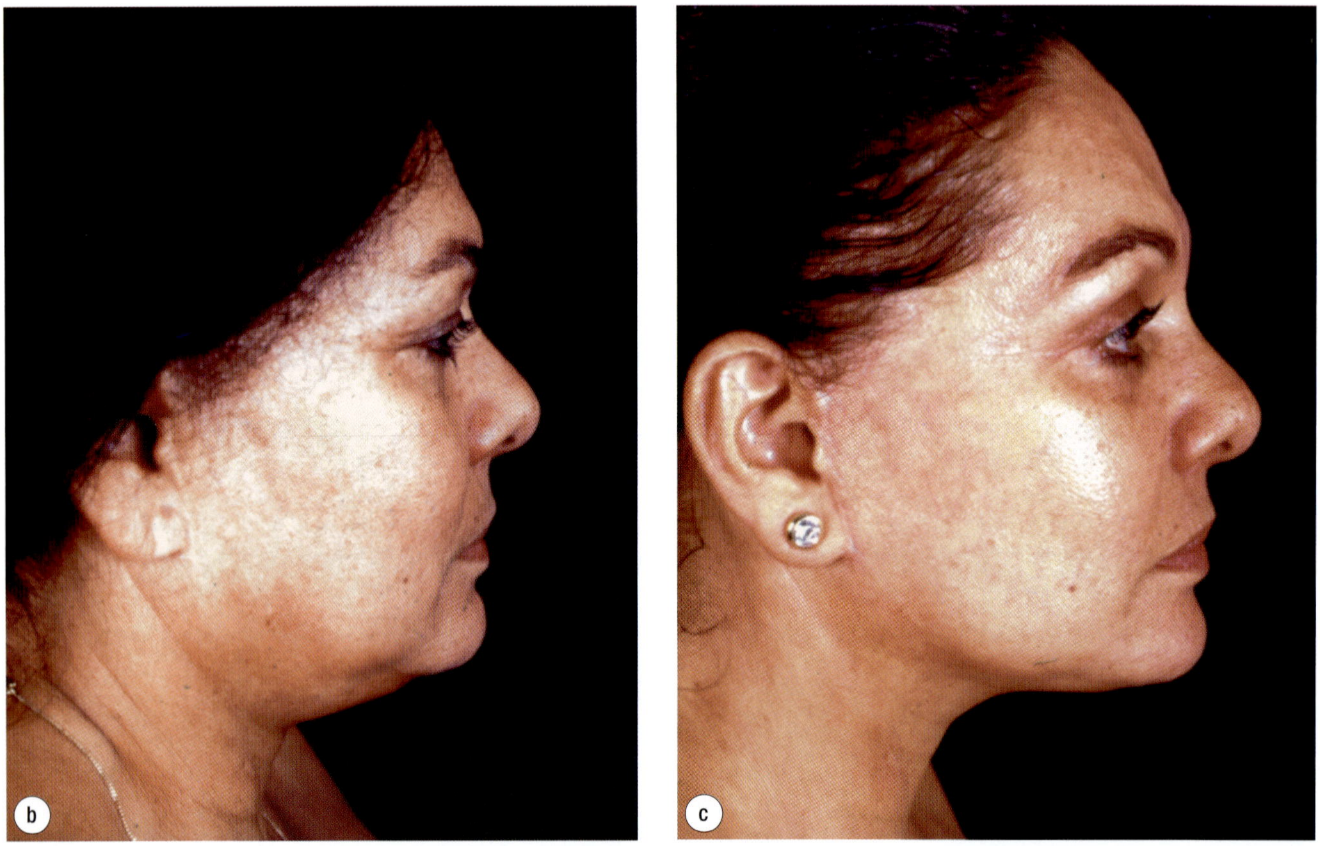

Finally, the plastic surgeon should be assured that the patient understands that the purpose of any procedure for the aging face is to help the individual cross with enhanced self-confidence the sometimes difficult path to a mature age, and not to return the patient to an earlier stage of life. Experience is necessary to investigate and appreciate these subjective motivations. This evaluation requires both empathy and openness toward the patient.

Acknowledgment

The authors are grateful to Natale Gontijo do Amorim, M.D., for her close collaboration in the preparation of this chapter.

FURTHER READING

Matarasso A. Botox injections for facial rejuvenation. In: Nahai, F. The art of aesthetic surgery: Principles and technique. St Louis: Quality Medical Publishing; 2005:195–221.

Matarasso A. Botulinum toxin. In: McCarthy J, Galiano R, Boutros S. Current therapy in plastic surgery. Philadelphia: Saunders; 2005:324–325.

Matarasso A, Elkwood A, Rankin M, Elkowitz M. National plastic surgery survey: face-lift techniques and complications. Plast Reconstr Surg 2000; 106:1185–1195.

Matarasso A. Elkwood AI, Rankin M, et al. National plastic surgery: Brow lifting techniques and complications. Plast Reconstr Surg 2001; 108(7):2143–2153.

Matarasso A, Rizk SS, Markowitz J. Short scar face-lift with the use of fibrin sealant. Dermatol Clin 2005; 23:495–504.

Matarasso A, Wallach SG, DiFrancesco L, Rankin M. Age-based comparisons of patients undergoing secondary rhytidectomy. Aesth Surg J 2002; 22:526–530.

Pitanguy I, Amorim NFG. Forehead lifting: the juxtapilose subperiosteal approach. Aesthetic Plast Surg 2003; 27:58–62.

Pitanguy I, Amorim NFG. Treatment of the nasolabial fold. Rev Bras Cir 1997; 87:231–242.

Pitanguy I, Brentano JMS, Salgado F, et al. Incisions in primary and secondary rhytidoplasties. Rev Bras Cir 1995; 85:165–176.

Pitanguy I, Ceravolo M. Hematoma post-rhytidectomy: how we treat it. Plast Reconstr Surg 1981; 67:526–528.

Pitanguy I, Ceravolo MP, Dègand M. Nerve injuries during rhytidectomy: considerations after 3,203 cases. Aesthetic Plast Surg 1980; 4:257–265.

Pitanguy I, Pamplona DC, Giuntini ME, et al. Computational simulation of rhytidectomy by the 'round-lifting' technique. Rev Bras Cir 1995; 85:213–218.

Pitanguy I, Pamplona DC, Weber HI, et al. Numerical modeling of the aging face. Plast Reconstr Surg 1998; 102:200–204.

Pitanguy I, Radwanski HN, Amorim NFG. Treatment of the aging face using the 'round lifting' technique. Aesth Surg J 1999; 19:216–222.

Pitanguy I, Radwanski HN. Rejuvenation of the brow. Matarasso SL, Matarasso A, eds. Dermatology clinics, vol 15. Philadelphia: Saunders; 1998:623–635.

Pitanguy I, Ramos A. The frontal branch of the facial nerve: the importance of its variations in face-lifting. Plast Reconstr Surg 1966; 38:352–356.

Pitanguy I, Salgado F, Radwanski HN. Submental liposuction as an ancillary procedure in face-lifting. Face 1995; 4(1):1–13.

Pitanguy I, Soares G, Machado BH, et al. CO2 laser associated with the 'round-lifting' technique. J Cutan Laser Ther 1999; 1:145–152.

Pitanguy I. Ancillary procedures in face-lifting. Clin Plast Surg 1978; 5:51–69.

Pitanguy I. Facial cosmetic surgery: a 30-year perspective. Plast Reconstr Surg 2000; 105:1517–1529.

Pitanguy I. Forehead lifting. In: Pitanguy I. Aesthetic surgery of head and body. Berlin: Springer Verlag; 1984:202–214.

Pitanguy I. Frontalis–procerus–corrugator apponeurosis in the correction of frontal and glabellar wrinkles. Ann Plast Surg 1979; 2:422–427.

Pitanguy I. Indication for and treatment of frontal and glabellar wrinkles in an analysis of 3,404 consecutive cases of rhytidectomy. Plast Reconstr Surg 1981; 67:157–166.

Pitanguy I. Les chemins de la beauté. Un maitre de la chirurgie plastique témoigne. Paris: JC Lattes; 1983.

Pitanguy I. The aging face. In: Carlsen L, Slatt B. The naked face. Ontario: General Publishing; 1979:27.

Pitanguy I. The face. In: Pitanguy I. Aesthetic surgery of head and body. Berlin: Springer Verlag; 1984:165–200.

Pitanguy I. The round-lifting technique. Facial Plast Surg 2000; 16(3):255–267.

APPROACH TO THE BREAST AFTER WEIGHT LOSS

4

J. Peter Rubin, James O'Toole and Siamak Agha-Mohammadi

> **Key Points**
> - Carefully assess parenchymal volume, amount of redundant skin envelope, and extent of lateral skin/fat roll.
> - Consider order of breast reshaping in association with other planned body-contouring procedures.
> - Plan Wise pattern marking to encompass lateral chest wall tissue in order to eliminate skin/fat roll and also allow for autologous volume augmentation.
> - Deepithelialization of entire Wise pattern and complete degloving of parenchyma preserves breast volume and provides broad dermal surface area.
> - Permanent suspension sutures secure dermis to rib periosteum, and multiple plication sutures in dermis allow precise control of breast shape.

INTRODUCTION

The nature of breast deformities after weight loss

Postbariatric patients manifest severe breast deformities that are very different from those seen in the traditional mastopexy candidate. Severe volume deflation with distortion of shape and inelastic skin is common. There are four problems.

1. There is a tendency toward significant and sometimes asymmetric breast volume loss with a deflated and flattened appearance.
2. There tends to be dramatic loss of skin elasticity, as well as tremendous skin excess relative to the parenchymal volume.
3. The nipples are usually too medial in position.
4. A final peculiarity, fairly unique to this population, is the presence of prominent axillary skin, or in many cases a fatty roll. This blurs the border between the lateral breast and chest wall, sometimes forming one continuous roll of tissue (Fig. 4.1).

The role of short scar techniques

To achieve an aesthetically pleasing breast in the setting of these deformities, there must be reshaping of the deflated breast parenchyma and augmentation with autologous tissue to restore superior fullness and projection. The skin envelope must be reduced and prominent axillary skin rolls eliminated. It is the authors' view that short scar techniques are inadequate in handling the redundant inelastic skin envelope in these patients. Moreover, short scar techniques cannot properly address the lateral skin excess.

Approach used by the authors

The authors have developed and refined a technique using the principles of dermal suspension and total parenchymal reshaping. An extended Wise pattern encompasses and eliminates lateral skin rolls, while at the same time providing additional tissue that may be used as necessary for volume augmentation. Deepithelialization of the entire Wise pattern creates a broad dermal surface area that can be plicated to precisely control breast shape and can be suspended to the chest wall.

Background

The technique developed by the authors for the weight loss patient is based on lessons learned from the historical development of breast-reshaping methods. Schwarzmann's early contribution demonstrating the importance of dermal blood supply was essential.[1] Beisenberger's conceptual revolution of total dissociation of the skin envelope from the glandular tissue was invaluable in the development of this and many other procedures.[2] While the Beisenberger technique had great support and longevity, surgeons continued to produce technical refinements. Thorek is credited with introducing the free nipple graft in the 1920s,[3] and this method provides a valuable lifeboat for breast surgeons who note poor nipple perfusion in the operating room. The 1950s saw Wise describe a technique to control the skin envelope in a manner that accentuates breast shape.[4] In 1960, Strombeck described a horizontal bipedicled procedure with enhanced nipple vascularity.[5] A significant contribution came from McKissock's vertical bipedicled flap, which facilitated the creation of a more natural-appearing breast.[6] In 1963, Skoog produced work supporting the transposition of the nipple areolar complex (NAC) on a unilateral vascular pedicle.[7] Eventually, Rubiero described,[8] and Courtiss and Goldwyn championed the inferior pedicle with the Wise pattern of scars.[9] The various approaches applied in the

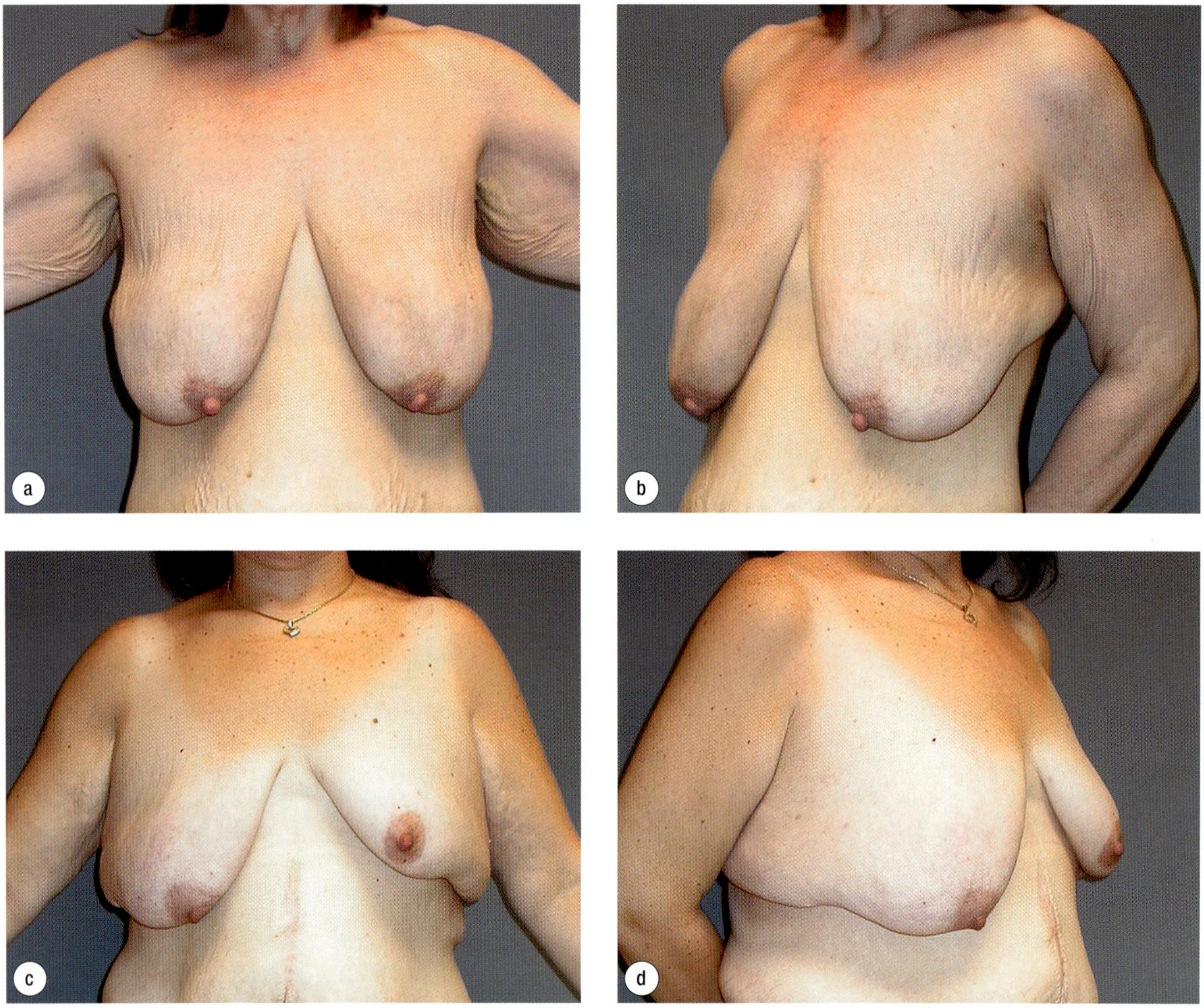

Figure 4.1 (**a** and **b**) Representative patient showing classic deformities of severe volume deflation and medial nipple position. (**c** and **d**) Representative patient demonstrating prominent lateral roll of skin and fat that distorts the border between breast and chest wall.

historical development phase of breast surgery demonstrated that safe and effective reshaping could be accomplished through multiple techniques based on sound principles.

Many techniques dictated that the shape of the breast was contingent on the pattern and amount of skin excised, and ultimately relied on skin support to maintain shape.[10] Untoward effects of this approach include parenchymal 'bottoming out', recurrent ptosis, and lengthy scars. Because of these realizations, surgeons sought to create ways to uplift and reshape the breast in a more durable fashion, while at the same time minimizing scar formation. Lassus pioneered the vertical mammoplasty, with volume control via a central wedge resection, transposition of the NAC on a superior pedicle flap, and a vertical scar to finish.[11,12] Lejour expanded on this by adding regional suction lipectomy, glandular undermining, and subsequent glandular fixation to the chest wall.[13] Chen and Wei preferred a variant of the vertical mammoplasty, the S approach.[14] To further pursue reliable parenchymal shaping with minimal scarring, Exner and Scheufler devised a vertical scar variant with segmental central parenchymal resection and concomitant dermal suspension via deepithelialized dermis caudal to the NAC and ultimately fixed to the chest wall.[15]

Progress toward desirable contour with minimal scarring was furthered by Benelli and his periareolar 'round block' technique.[16] Hammond utilizes a technique with fixation of the pedicle to the chest wall with permanent sutures, and closure with a periareolar scar with a variable-length vertical component.[17] Goes described a 'double skin technique' and ultimately utilized mesh to achieve desirable breast contour with greater support.[18]

Many surgeons focused on strategies to improve and maintain upper pole fullness, and these techniques often involved fixation of breast tissue to adjacent structures. Pitanguy restricted resection to only the inferior pole, and utilized a 'straight resection' or 'inverted keel' for firmer breast tissue. Closure of medial and lateral pillars of parenchyma and an inverted T incision finished his procedure.[19] Cerqueira's approach was to create a superior pedicle, resect a central block of parenchyma, and subsequently secure the dermoglandular pedicle under the pectoralis.[20] Frey's contribution allowed for parenchymal contouring and suspension via a dermal brassiere fixated to the anterior thoracic wall with non-absorbable suture, and complete elimination of the medial component of the scar.[21] Building upon the concept of a dermal bra, Qiao et al. devised an approach that resected a crescent of glandular tissue superolaterally, with dermal fixation to the pectoralis fascia.[22] Gulyas's periareolar techniques also relied on manipulation of the 'dermal cloak' to support and shape the breast.[23] Graf and Biggs created an inferior dermoglandular pedicle that they passed under a loop of pectoralis and secured to the pectoralis fascia. The NAC is carried on the elevated breast, and the inferior flap is fixed to the pectoralis fascia in the upper pole to ensure upper pole fullness with closure of medial and lateral pillars behind the flap.[10] Lockwood achieved his results via a modification of the Wise pattern, with the primary supportive element being non-absorbable sutures in the superficial fascial system to decrease dermal tension and subsequent scarring.[24]

Many important principles are embodied in the techniques described. However, when considering the complex deformity seen in the massive weight loss patient, none of the above procedures seem to be ideal. Moreover, it becomes obvious that short scar techniques are of limited value in this patient population. What is required is a technique that allows for:

- precise and symmetric NAC positioning,
- precise control of parenchymal breast shape and contour,
- possible autoaugmentation in the volume-deficient patient, and
- control of the remaining skin envelope.

In our technique, we make use of a well-vascularized central dermoglandular pedicle.[2,16] A modification of the traditional Wise pattern allows for precise control of the skin envelope and NAC position.[4] The dermal suspension techniques of Qiao, Frey, Cerqueira, and others prompted our use of parenchymal suspension and extensive sculpting via dermal plication and fixation to the chest wall.[15,18,20–23] Holmstrom's lateral thoracodorsal transposition flap for breast reconstruction after mastectomy facilitated the notion of autoaugmentation via recruitment of redundant axillary tissue.[25] Medial fullness is assured via the elevation and manipulation of a medial breast flap.

The technique described below has the advantages of correcting, with a low complication rate, the severe breast deformities associated with weight loss. Notably, the deformity of a lateral axillary roll can be eliminated and used to augment breast volume. The disadvantages of this technique include:

- a lengthy scar,
- considerable time in the operating room for the extensive deepithelialization, and
- a high degree of 'intraoperative tailoring' that cannot be premarked.

Despite the disadvantages, this technique is safe and reliable for restoring a youthful breast shape in the massive weight loss patient. Great control over both skin envelope and parenchymal shape may be gained with this procedure.

PREOPERATIVE EVALUATION

Patients with mild breast deformities following weight loss should be considered for traditional mastopexy techniques, including short scar approaches. However, existing mastopexy techniques are not always adequate to achieve a good aesthetic result with these deformities when faced with the following clinical findings.

- Profound breast volume loss with flattening of the parenchyma against the chest wall.
- A redundant, inelastic skin envelope.
- Grade 3 nipple ptosis.
- Medialization of the NAC.
- The presence of a prominent axillary roll of skin that extends from the lateral breast.

We have identified few contraindications for the use of this technique. Because of the extensive flap dissection, we have avoided performing this procedure on active tobacco users. As with all breast reshaping patients, we perform a thorough history and physical examination for breast disease, as well as require mammography imaging consistent with the American Cancer Society screening guidelines. Scars from previous breast surgery may present a relative contraindication if they pose a risk to perfusion of undermined tissues. Careful evaluation for parenchymal volume is undertaken, as well as asymmetry. The lateral breast region is inspected for a significant skin roll, and an assessment is made regarding the amount of tissue that may be mobilized from the lateral chest wall for autologous breast augmentation. In the case of significant asymmetry, we will either selectively augment the smaller breast using lateral chest wall tissue or, if this is not possible, reduce the larger breast to match the smaller one.

The surgical goals for breast reshaping in the face of these deformities are to:

- use all available breast tissue, and also have the ability to recruit additional autologous tissue;
- address the nipple position;
- restore superior pole projection;
- reshape the skin envelope without relying on it for support;
- eliminate the lateral skin roll; and
- create a discrete 'lateral sweep' to the breast shape.

The technique we describe, using the principles of controlled parenchymal reshaping and dermal suspension, will meet these goals. This safe and reproducible technique yields a youthful breast shape in a very challenging population.

SURGICAL TECHNIQUE

Marking

The surgical technique is based on a Wise pattern with preservation of a central pedicle. The nipple position is referenced to the inferior mammary fold, and moved to a more lateral position along a symmetrically drawn breast meridian. The vertical limbs are marked at 5 cm. The lateral portion of the Wise pattern is extended posteriorly to encompass the axillary skin roll and provide additional autologous tissue for breast volume. The Wise pattern can be extended to the posterior axillary line and beyond, depending on the extent of the lateral skin roll and the amount of tissue desired for autologous breast augmentation (Fig. 4.2). The robust blood supply of the lateral thoracic region allows for a significant amount of tissue to be safely mobilized to the breast.

We must make an important point here: The area of skin resection to alleviate the lateral skin roll may extend beyond the portion of the Wise pattern to be deepithelialized (i.e. a portion of the lateral 'wing' of the Wise pattern may be deepithelialized and saved to assist in the reshaping and add volume, while the remainder is simply excised to eliminate the skin roll). This flexibility in design allows the surgeon to control the skin envelope and titrate the amount of lateral tissue to mobilize to the breast.

Technique

The entire region within the Wise pattern is deepithelialized (Figs 4.3 and 4.4). The breast parenchyma is then completely degloved by raising a 1 cm-thick flap overlying the breast capsule. Once the chest wall is reached, undermining continues over the pectoralis major fascia to the level of the clavicle. Medial and lateral flaps of breast tissue are mobilized by undermining over the chest wall. Care is taken to preserve significant perforating vessels that enter the tissue flaps near the base. The lateral flap is trimmed to desired size, as necessary. The nipple survives on a healthy central pedicle.

The next step is suspension of the central dermal extension to the chest wall. This is performed with a 0 braided permanent suture in a mattress fashion. The dermis is firmly tacked to the periosteum of a selected rib along the breast meridian. This carefully placed suture must pass through the pectoralis muscle, and relies on palpation of the rib with the non-dominant hand to guide the needle pass. The choice of rib level for fixation is made intraoperatively based on the distance between the dermal edge and the nipple (i.e. how NAC position is affected by height of suspension). This is most often the second rib. The suspension should raise the level of the nipple close to the intended final position. The lateral breast flap is then suspended and secured to the chest wall by tacking to rib periosteum in a similar manner. The lateral flap dermal suspension suture will be very close to the central suspension suture, although a lower rib level may be selected to provide the desired shape. This will create a discrete lateral curvature to the breast shape and replace the unsightly blending of breast tissue with the lateral chest (Fig. 4.5). The medial breast flap is then suspended and secured to the chest wall.

With the suspension points established, control of the parenchymal shape is then gained. The broad surface area of dermis is meticulously plicated with running absorbable sutures to adjust the shape. Braided absorbable 2–0 sutures are used. The process starts with approximation of the dermis of the lateral flap to the central dermal extension. This is followed by plication of the medial flap dermis to the central dermal extension. The inferior pole of the breast is then plicated to shorten the nipple to inframammary fold (IMF) distance and to increase projection. The authors have learned to do each suspension and plication step simultaneously on both breasts rather than completing one breast and moving to another. This permits better symmetry.

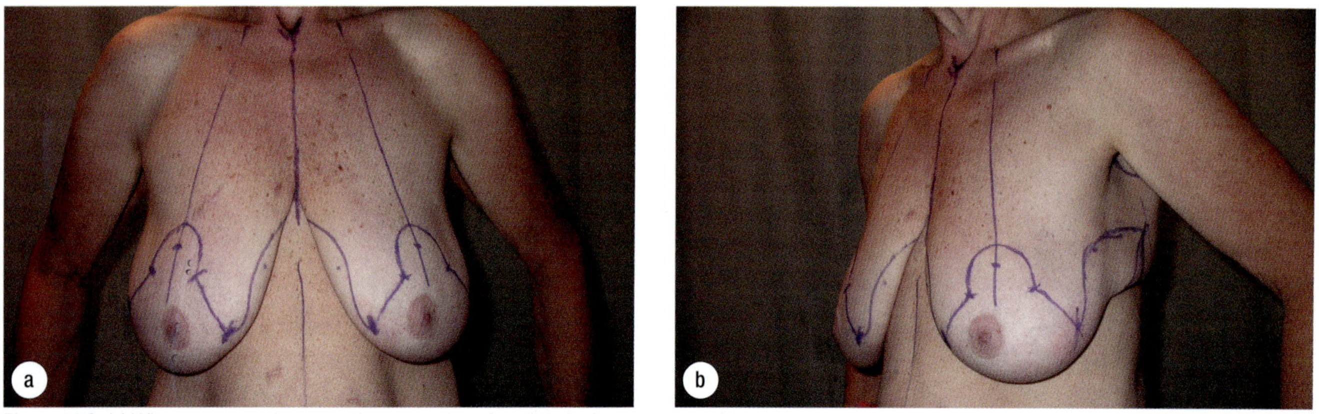

Figure 4.2 (**a**) Wise pattern marking showing correction of medial nipple position and (**b**) extension of pattern to address lateral skin roll and provide additional tissue for autoaugmentation.

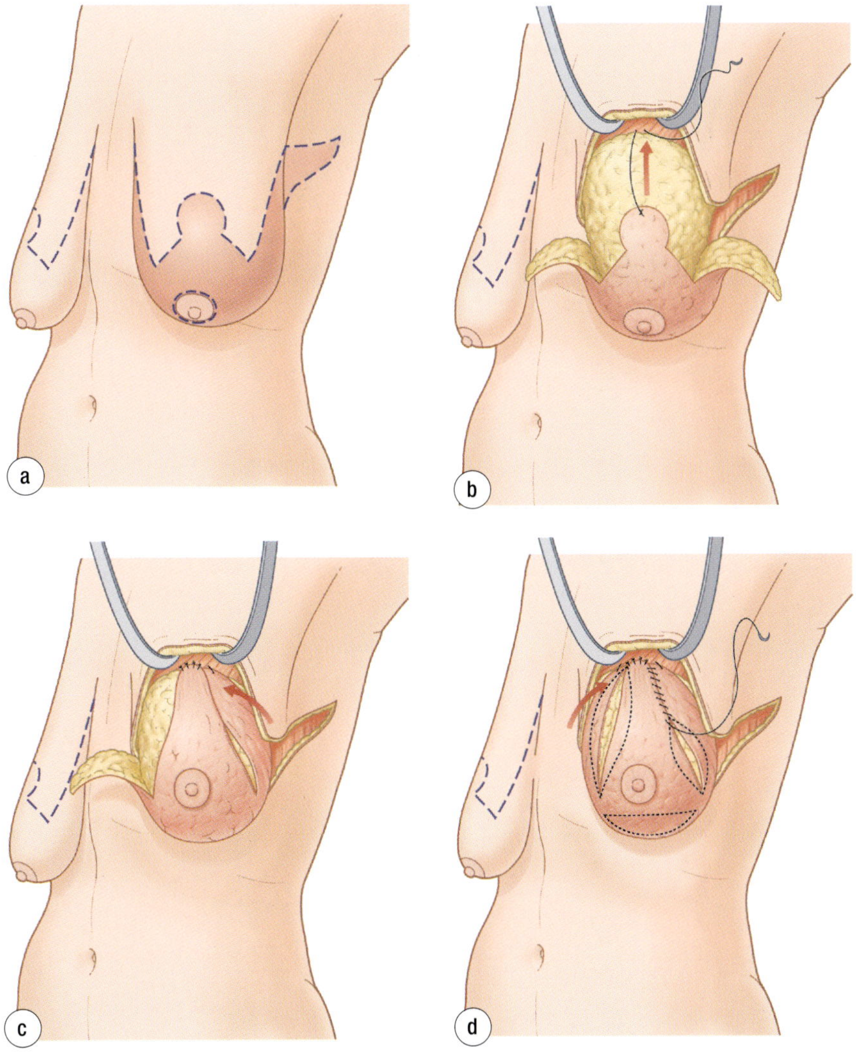

Figure 4.3 (a) The patient is marked with a Wise pattern that extends laterally to encompass the redundant axillary roll. The entire area of the Wise pattern is deepithelialized, preserving an extensive dermal surface. (b) The breast parenchyma is degloved by raising a 1 cm-thick flap and then continuing the dissection superiorly just superficial to the pectoralis fascia. Medial and lateral flaps of dermis/breast tissue are mobilized from the chest wall. The central dermal extension is elevated and secured to the chest wall (usually rib periosteum) using braided nylon suture. (c) The lateral breast flap is elevated to create the lateral curvature of the breast mound, and the dermis secured to the chest wall near the previous fixation point. The lateral flap can be extended posteriorly on the chest wall to provide extra tissue for autologous volume augmentation. (d) The dermal edge of the medial breast flap is fixed to the chest wall. A running braided suture is used to approximate the dermal edges of the lateral flap and central dermal extension. Dashed lines show the pattern of plication used. The pattern of plication may be individualized to achieve the best breast shape in each patient. In general, there is a later component, a medial component, and an inferior component that corrects the "bottomed out" appearance and increases projection.

After initial placement of plication sutures, a fine-tuning process follows in which additional plication sutures are added. Sutures may be necessary to secure the lateral breast flap to the lateral chest wall fascia. Constant redraping of the skin flap during the shaping process helps guide both major and minor adjustments to breast form. If the abdominal wall tissues are very loose, a decision may be made to secure the superficial fascial system layer of the dissected edge of the abdominal wall to the periosteum of the fifth rib. This will restore IMF position.

For closure, the authors favor using a half-buried mattress suture to secure the dermal edges at the 'triple point' along the IMF. The dermis around the nipple may be incised part-way around the circumference to release any tethering as necessary. Intradermal sutures are then used to complete the closure, and suction drains placed in each lateral breast. A lightly compressive chest wrap is then placed.

Restoration of breast shape and symmetry can be achieved in difficult cases with this technique. Patient satisfaction has been high in all cases. Pre- and postoperative results are shown in Figures 4.6–4.8.

Optimizing outcomes

- Extend the Wise pattern as far lateral as is necessary to eliminate the skin rolls.

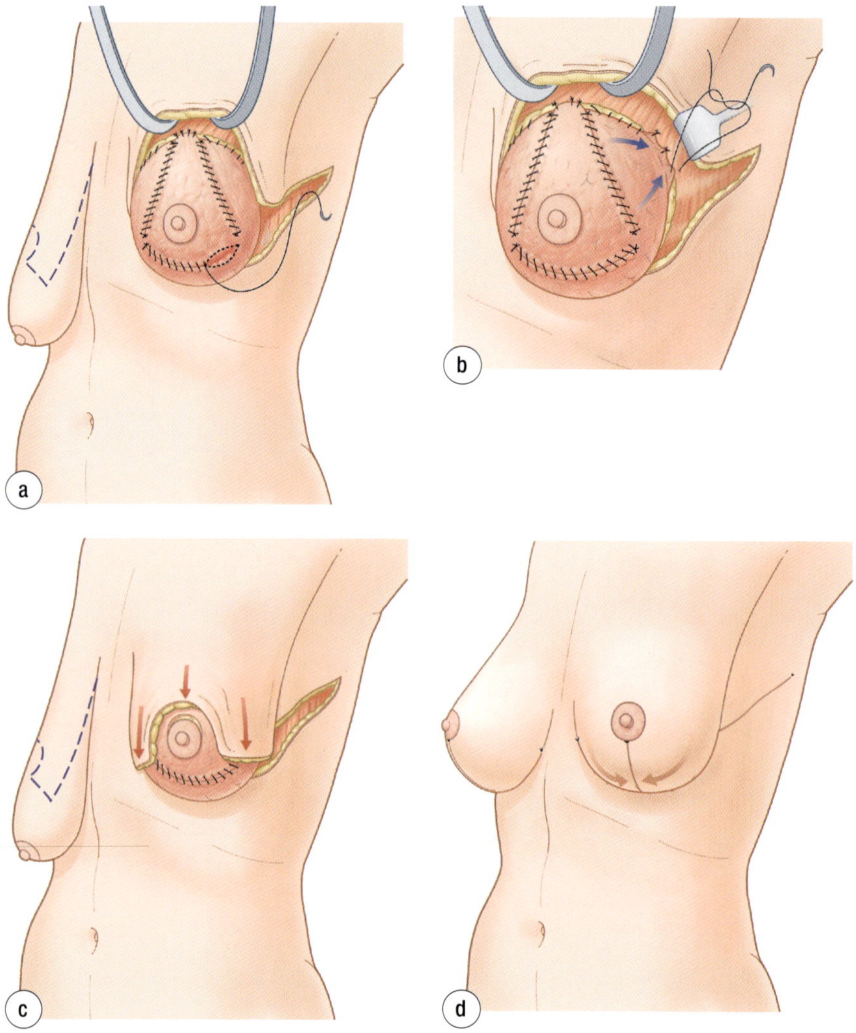

Figure 4.4 (**a**) The dermis of the medial breast flap is approximated to the central dermal extension using a running suture. The dermis on the inferior pole of the breast is plicated with a running suture to shorten the distance between areola and inferior mammary fold to approximately 5 cm. (**b**) The dermis along the lateral breast is secured to the lateral chest fascia (not rib pereostium) with permanent sutures to increase projection and accentuate the lateral curve of the breast. The breast parenchyma is now firmly secured to the chest wall, and the shape has been adjusted using the plication sutures. (**c** and **d**) The breast skin flap is redraped and closed with absorbable intradermal sutures over a drain. If the nipple is tethered and pointing in an inappropriate direction, the dermis adjacent to the nipple is scored to release the tension. Because of the robust pedicle, scoring of the dermis can be safely performed along part of the circumference, if necessary.

- The entire lateral wing of the Wise pattern may be deepithelialized and preserved to add volume to the breast, as needed. Conversely, a smaller portion may be preserved and the remainder excised.
- Keep the breast flap approximately 1 cm thick (or greater), and once at the level of the pectoralis fascia, continue undermining superiorly above the level of the second rib.
- Avoid performing this operation on smokers because of the risk of flap necrosis.
- Plication of the dermis is most effective on the lateral and inferior aspects of the breast, where it serves to increase projection and create a distinct lateral curvature to the breast mound.
- If the nipple is tethered, the surrounding dermis may be partially incised to release it. A robust central pedicle supports the nipple and allows this to be done safely.

Postoperative care and course

- The authors use a lightly compressive breast dressing for the first 5 days, and then ask the patient to wear a sports bra with no wires for the next month.
- Drains are maintained for the first 48 h and then discontinued if the output is decreasing.
- Heavy lifting and exercise is prohibited until 4 weeks after surgery.

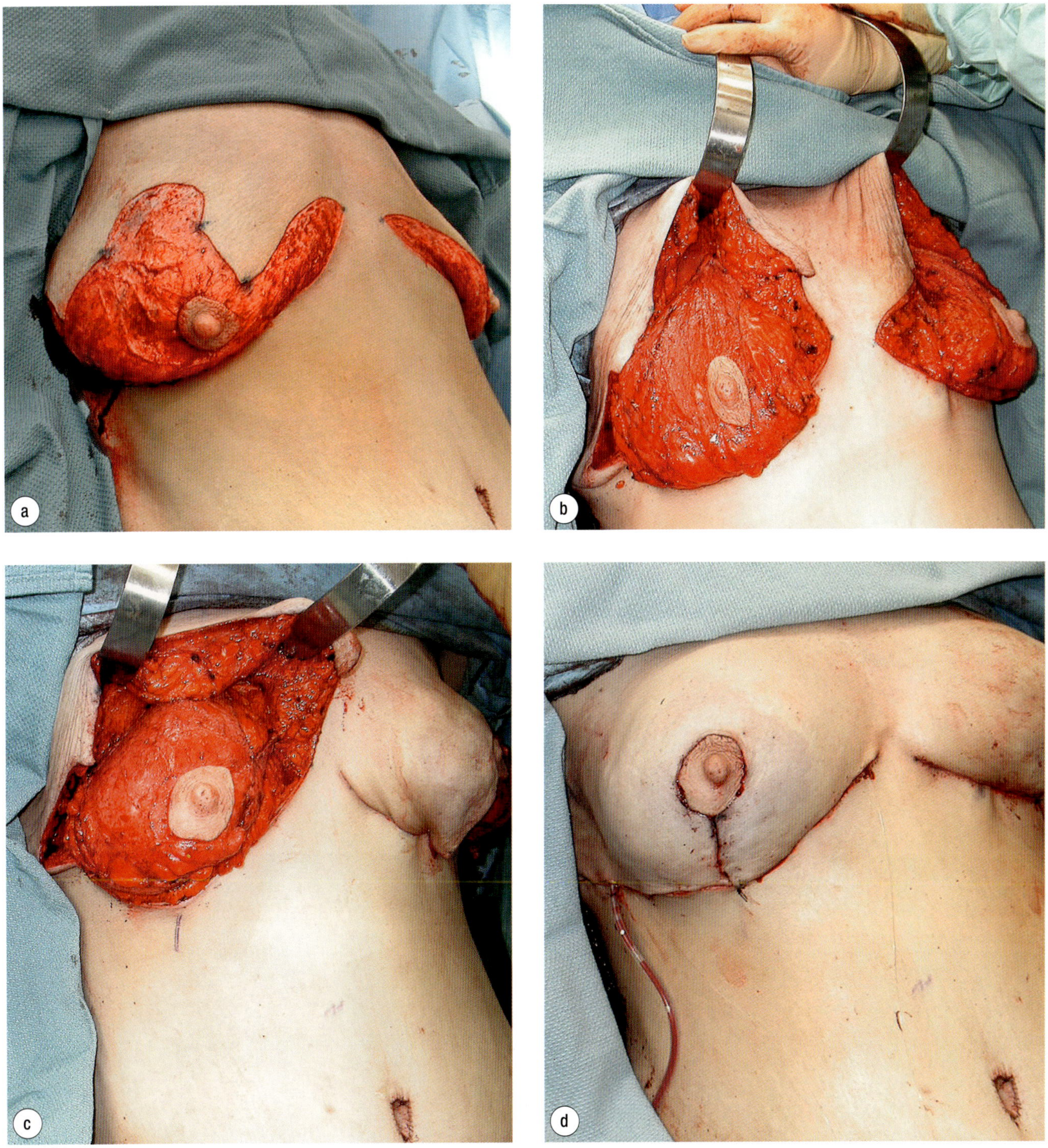

Figure 4.5 (**a**) Intraoperative photographs showing extensive de-epithelialization. (**b**) Suspension of the central dermal extension bilaterally. (**c**) Plication sutures in place. (**d**) Redraping of skin flap. Pre- and postoperative photographs of this patient are shown in Figure 4.6.

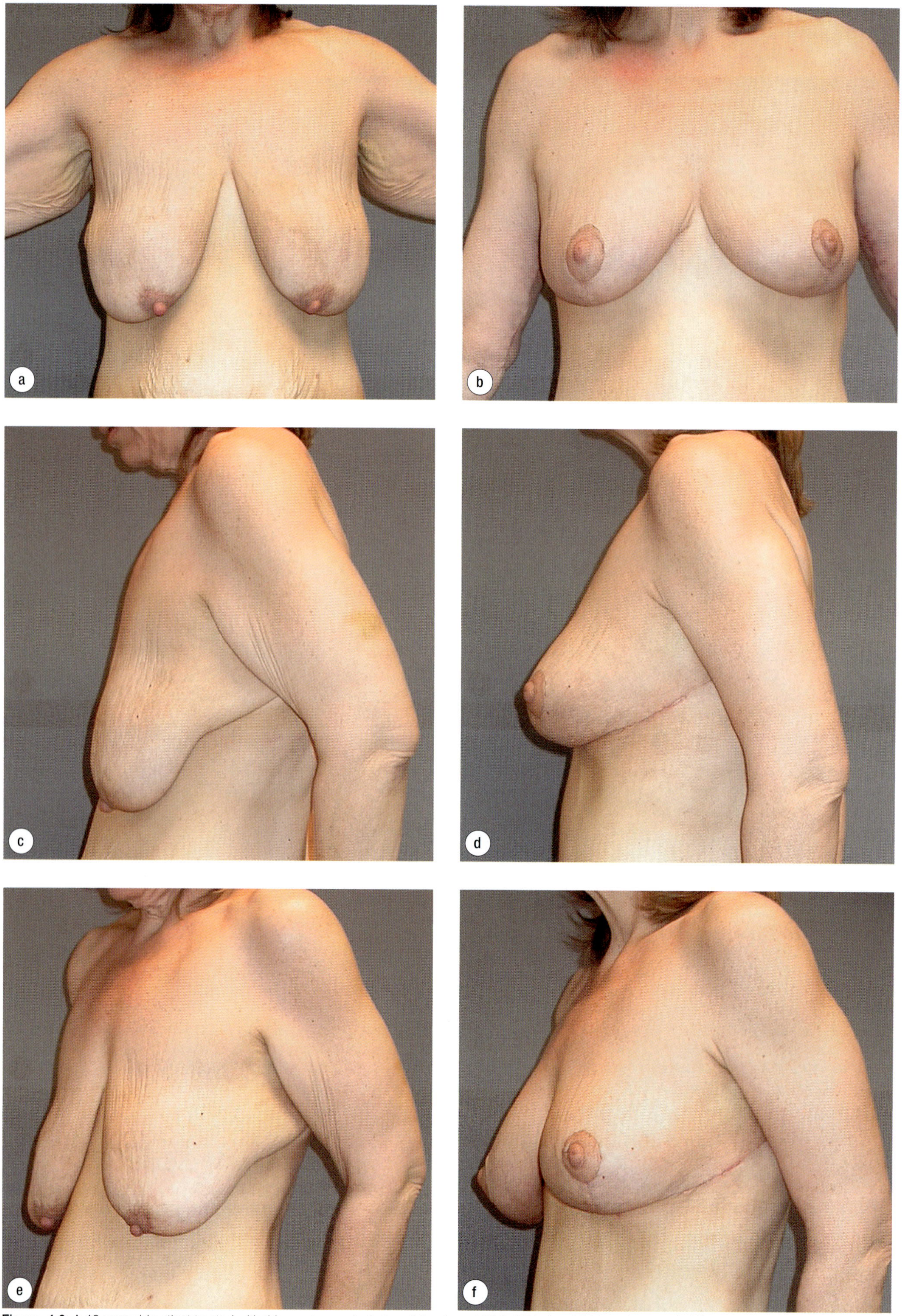

Figure 4.6 A 46-year-old patient treated with this mastopexy technique following a 160-lb (73 kg) weight loss. (**a**, **c**, and **e**) Preoperative and (**b**, **d**, and **f**) 6-month postoperative views.

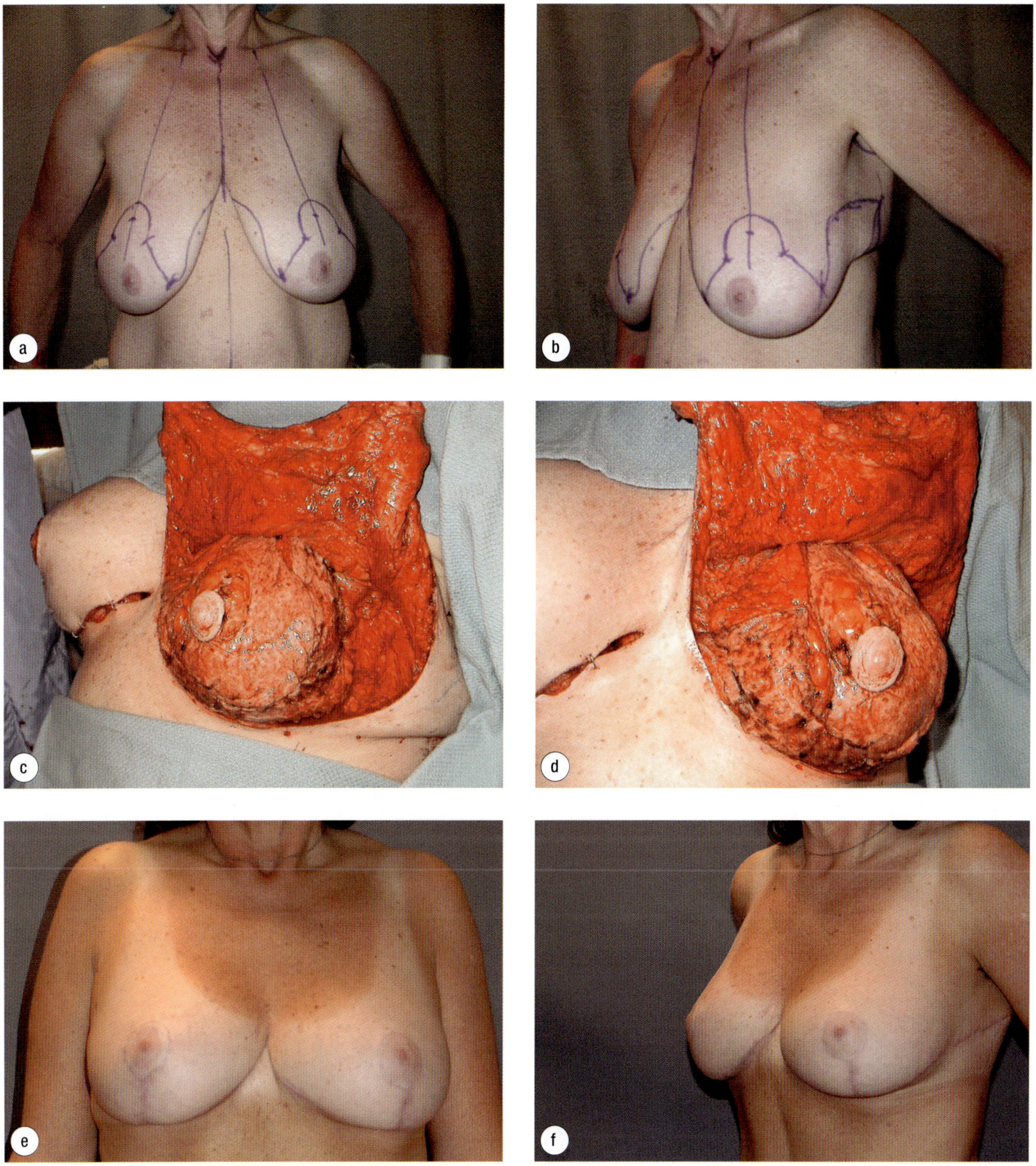

Figure 4.7 A 57-year-old patient following 130-lb (60 kg) weight loss. Preoperative views (**a** and **b**) show severe ptosis with lateral roll. Intraoperative views (**c** and **d**) demonstrate control of parenchymal shape with this technique, which is translated into restoration of aesthetic shape at 6 months postoperatively (**e** and **f**).

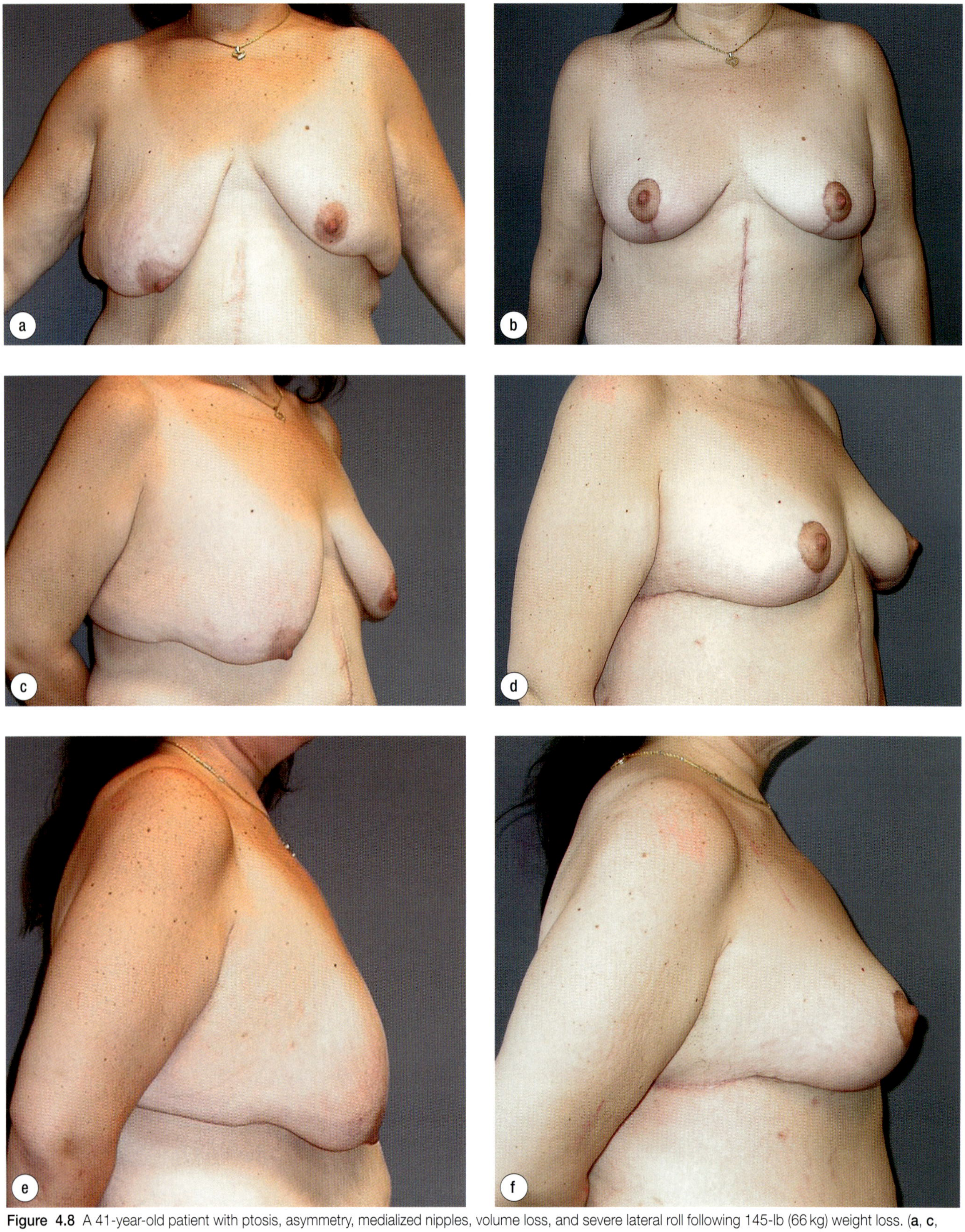

Figure 4.8 A 41-year-old patient with ptosis, asymmetry, medialized nipples, volume loss, and severe lateral roll following 145-lb (66 kg) weight loss. (**a**, **c**, and **e**) Preoperative and (**b**, **d**, and **f**) 6-month postoperative views demonstrate improvement in breast shape.

Complications

Complications have been infrequent. In 48 cases, the following complications occurred.

- One patient suffered a small postoperative hematoma in the lateral right breast during the early postoperative course; this was treated non-operatively.
- One patient had a minor wound dehiscence (less than 1 cm) at the confluence of incisions along the IMF; this healed rapidly with local wound care.
- One patient underwent scar revision of a portion of the right breast medial incision in a minor procedure suite.

There were no occurrences of major skin necrosis or nipple loss. Breast shape is shown to be fairly durable at 1 year (Fig. 4.9), with some settling of the inferior pole noted.

REFERENCES

1. Schwarzmann E. Die Technik der Mammaplastik. Chirurg 1930:932–943.
2. Beisenberger H. Eine neue Methode der Mammaplastik. Zentrabl Chir 1928; 55:2382–2387.
3. Thorek M. Plastic reconstruction of the female breasts and abdomen. Springfield: Thomas; 1942:1–356.
4. Wise RJ. A preliminary report on a method of planning the mammaplasty. Plast Reconstr Surg 1956; 17:365–370.
5. Strombeck J. Mammaplasty: report of new technique on the two pedicle technique. Br J Plast Surg 1960; 13:79–84.
6. McKissock PK. Reduction mammaplasty with a vertical dermal flap. Plast Reconstr Surg 1972; 49(3):245–252.
7. Skoog T. A technique of breast reconstruction: transposition of the nipple areolar complex on a cutaneous vascular pedicle. Acta Chir Scand 1963; 126:453.

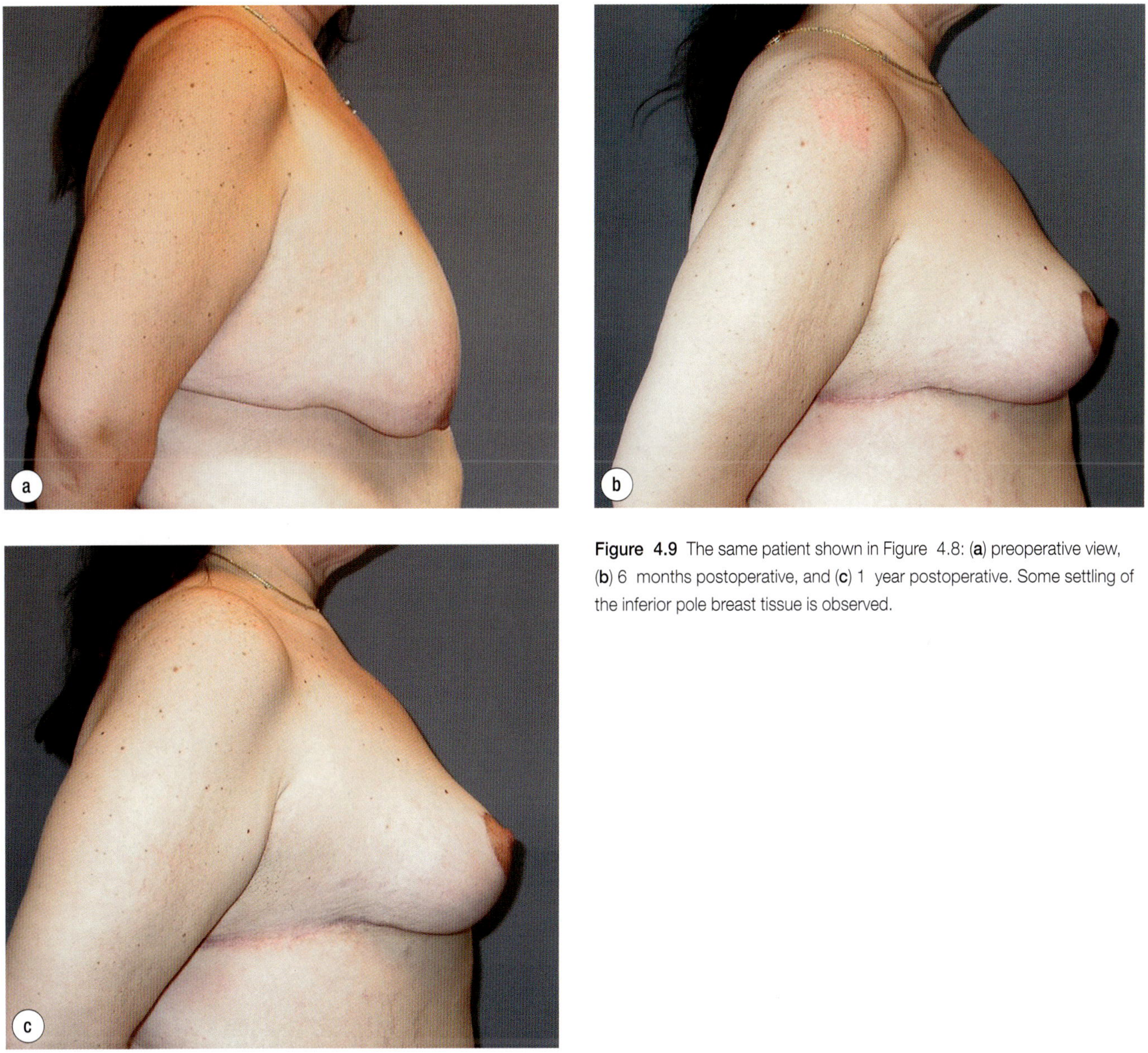

Figure 4.9 The same patient shown in Figure 4.8: (**a**) preoperative view, (**b**) 6 months postoperative, and (**c**) 1 year postoperative. Some settling of the inferior pole breast tissue is observed.

8. Rubiero L. A new technique for reduction mammaplasty. Plast Reconstr Surg 1975; 55:330–334.
9. Courtiss EH, Goldwyn RM. Reduction mammaplasty by the inferior pedicle technique. Plast Reconstr Surg 1977; 59:64–67.
10. Graf R, Biggs TM. In search of better shape in mastopexy and reduction mammoplasty. Plast Reconstr Surg 2002; 110(1):309–317.
11. Lassus C. A 30 year experience with vertical mammaplasty. Plast Reconstr Surg 1996; 97:373–380.
12. Lassus C. A technique for breast reduction. Int Surg 1970; 53:69–72.
13. Lejour M. Vertical mammaplasty without inframammary scar and with breast liposuction. Perspect Plast Surg 1990; 4:64–67.
14. Chen T, Wei F. Evolution of the vertical reduction mammaplasty: the S approach. Aesthetic Plast Surg 1997; 21:97–104.
15. Exner K, Scheufler O. Dermal suspension flap in vertical-scar reduction mammaplasty. Plast Reconstr Surg 2002; 109:2289–2300.
16. Benelli L. A new peri-areolar mammaplasty: the 'round block' technique. Aesthetic Plast Surg 1990; 14:93.
17. Hammond D. Short scar peri-areolar inferior pedicle reduction (SPAIR) mammaplasty. Plast Reconstr Surg 1999; 103:890–901.
18. Goes J. Periareolar mammaplasty with mixed mesh support: the double skin technique. Oper Tech Plast Reconstr Surg 1996; 3:197–199.
19. Pitanguy I. Evaluation of body contouring surgery today: a 30 year perspective. Plast Reconstr Surg 2000; 105:1499–1514.
20. Cerqueira A. Mammaplasty: breast fixation with dermoglandular mono upper pedicle flap under the pectoralis muscle. Aesthetic Plast Surg 1998; 22:276–283.
21. Frey M. A new technique of reduction mammaplasty: dermis suspension and elimination of medial scars. Br J Plast Surg 1999; 52:45–51.
22. Qiao Q, et al. Reduction mammaplasty and correction of ptosis: dermal bra technique. Plast Reconstr Surg 2003; 111:122–1130.
23. Gulyas G. Mammaplasty with a periareolar dermal cloak for glandular support. Aesthetic Plast Surg 1999; 23:164–169.
24. Lockwood T. Reduction mammaplasty and mastopexy with SFS suspension. Plast Reconstr Surg 1990; 5:1411–1420.
25. Holmstrom H. The lateral thoracodorsal flap in breast reconstruction. Plast Reconstr Surg 1986; 77:933–943.

APPROACH TO THE ABDOMEN AFTER WEIGHT LOSS

5

Susan E. Downey

Key Points

A lower abdominal incision may not adequately address the redundancy of the abdomen in a post–massive weight loss patient; vertical or lateral abdominal incisions may need to be utilized.

- Contouring of the mons should be considered in most weight loss patients.
- Postoperative seromas are an increased risk in this population, and intraoperative techniques may need to be altered to minimize this occurrence.
- Hernias may be addressed safely at the time of panniculectomy.

DEFINITIONS

- **Abdominoplasty.** Removal of skin and fat of the abdominal wall with tightening of the underlying musculature. In general, this is considered a cosmetic procedure.
- **Belt lipectomy.** A method designed to circumferentially reduce truncal excess combining an abdominoplasty, lateral thigh lift, buttocks lift, and sometimes liposuction of select areas.
- **Lower body lift.** Described initially by Lockwood and refers to a combined transverse thigh/buttock lift with a high-tension abdominoplasty.
- **Panniculectomy.** Removal of skin and fat of the abdominal wall. In general, this is considered a reconstructive procedure.

As early as 1899, the term *abdominal lipectomy* was devised by Kelly to describe a transverse resection of a large pendulous abdomen.[1] In 1910, Dr. Kelly described his experience with eight patients.[2] Thorek in 1939 described his technique, which he called 'plastic adipectomy' for resecting 'fat aprons'.[3] These early operations were designed to relieve the functional problems associated with large fat aprons. However, early on the cosmetic benefits were noted. Kelly stated in 1910 that 'quite apart, however, from the tremendous physical and, in some cases psychical benefit, I personally recommend and would do the operation in extreme cases for the cosmetic benefit'.[2]

From these early efforts have come the techniques known as abdominoplasty. Although abdominoplasty is a procedure well known to plastic surgeons, the management of the post–massive weight loss abdomen is much more complicated. Although variation can be seen in the traditional abdominoplasty patient, the post–massive weight loss patient presents with a wider range of anatomical variables as well as a higher rate of complications.

As patients lose weight following bariatric surgery, they begin to develop loose and overhanging skin in many areas. Universally, the abdomen is a prime focal area of concern in post–massive weight loss patients. Various techniques have been described. The goals of all these techniques are to:

- allow excision of excess skin and fat, and
- tighten the diastasis recti and/or repair hernias if present.

In traditional abdominoplasty patients, the third goal is to have minimum scarring.[4] This is not the case for the massive weight loss patient. Contour is a more important goal than minimum scarring in this population, and several scars may be necessary to give the patient the desired contour.

Panniculectomy and abdominoplasty have been used interchangeably to describe surgical procedures to remove excess skin and fat of the abdominal wall. Panniculectomy describes procedures removing only skin and fat—i.e. a functional operation that removes a symptomatic apron of skin—while abdominoplasty refers to not only the removal of skin and fat but also the tightening up of the muscles of the abdominal wall (it is a term that connotes aesthetic goals). Often, the abdominoplasty may be considered a cosmetic procedure while a panniculectomy refers to a more reconstructive type of operation. A panniculcetomy may be done in patients who have not yet begun their weight loss to remove a large apron, or in patients who have an extremely large overhanging apron after massive weight loss and have interference with activities of daily life or a history of recurrent rashes. For the massive weight loss patient, an abdominoplasty is commonly done after weight loss is complete, and is performed to recontour the abdominal wall with removal of excess skin and fat as well as tightening up of the muscles underneath.

As a general rule, more attention can be safely given to aesthetic goals as the BMI of the patient decreases. Wound complications tend to be higher when contouring operations are performed in patients who are still obese, and a more aggressive approach can invite greater risk of local and even systemic sequelae.

A belt lipectomy refers to a circumferential resection of skin and fat that often also includes the tightening of the abdominal musculature within the same procedure. Patients who have undergone an abdominal procedure, either an abdominoplasty or a panniculectomy, may then elect to undergo a belt lipectomy at a later time. For these patients, the resection is begun in the posterior aspect and the dog ears are excised anteriorly, thereby revising the abdominal portion of their previous procedure.

PREOPERATIVE PREPARATION

Following massive weight loss, patients may present with redundancy all over the face and torso. The decision-making process should involve consideration of the patient's:

- priorities,
- aesthetic goals,
- body contour,
- finances, and
- overall health.

Plastic surgery after massive weight loss may be, and indeed is often, a multiple-staged procedure. Given the opportunity to prioritize which parts of their bodies they would like to have addressed first by a plastic surgeon, the abdomen is usually at the top of the list. Even with a discussion of the belt lipectomy, patients may opt to just do their abdomen initially. This decision may be due to financial constraints. For patients whom the plastic surgeon feels would benefit most from a belt lipectomy, the discussion needs to be had with the patient comparing doing an abdominoplasty versus doing a belt lipectomy. Although an abdominoplasty can be converted to a belt lipectomy, some surgeons feel that the best result in selected patients may be achieved only when a complete belt lipectomy is done as the first stage. Proponents of the belt lipectomy for the initial stage feel that lateral excess can be accentuated by abdominoplasty alone.[5,6]

The assessment of the massive weight loss patient who presents for abdominoplasty should involve a close evaluation for possible hernias. If the patient has had an open procedure, there is a high incidence of incisional hernias. These can be safely repaired at the same time as the panniculectomy (Figs 5.1 and 5.2).[7] In addition, patients who were previously very heavy often have umbilical hernias. These can sometimes be difficult to assess preoperatively. Certainly, if a hernia is present and in close proximity to the umbilicus the patient should be cautioned that the umbilicus may need to be sacrificed to get an optimal repair of the hernia. The stalk of the umbilicus in patients who were previously very heavy can be very long, and in some cases it might be necessary to create a neoumbilicus rather than utilize the patient's original umbilicus.

Many patients after massive weight loss have had previous procedures done with the resulting scars. Common and concerning scars are any scars above the umbilicus, including subcostal scars resulting from an open cholecystectomy. If a midline incision is to be used, this scar will not only be brought inferiorly but also medially, and will be resected in part. In general, this previous subcostal scar will end up at the level of the umbilicus (Figs 5.3 and 5.4). Despite this shortening of the scar, there is still concern about the viability of the skin and fat inferior to this scar. The potential risk of loss of tissue below this old scar should be raised with the patient. In general, perhaps due to the increased vascularity that developed when the patient was heavy, this tissue can survive without a problem. However, patients with other disease processes (such as cardiac disease) or patients who smoke will be at higher risk for tissue loss. Moreover, unconventional incisions can be designed to incorporate or accomodate upper abdominal scars.

Many patients want to do several procedures under the same anesthetic. Abdominoplasty in the post–massive weight

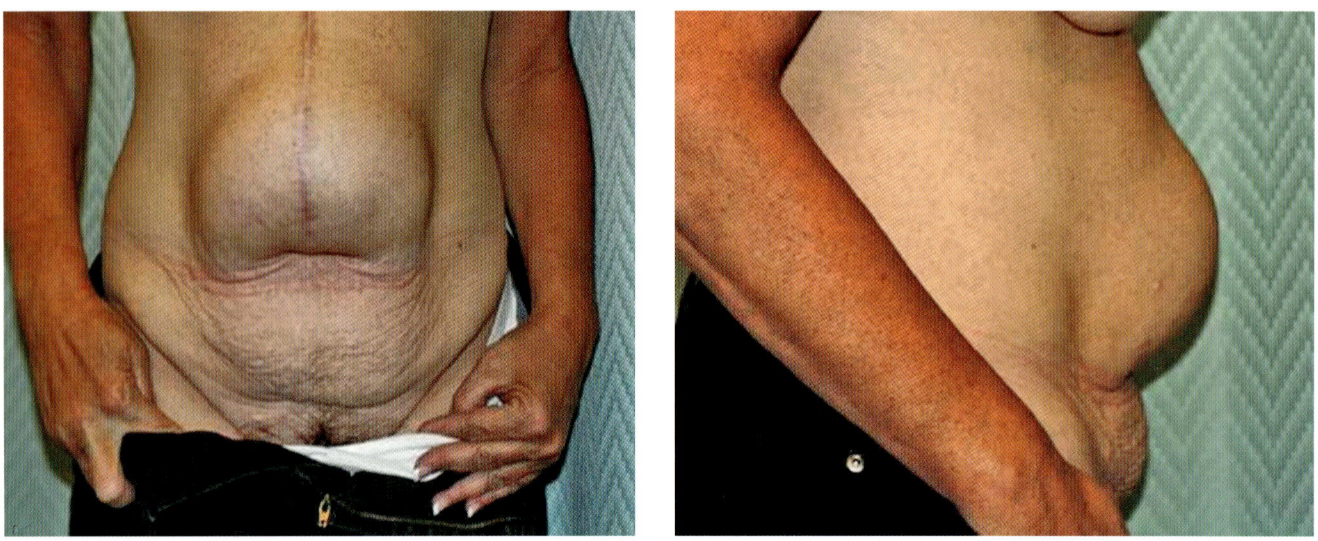

Figure 5.1 Incisional hernia following open bariatric surgery. Total weight loss: 120 lbs (54 kg).

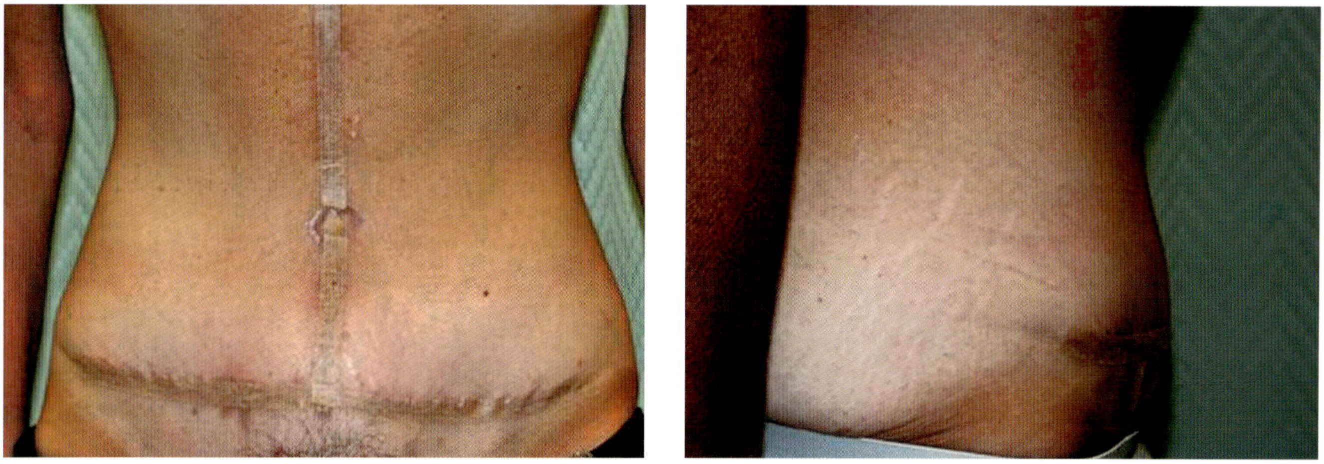

Figure 5.2 Postoperative views after incisional hernia repair and resection of abdominal pannus, utilizing lower abdominal and midline incisions.

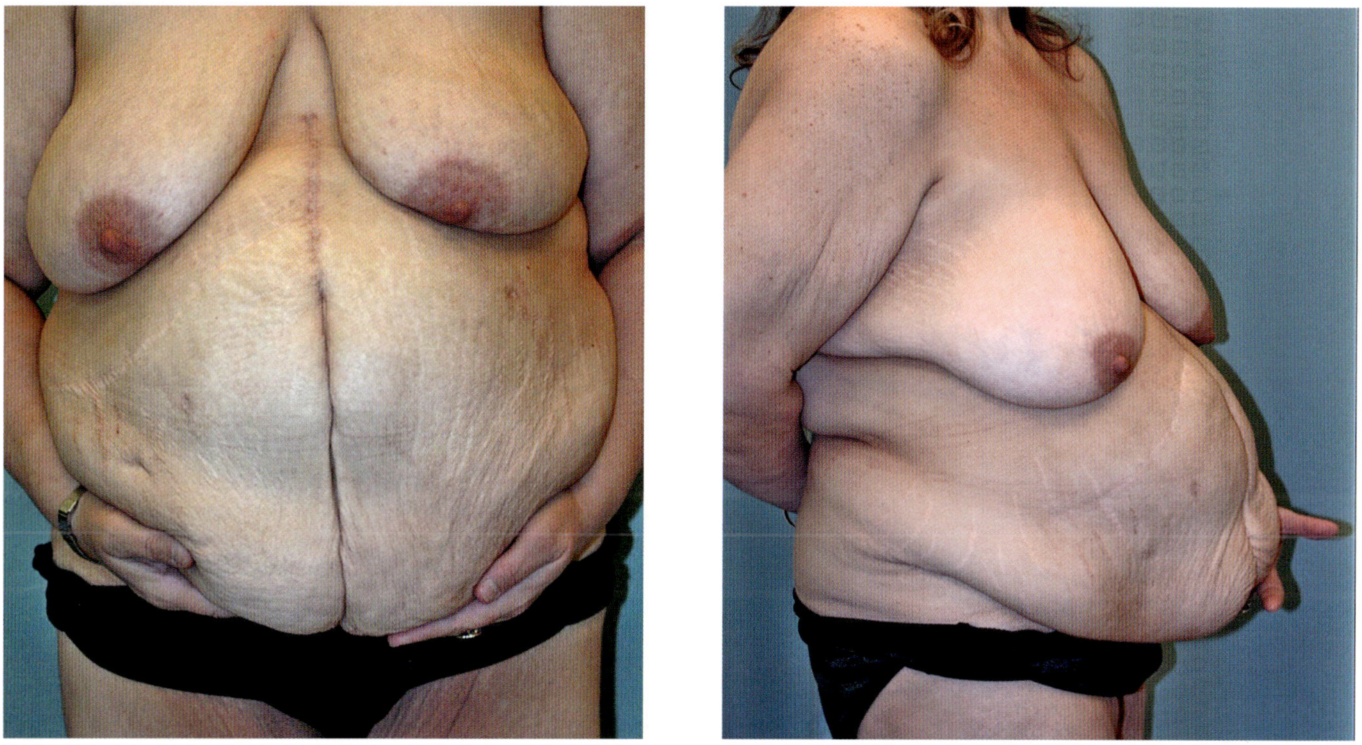

Figure 5.3 Subcostal midline incision after open bariatric procedure. Total weight loss: 111 lbs (50 kg).

loss population can often be combined with other procedures, while considering each patient individually and taking into consideration safety issues such as:

- the total length of surgery planned,
- the patient's overall health, and
- the length of time the surgery will take.

In a review of 73 consecutive procedures, it was found that additional dermolipectomies do not increase abdominoplasty-related morbidity and actually demonstrated better long-term results.[8]

Markings for resection of the abdominal panniculus are best done in the preoperative area with the patient in the standing position or prior to admission. Avoidance of dog ears is critical (Figs 5.5 and 5.6); marking the end of the overhanging panniculus is key to the avoidance of dog ears (Fig. 5.7). When the patient lies down, this lateral overhang is lost (Fig. 5.8). The inferior marking can be done on the operating table. The inferior marking should take into consideration the excess that may be present in the mons area and adjusted accordingly (Fig. 5.9). Many women will present with ptosis and/or exces-

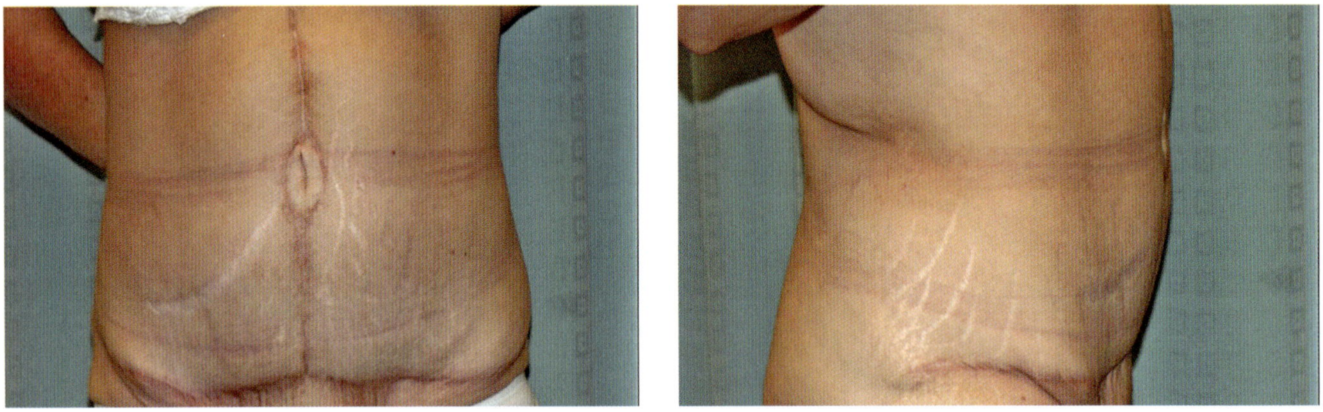

Figure 5.4 Subcostal incision scar postoperatively after resection of skin and fat in horizontal and vertical directions.

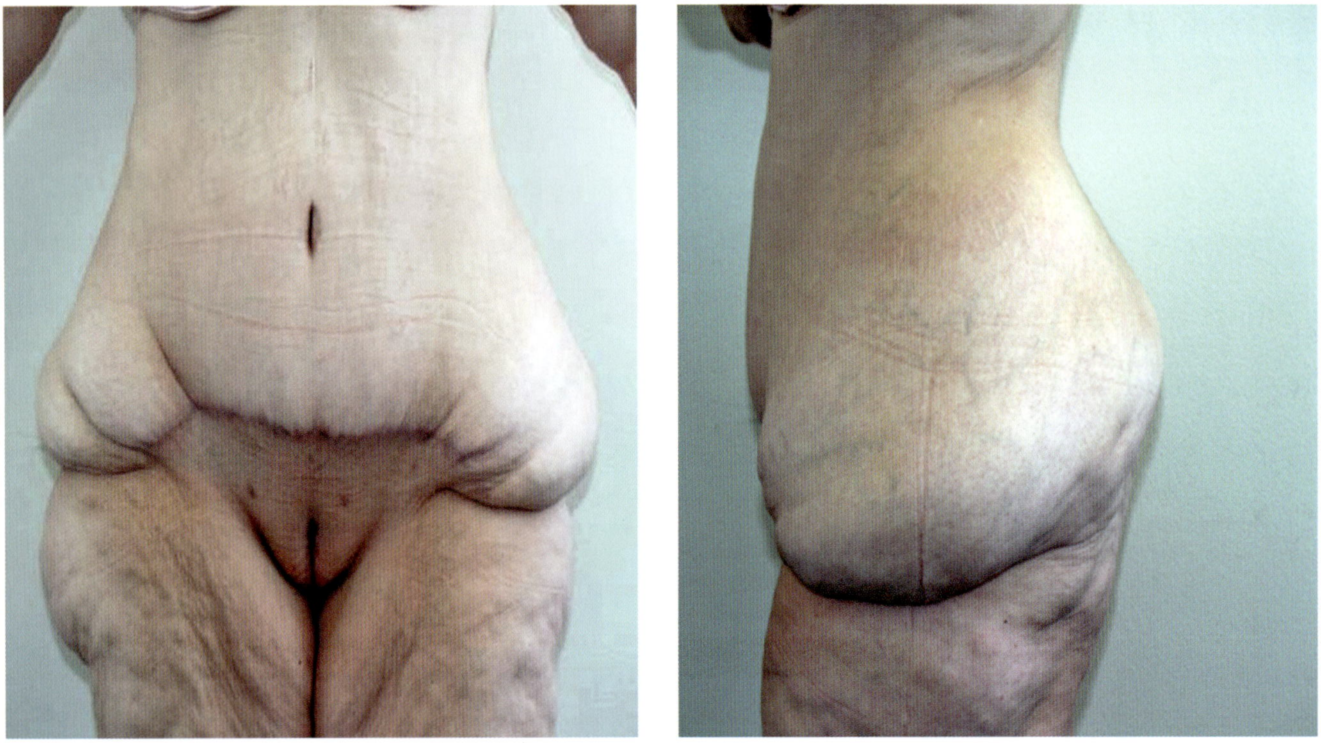

Figure 5.5 Dog ears after abdominal panniculectomy.

sive fullness of the mons. While the patient may not specifically draw attention to these deformities, correction of mons shape and position should factor into any abdominal-contouring strategy. Patients will be very unhappy if a resection of their excess mons area is not done either at the time of a panniculectomy before weight loss (Fig. 5.10) or at the time of the panniculectomy after massive weight loss (Fig. 5.11).

The resection of the abdominal panniculus will address the anterior abdomen, but will not address areas such as back rolls or excess fat in the posterior hip area. Preoperative evaluation of the patient needs to include discussion of the patient's anatomy and the extent of the panniculectomy, and areas that will not be addressed during this surgery. If the patient wishes to have these areas addressed, alternative procedures—such as a belt lipectomy, liposuction, or even wedge resections of these additional areas—should be discussed. Reviewing photos of patients with similar anatomical variations can make the discussion and the expectations easier (Figs 5.12–5.17).

In patients who have undergone an open bariatric procedure, the previous midline scar is utilized to resect the excess skin and fat in both a horizontal and a vertical direction. In patients who have had a laparoscopic procedure or who have

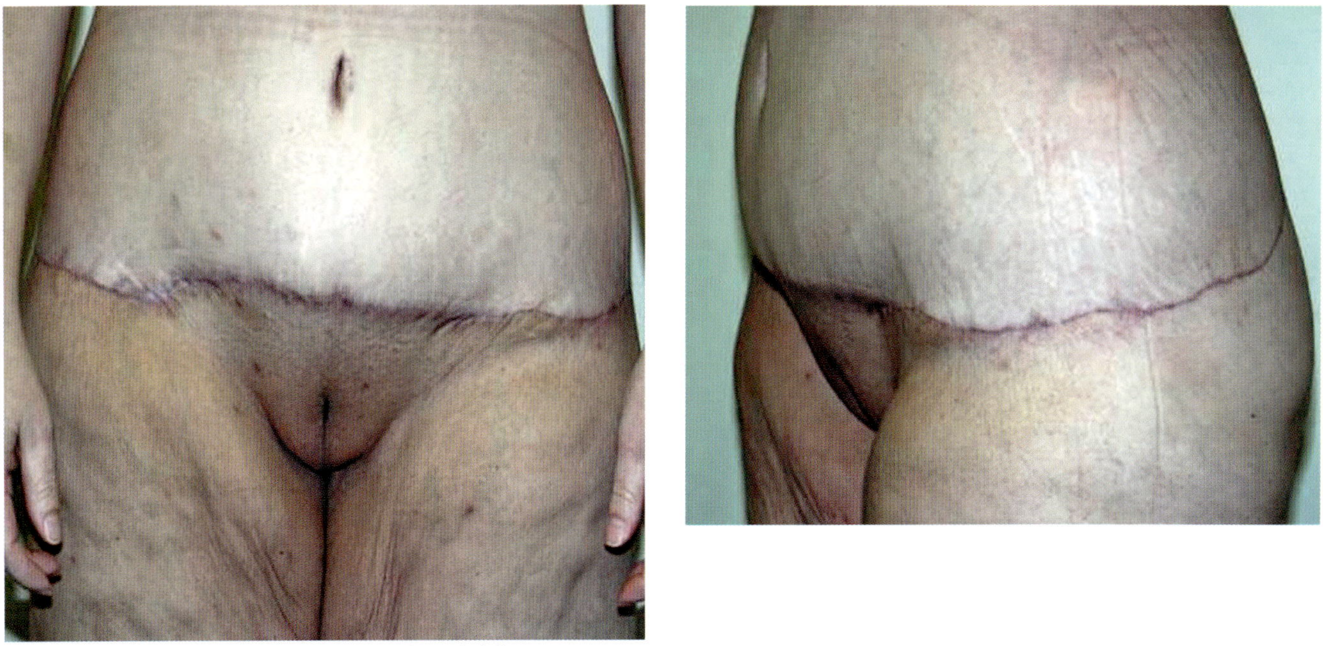

Figure 5.6 Correction of dog ears with conversion to belt lipectomy.

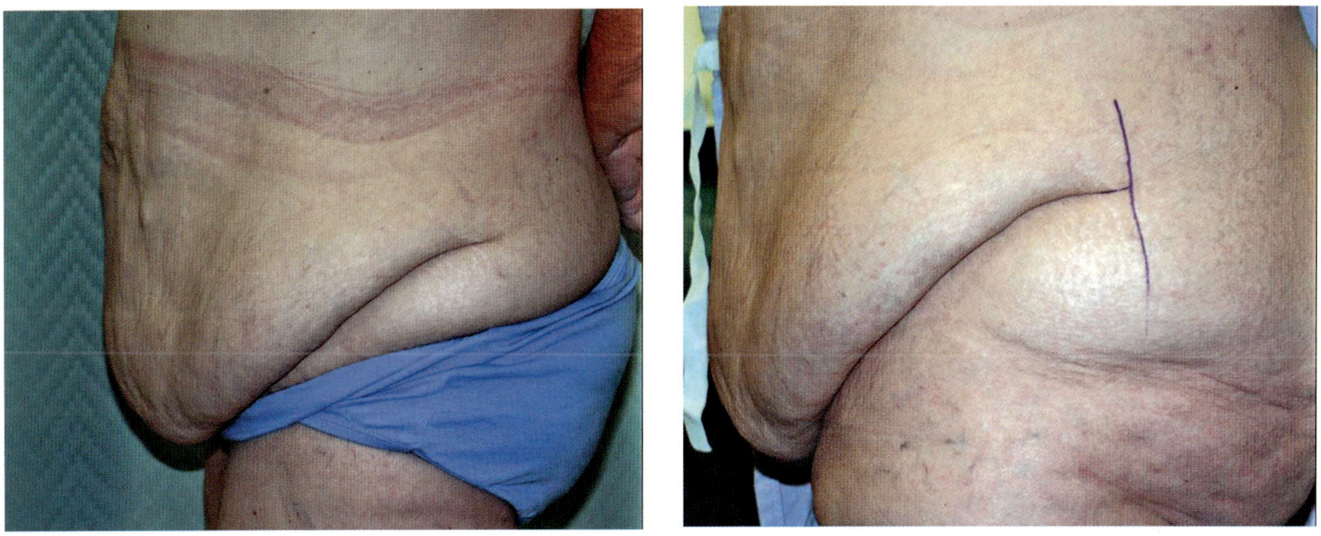

Figure 5.7 Abdominal markings with the patient standing.

lost their excess weight through diet and exercise, an evaluation of the redundancy of the skin and fat in the upper abdomen should be done. If there is an excess of skin and fat in the upper abdomen, the possibility of a midline scar should be considered (Figs 5.18 and 5.19). Vertical incisions have been utilized to address the upper abdomen as early as 1916, when Babcock described vertical ellipses of fat and skin with wide undermining and midline approximation to contour the waist and lower abdomen.[9] If a midline scar is not utilized, there may still be redundancy in the upper abdomen that the patients may not be happy about postoperatively.

The goal, as described by Savage,[10] should be the removal of the greatest amount of skin and fat rather than concern about scars. A mixture of horizontal and/or vertical scars may be necessary to get the desired contour. The upper abdominal area may also be addressed at a later stage with the addition of a midline scar,[11] or even, in some patients, a lateral scar may be used as a continuation of a brachioplasty scar, addressing the lateral folds of the breast as well as the residual laxity of the upper abdomen all in one incision. Some surgeons have even suggested an upper abdominal incision or 'melon slice' type of excision to remove upper abdominal excess.[12]

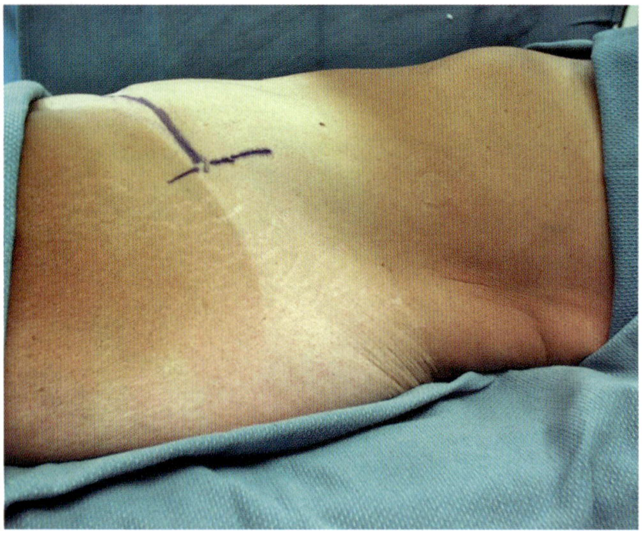

Figure 5.8 Abdominal markings with the patient supine on the operating room table.

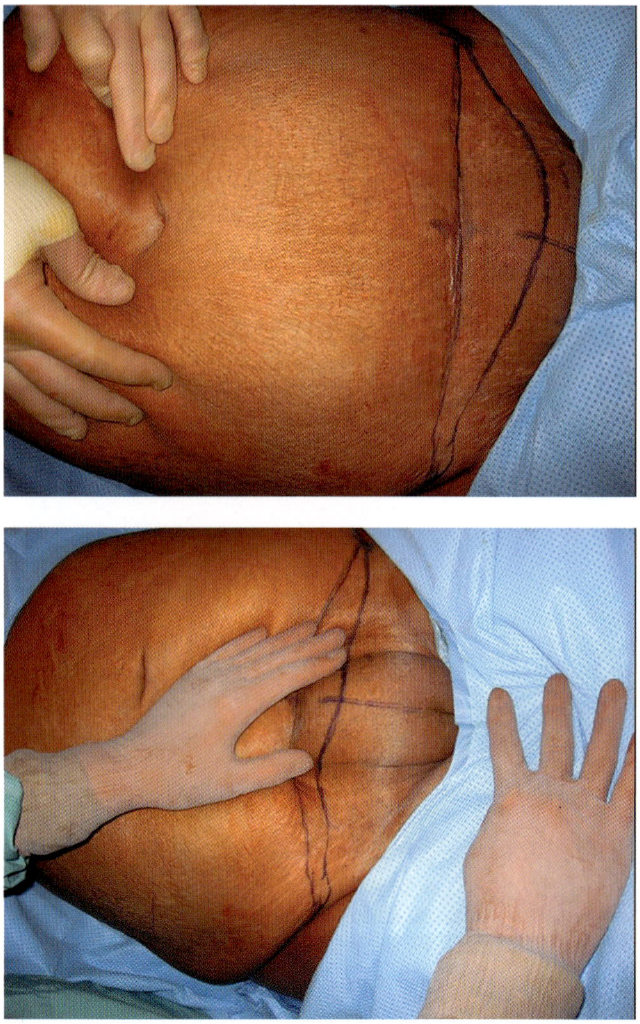

Figure 5.9 Markings on the operating room table for resection of mons.

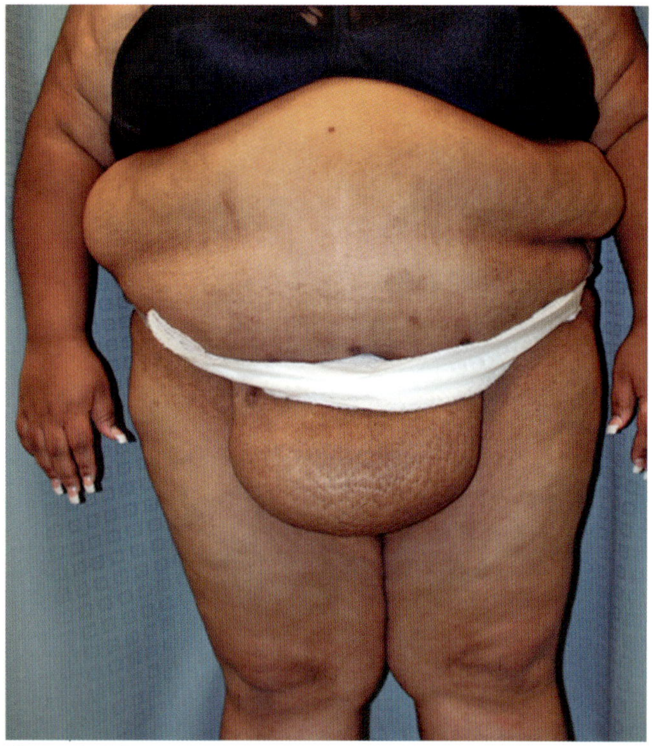

Figure 5.10 Panniculectomy done before bariatric surgery without resection of mons.

ABDOMINOPLASTY IN THE MASSIVE WEIGHT LOSS PATIENT

Once the patient has been marked in the standing position, she or he can be taken to the operating room. Vertical marks should be made at the lateral aspect of the overhanging pannus while the patient is in the standing position. This then delineates the lateral extent of the resection and will help avoid dog ears (Fig. 5.7). The lower abdominal incision can be marked when the patient is supine on the operating table.

The procedure is best done under general anesthesia with the patient in the supine position. Intermittent compression devices are placed on the patient as soon as he or she is on the operating table or earlier, and a Foley catheter is inserted. The abdomen is prepared from above the costal margin, laterally to the operating table and including the pubic area. Shaving of body hair may be done as indicated. Markings for the lower abdominal incision should be done at this time. The marking should take into consideration any excess of the mons area that exists. The lower incision should be placed 2–3 cm above the labial cleft to place the final scar at this level and to adequately address the mons excess (Fig. 5.9).

Once the patient is prepared, the surgery begins through the midline incision, if present. Incisional hernias, if present, are dissected out. The umbilicus is dissected out and left attached to its stalk. The incision is carried down to the pubic area and out to the lateral extent of the lower abdominal incision

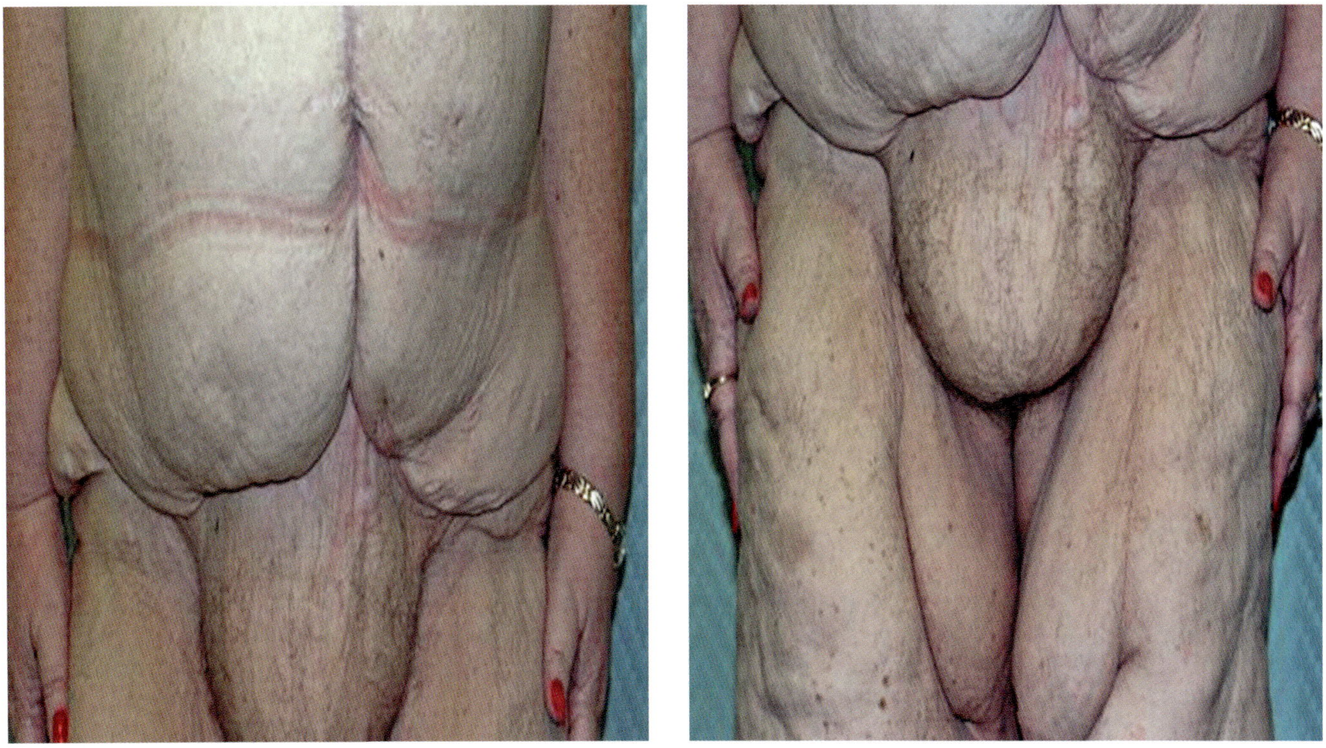

Figure 5.11 Panniculectomy done after bariatric surgery without resection of mons.

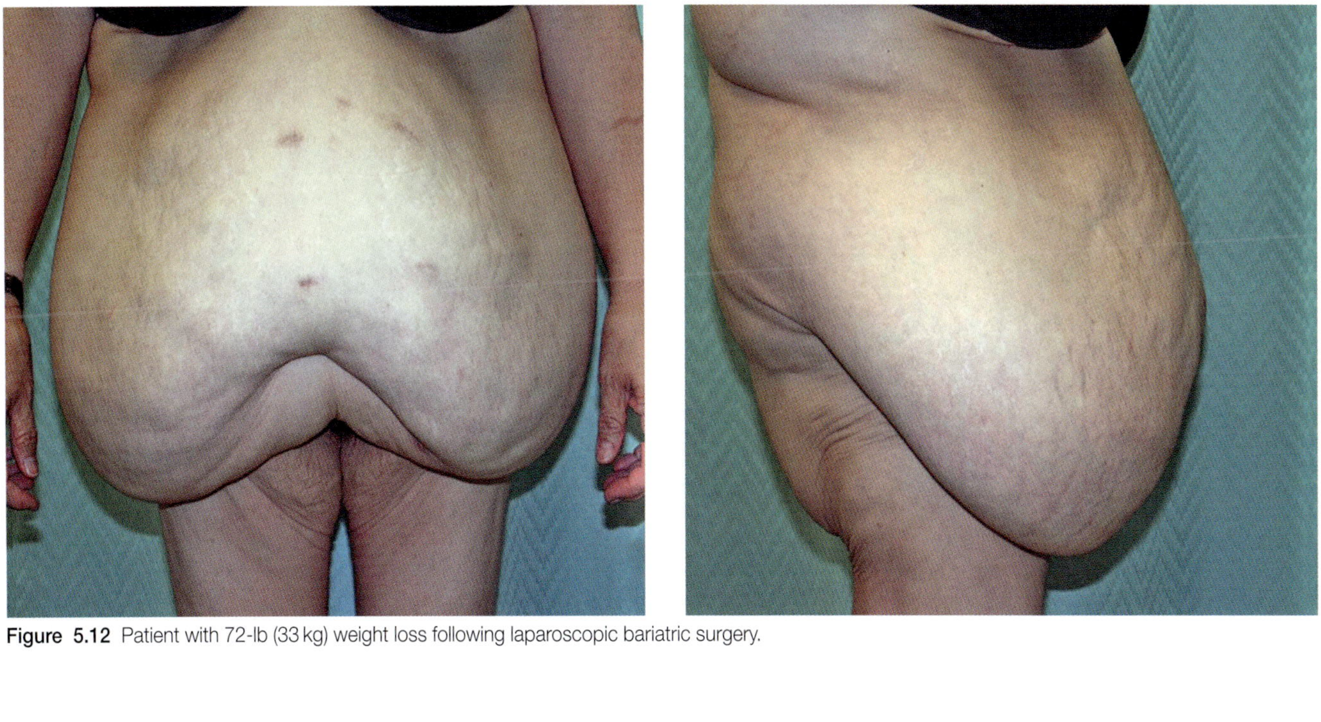

Figure 5.12 Patient with 72-lb (33 kg) weight loss following laparoscopic bariatric surgery.

(Fig. 5.20). The skin and fat are then mobilized and rotated medially and inferiorly, and the excess skin and fat are resected. Tension should be applied to the skin and fat being resected in the upper abdomen to resect as much as possible in this area and to avoid upper abdominal fullness in the postoperative period (Figs 5.21 and 5.22).

Concern is always raised about elevating flaps under previous incisions. In patients in whom there is a lot of concern about tissue viability, such as nicotine users, undermining might be limited to the level of the previous surgery; in most patients, this area can safely be elevated and the tissue will survive.

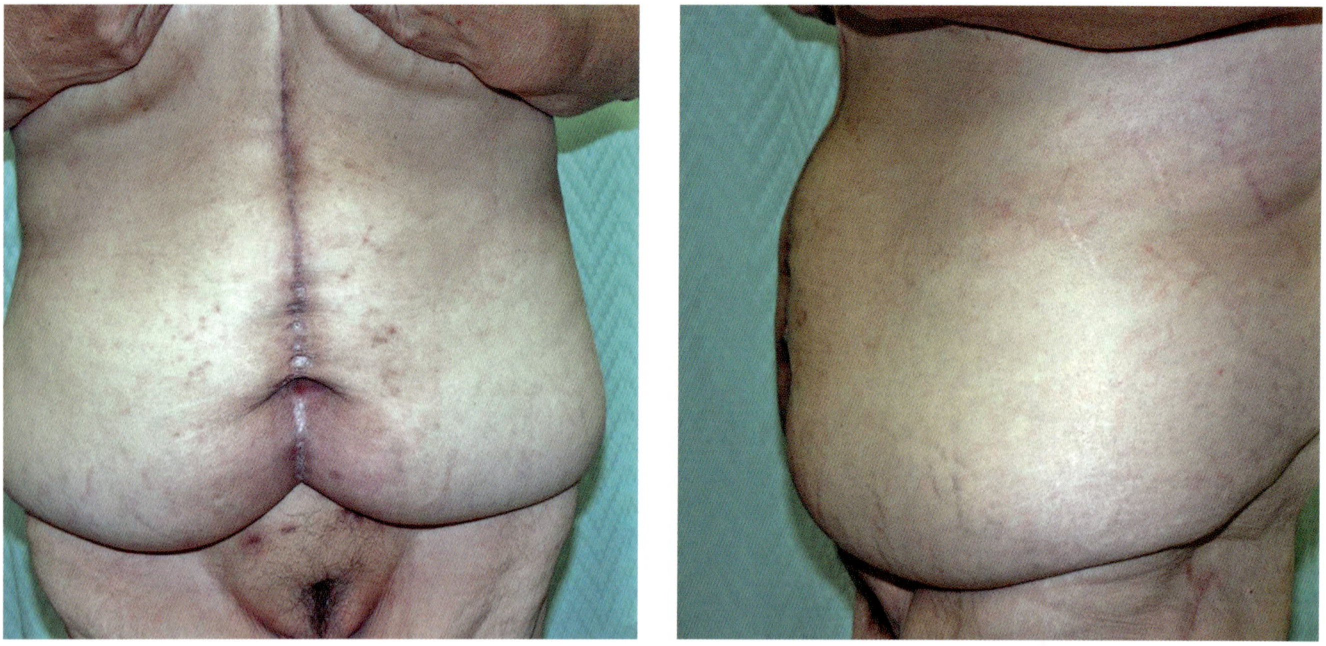

Figure 5.13 Resection of 11.4-lb (5185 g) pannus, utilizing midline and lower abdominal incisions.

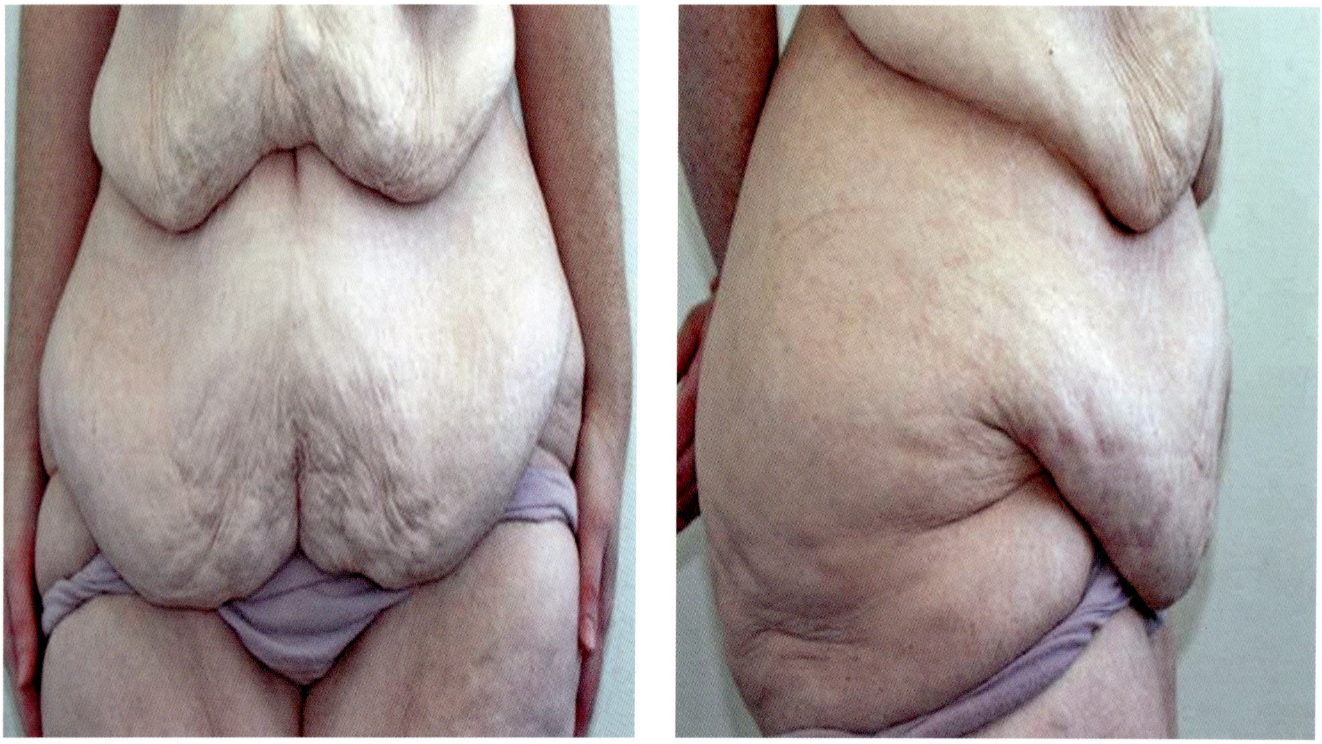

Figure 5.14 Patient with 200-lb (91 kg) weight loss following placement of an adjustable gastric band.

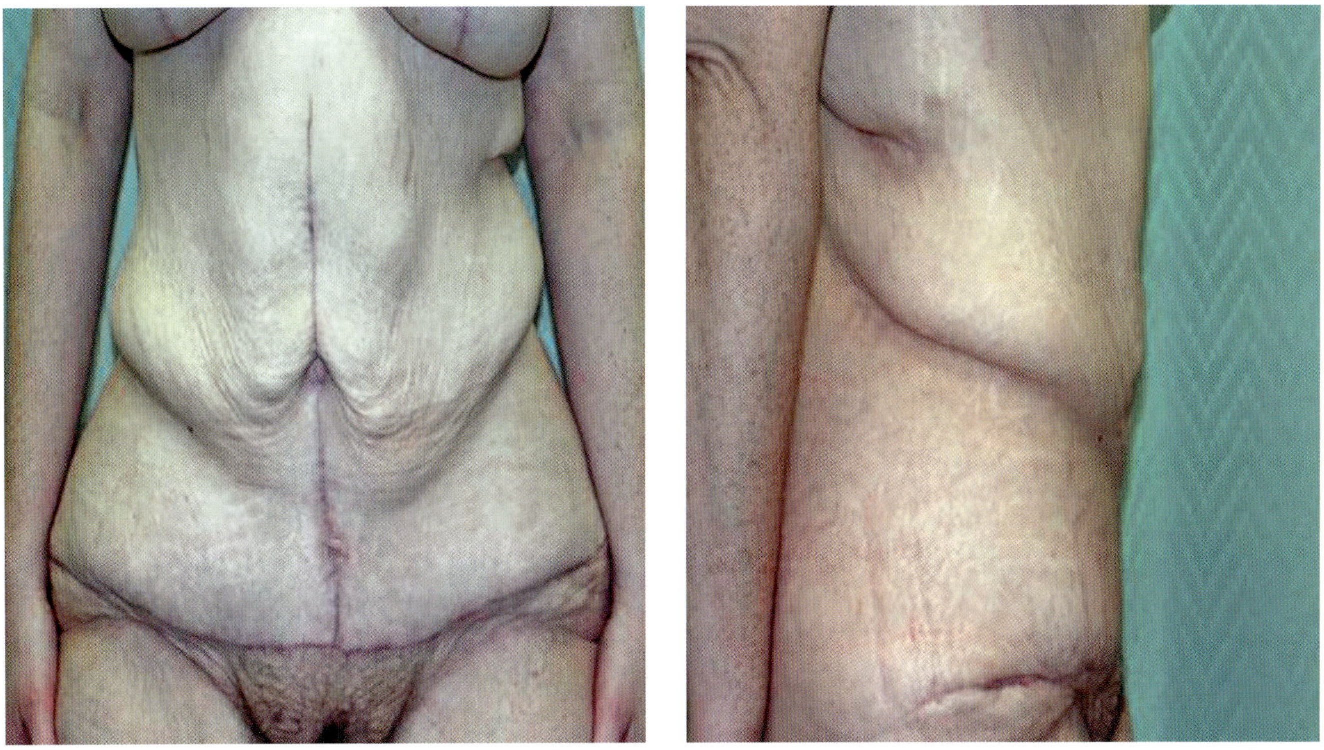

Figure 5.15 Postoperative views after resection of abdominal pannus with midline and lower abdominal incisions in a patient with an adjustable gastric band.

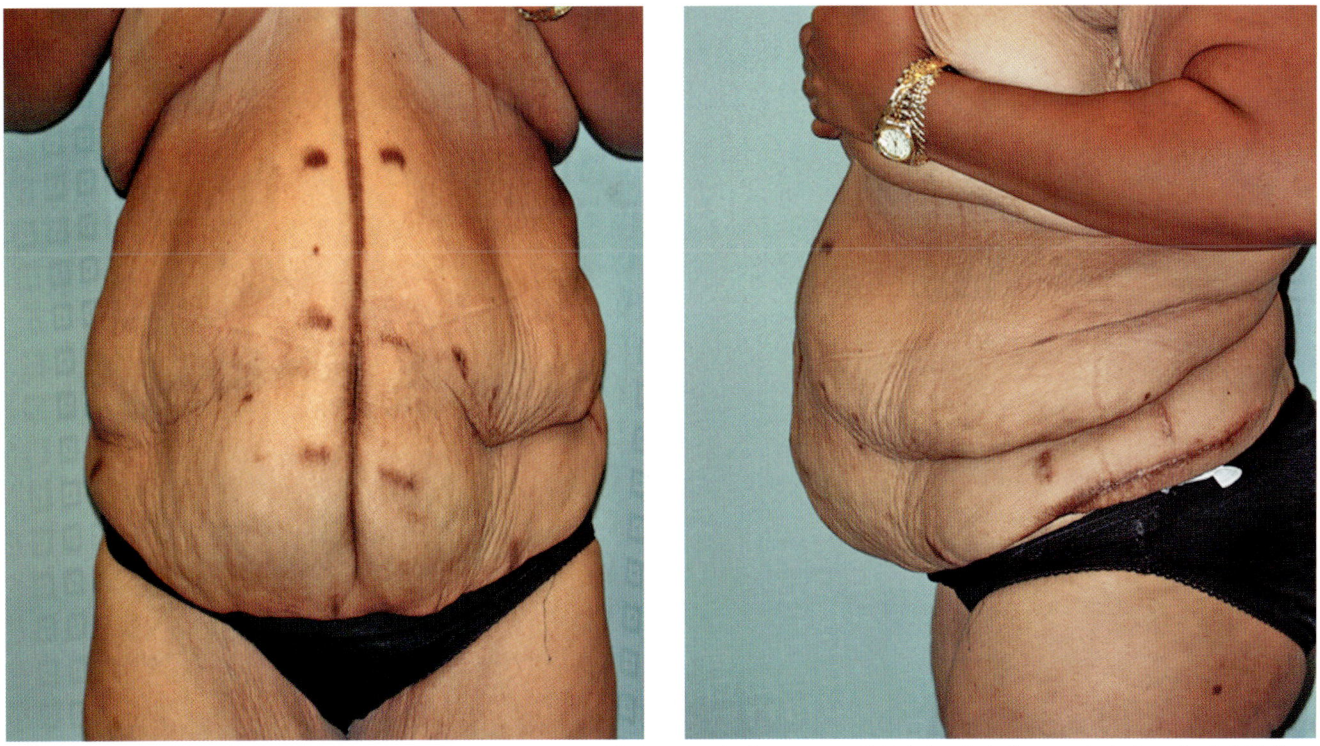

Figure 5.16 This patient had undergone a 27-lb (12 kg) panniculectomy before open bariatric surgery. Weight loss including panniculectomy totaled 157 lbs (71 kg).

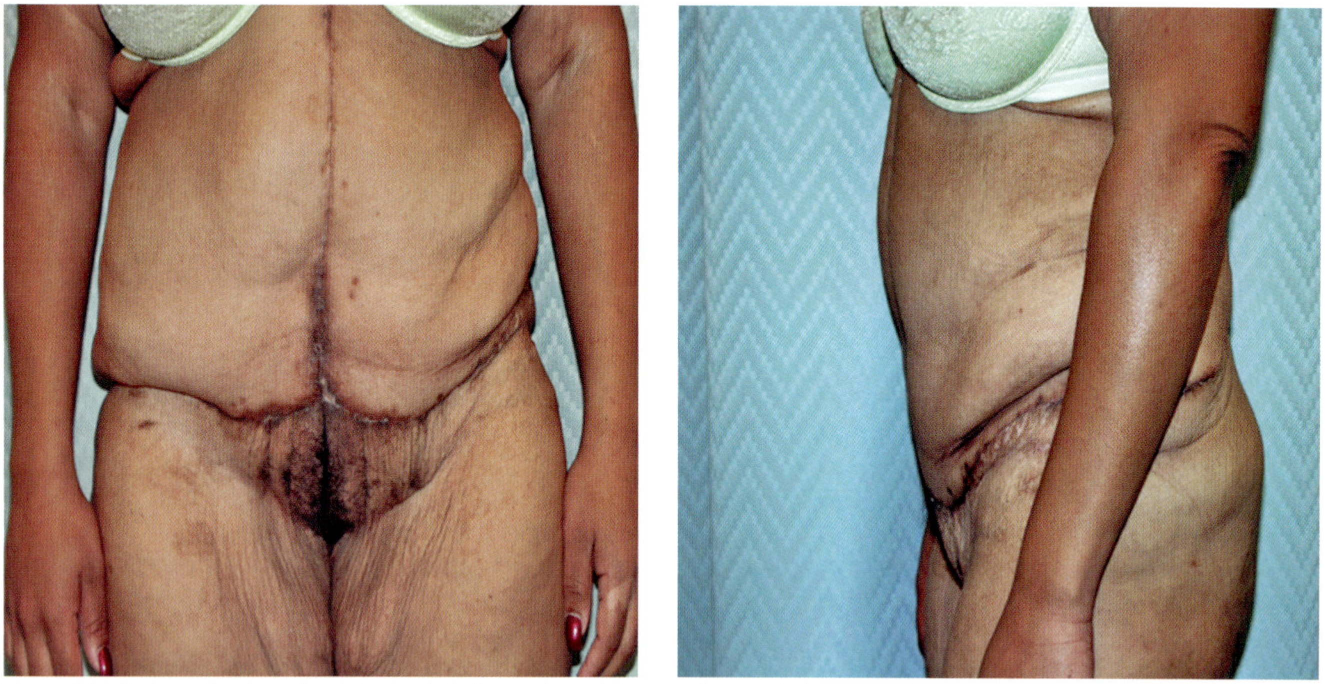

Figure 5.17 Postoperative views after abdominoplasty. The previous midline scar after open bariatric procedure was utilized to resect excess skin in both a horizontal and a vertical direction.

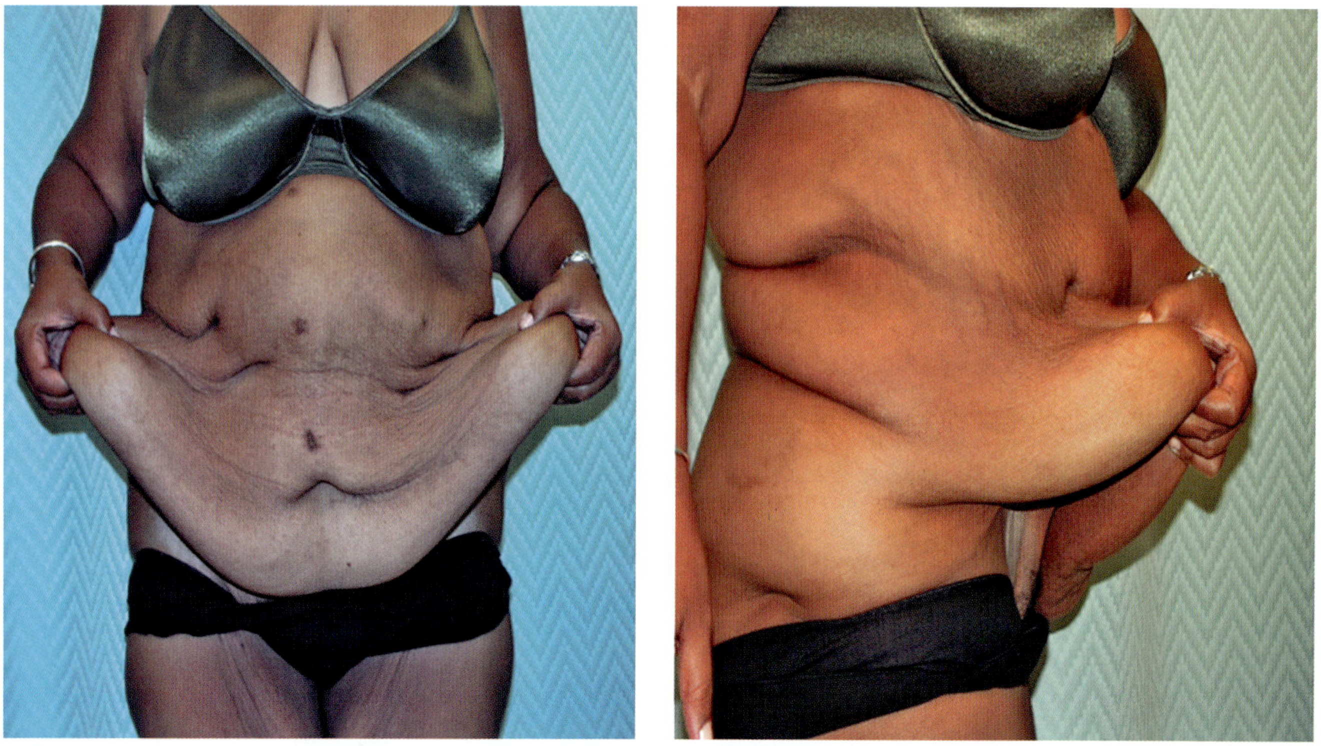

Figure 5.18 Excess skin and fat after weight loss from laparoscopic procedure with 120-lb (54 kg) weight loss.

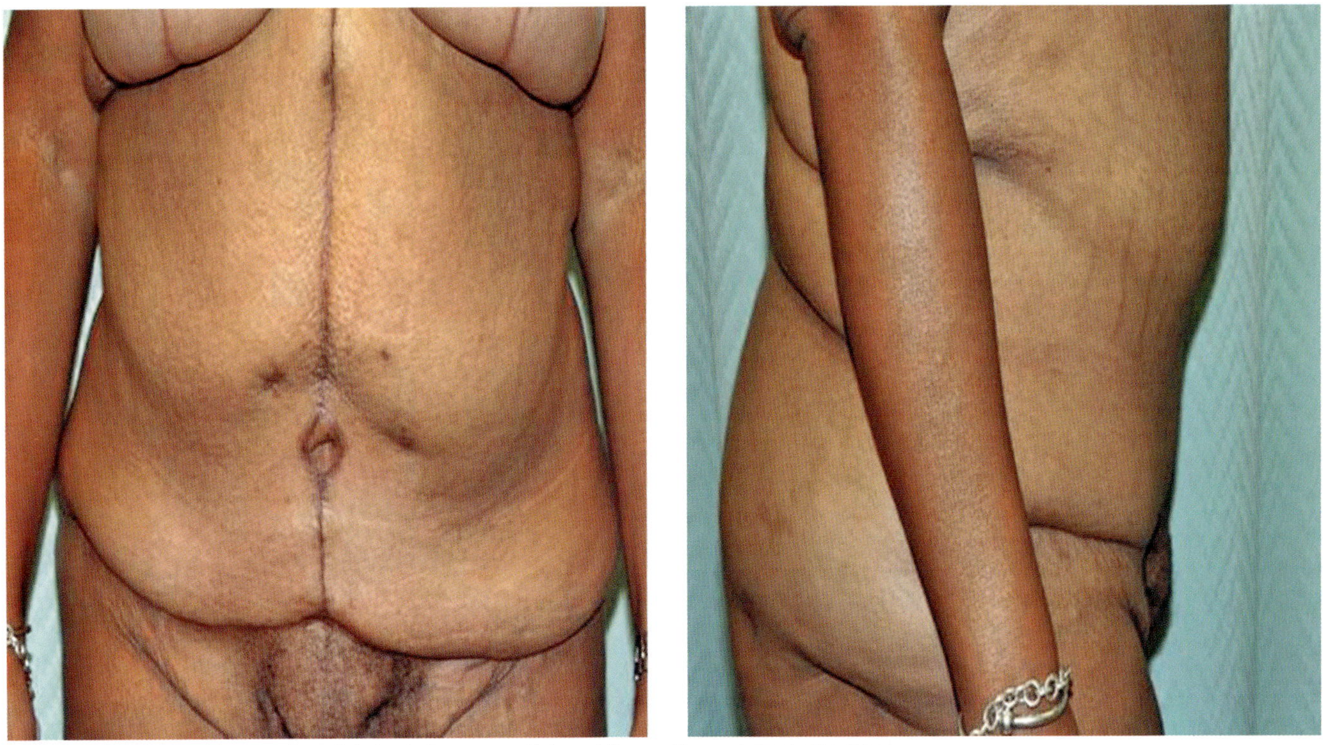

Figure 5.19 Postoperative resection of abdominal pannus, utilizing midline and lower abdominal incisions.

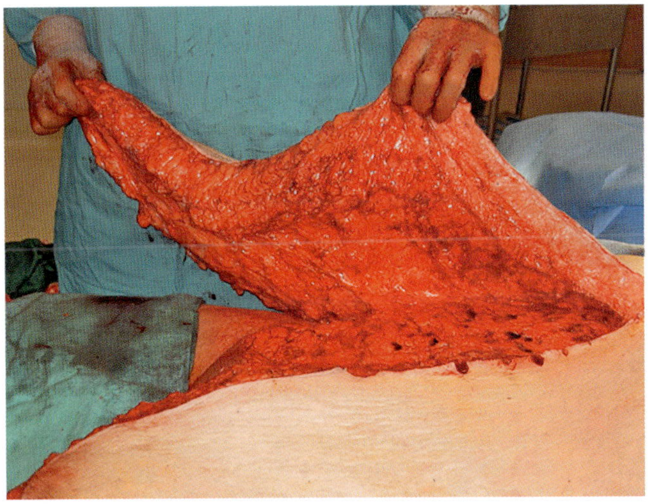

Figure 5.20 Elevation of skin flaps.

Once the skin and fat have been mobilized, the hernias (if present) or the diastasis recti can be addressed. A technique that has been very successful in these patients involves a hernia repair without opening the hernia sac and utilizing onlay mesh.[7]

The hernia sac is dissected free without opening the sac, and then the hernia repair is done by primary imbrication of the fascia. This avoids potential complications from opening the hernia sac and entering the peritoneal cavity, such as bowel perforation or other intraabdominal problems. Ethibond suture (Ethicon, Inc., Somerville, New Jersey) is the preferred suture, as Prolene suture can leave long knots that in thinner patients can be palpable under the skin. The Ethibond suture is left long, and then the suture is passed through a soft mesh and tied over the mesh. A running Ethibond suture is then sewn around the periphery of the mesh. The umbilicus is then brought through a slit in the mesh (Figs 5.23–5.26). If the hernia involves the umbilicus, the umbilicus is amputated, and either the patient is closed without an umbilicus (Fig. 5.27) or a neoumbilicus can be constructed.

Below the hernia, there will still be a diastasis recti; this should be repaired. In patients without a hernia, imbrication should still be undertaken. Various techniques have been proposed. Because of the extensive laxity, some surgeons have advocated a double-layer imbrication, first doing a standard imbrication, as in a non–massive weight loss patient, and then a second imbrication to tighten the hernia again and adequately tighten the fascial layer.[5]

If a continuous infusion pain pump is to be used, it should be placed at this time. The area of maximal pain would be expected to be along the hernia/diastasis recti repair, and so the catheters should be placed along this area. To avoid having the pain pump catheters being pulled out when the drains are emptied, it is advantageous to insert the pain pump catheters from the upper abdomen (Fig. 5.28).

Seromas are a big concern in this abdomen following massive weight loss, and four drains are commonly used in this

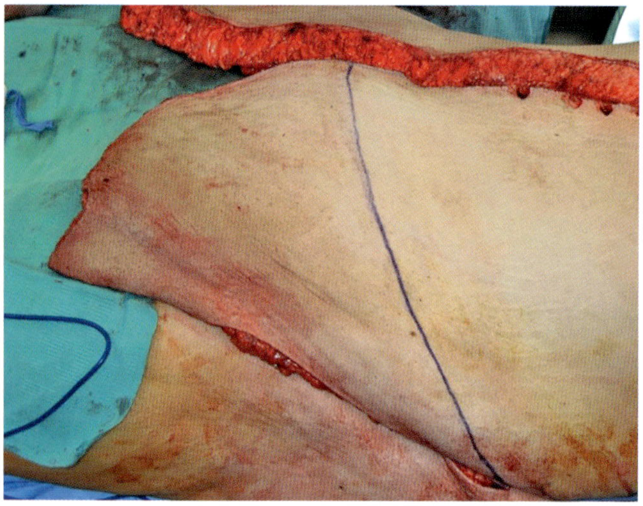

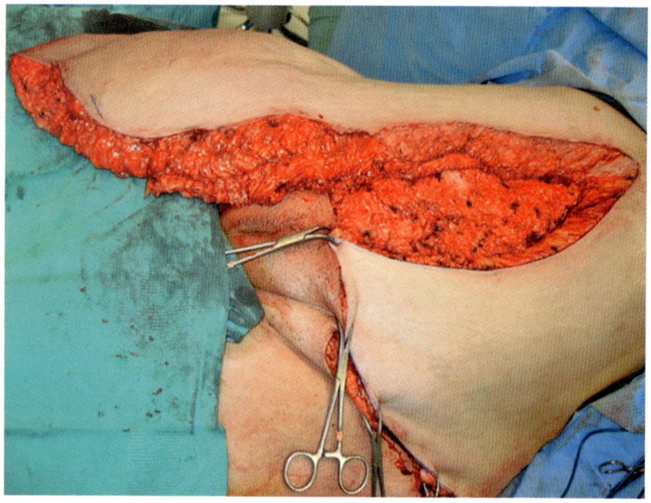

Figure 5.22 Comparison of flaps before and after resection.

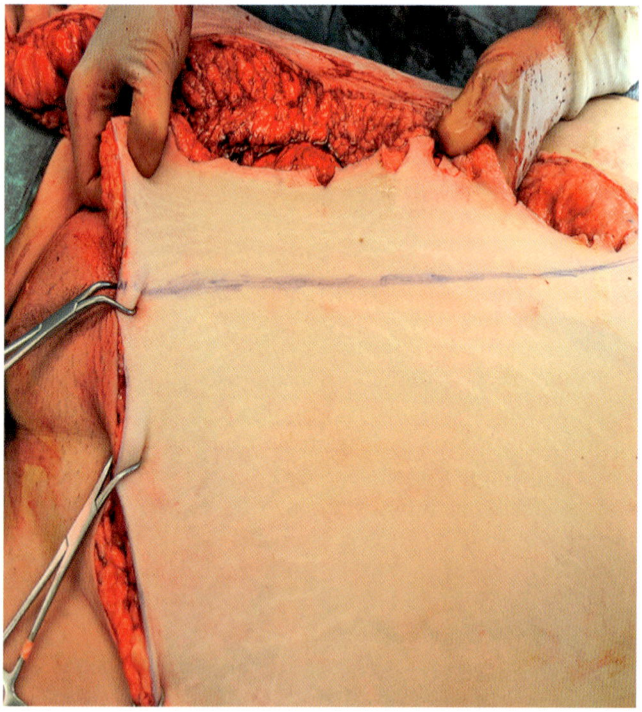

Figure 5.21 Resection of horizontal and vertical flaps.

population (Fig. 5.29), as opposed to two drains in the non–weight loss patient. These drains can be brought out in the standard manner in the pubic area. Our practice has been to leave the drains in place until the drainage is less than 40 cc from each for a 24-h period, which usually is about 2 weeks. Closure of the abdomen can be carried out as the surgeon prefers. Our current closure is 2:0 Vicryl Plus for Scarpa's fascia and 3:0 Vicryl Plus as a buried subdermal closure, and Dermabond as a skin sealant. Abdominal binders are used for patient comfort.

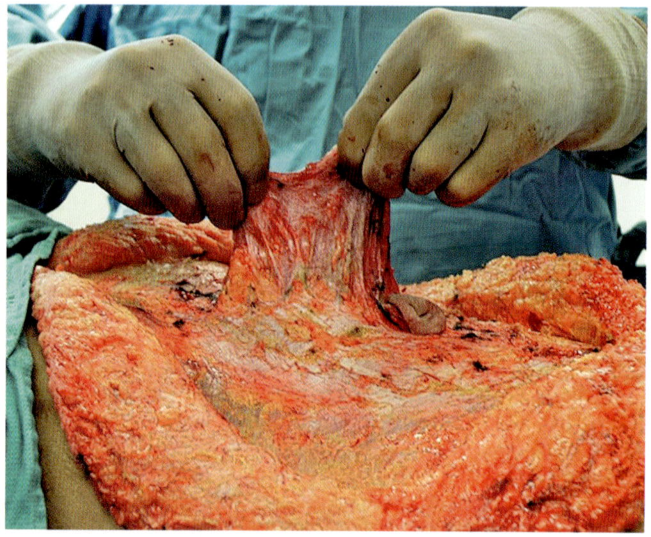

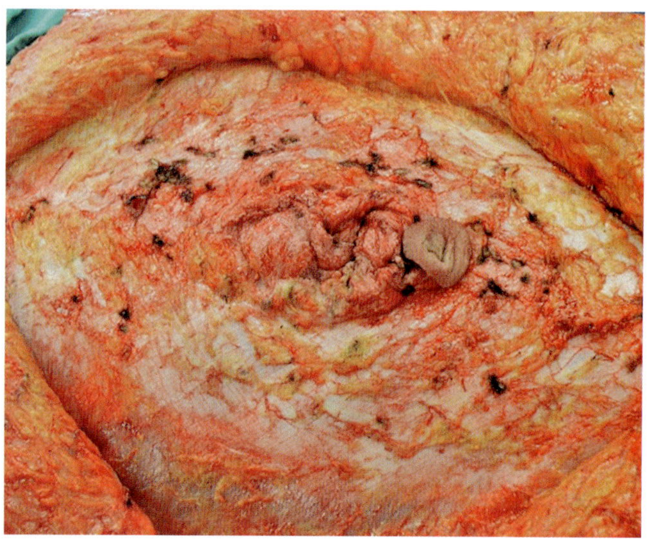

Figure 5.23 Incisional hernia sac after weight loss from open bariatric surgery.

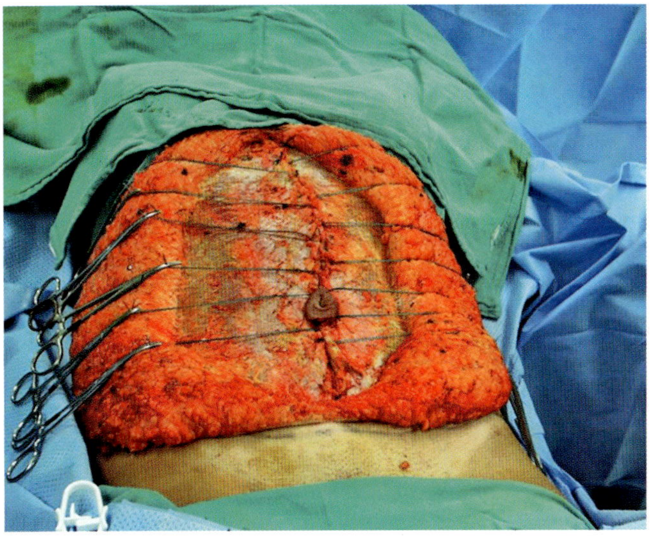

Figure 5.24 Imbrication of hernia.

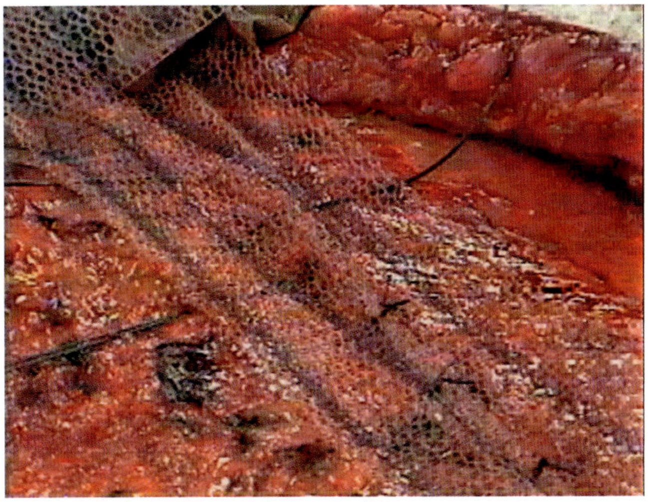

Figure 5.25 Anchoring of mesh through midline sutures.

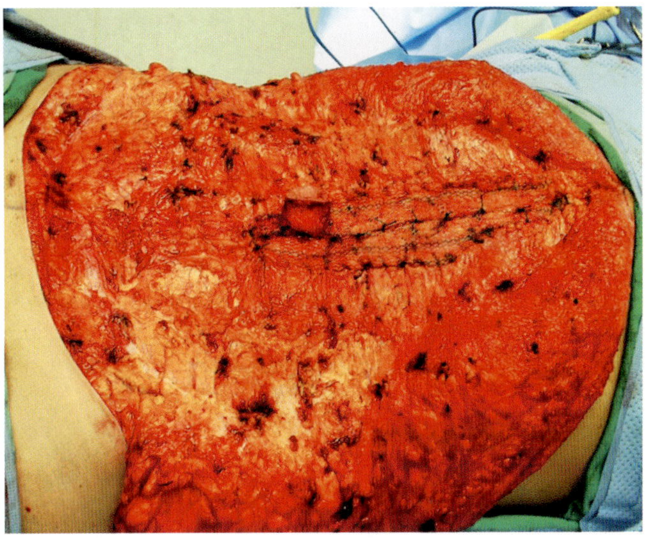

Figure 5.26 Repaired hernia with primary imbrication and onlay mesh.

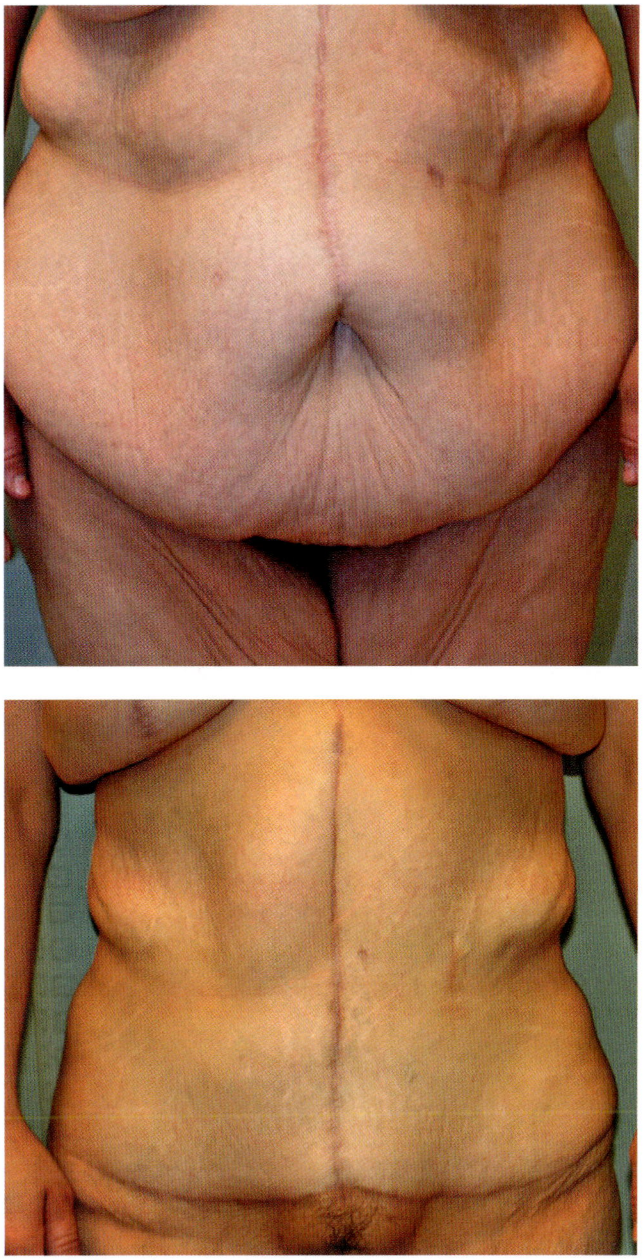

Figure 5.27 (**a**) Pre- and (**b**) postoperative hernia repair necessitating amputation of umbilicus.

SUMMARY OF SURGICAL TECHNIQUE
(Figs 5.20–5.26)

1. Mark the lateral extent of the overhanging pannus in the standing position.
2. Mark for lower abdominal incision and mons resection when patient is on the table.
3. Elevate the skin and fat to the costal margins and to the anterior axillary line.
4. Repair hernia (if present) or diastasis recti.
5. Resect excess skin and fat in both vertical and horizontal directions (if utilizing midline incision).
6. Close over four drains.

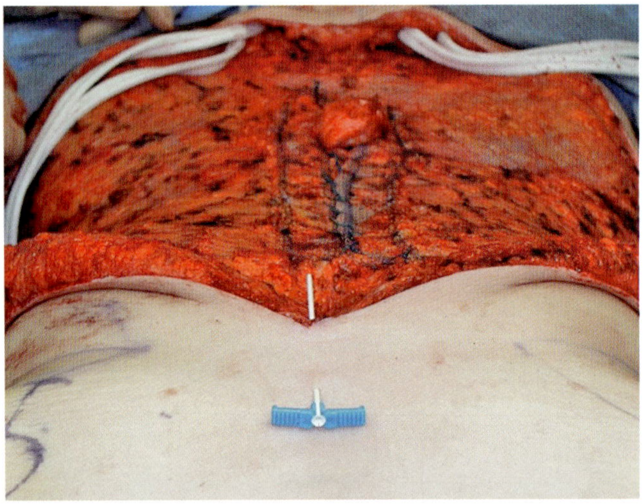

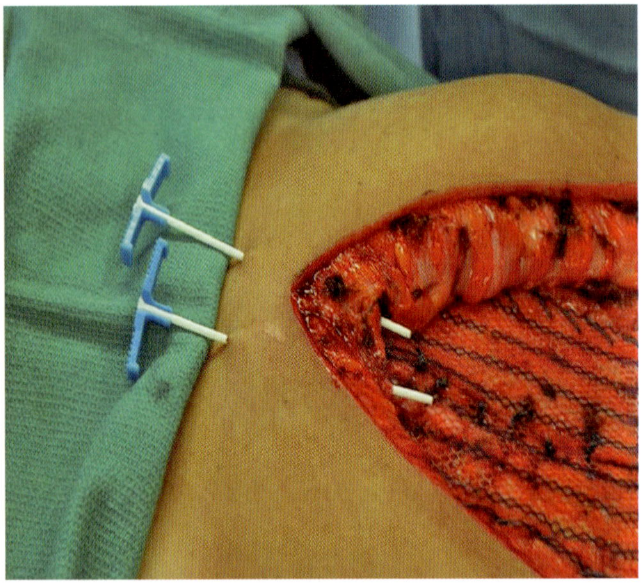

Figure 5.28 Insertion of pain pump catheters through the upper abdomen.

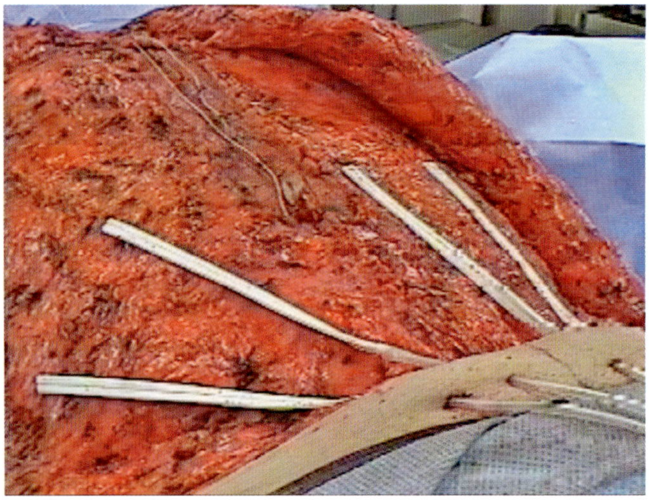

Figure 5.29 Insertion of four drains.

MANAGEMENT OF THE MASSIVE ABDOMINAL PANNUS BEFORE BARIATRIC SURGERY

For several reasons, a patient may present to a plastic surgeon for removal of an extremely large pannus without having undergone any weight loss. In some patients with a large overhanging panniculus that impedes ambulation and makes hygiene difficult, some surgeons will combine bariatric surgery with panniculectomy.[13,14] Our experience has been that there is a very high complication rate with combining the panniculectomy with the bariatric surgery. Our current practice is to do the panniculectomy first and allow the patient to recover fully before proceeding with the bariatric surgery (Figs 5.30 and 5.31). Other morbidly obese patients will require removal of their massive pannus in order to give gynecologists access to the abdomen for gynecologic procedures, such as hysterectomy for uterine cancer, or to give colorectal surgeons access to the abdomen for the surgical treatment of colorectal cancer.

The weight of the pannus can make surgical dissection difficult as well as lead to significant blood loss. In addition, the difficulty in preparing below the pannus can increase the risk of wound infection in patients who already have increased risk of infection due to other comorbidities. For these reasons, the use of a suspension-type system can be useful, especially when combined with an open wound management technique. Several suspension-type devices have been used, and some surgeons have even had specialized cranes built.[13,15,16] In our experience, orthopedic devices are readily available in the operating room (Hoyer crane or shoulder suspension device) and can be used to lift the weight of the pannus off the patient's abdomen. The lateral extent of the pannus is marked preoperatively with the patient standing (Fig. 5.32).

After attainment of general anesthesia, the patient is prepared and draped. The suspension device is then draped with a sterile drape (microscope drape, laparoscopic camera drape, and impervious stockinet) and large clamps (Adair clamps) are placed along the extent of the panniculus. A sterile rope is then passed through the clamps and attached to the suspension device. The suspension device can then be raised to suspend the pannus (Fig. 5.33).

The dissection is then started at the most lateral sides of the pannus, and it is carried down to the fascia. The dissection is carried out at this level toward the midline. The task can be carried out by two teams, both working simultaneously toward the midline. As the dissection progresses, the crane is elevated, lifting the pannus off the abdominal wall and helping delineate the desired plane of dissection at the fascial level (Fig. 5.34). This elevation has the effect of draining some of the blood from the pannus into the patient, as well as increasing visibility of the desired surgical plane. Care should be taken as the umbilicus is approached, as some patients may have an umbilical hernia that may not have been palpable due to the patient's

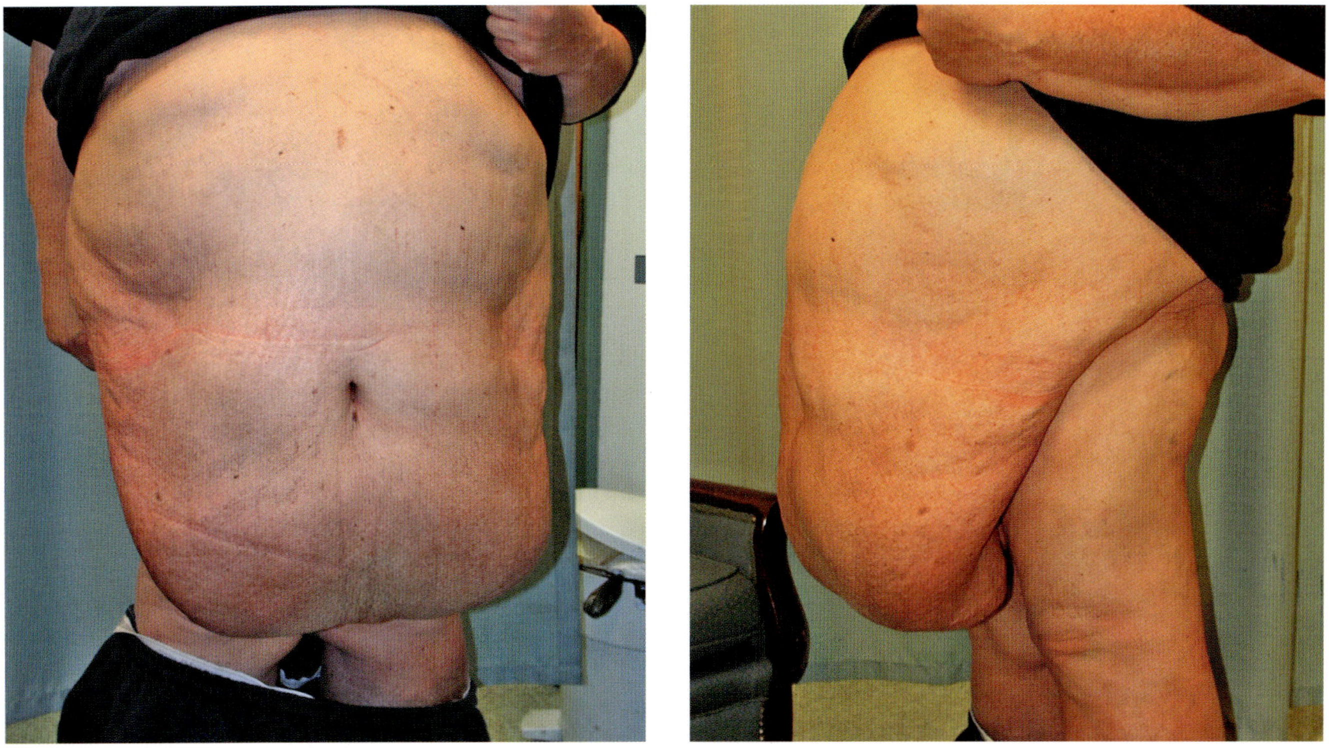

Figure 5.30 Preoperative view before panniculectomy, prior to bariatric surgery.

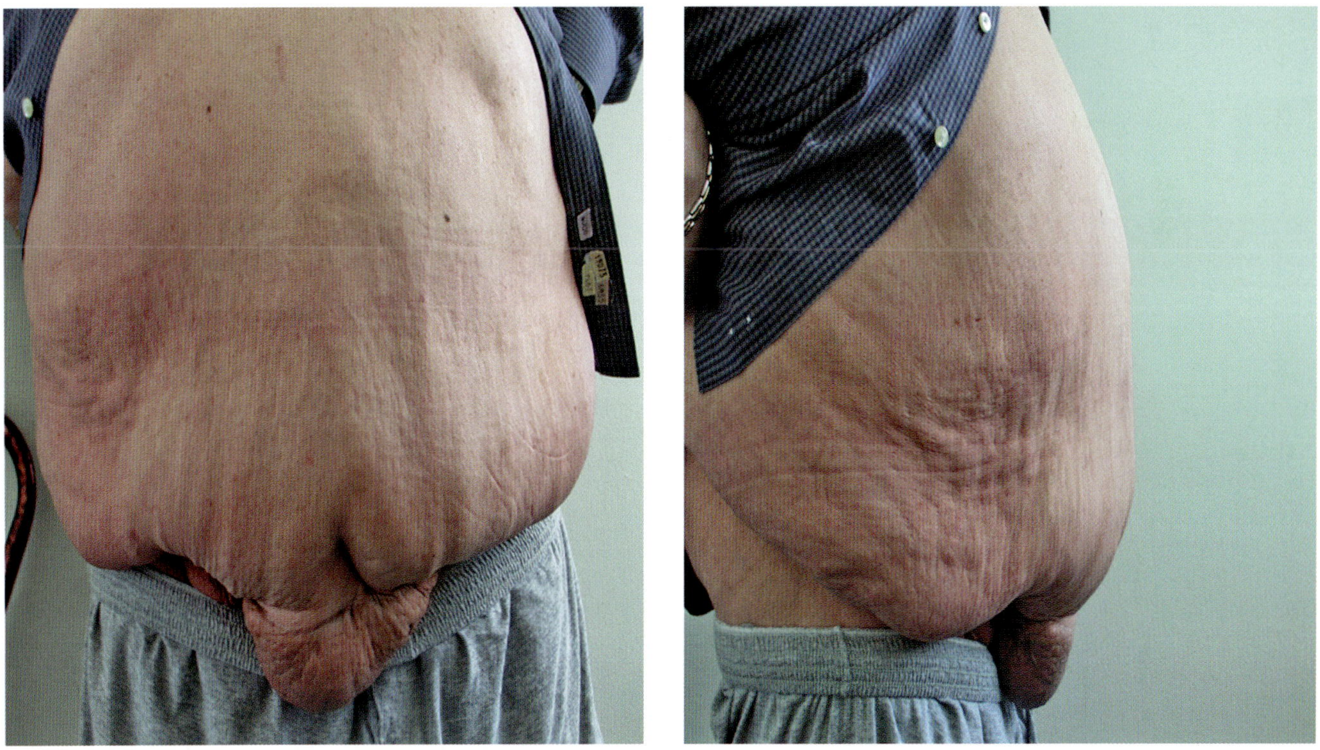

Figure 5.31 Postoperative view after resection of 22-lb (10 kg) pannus.

size before surgery. The patient's umbilicus is usually amputated during this procedure.

The risk of infection is increased in morbidly obese patients, and the preparation of a large pannus is difficult. Despite this, some surgeons report success with closing the wound and report an acceptable infection rate.[17] Our experience has been different, and therefore we have developed an open wound management technique to minimize the risk of infection. Large mattress sutures using #2 nylon are placed at approximately 6-inch intervals. For patient comfort, it is preferable to put the knot of the suture above the incision rather than on the lower flap. This is to facilitate later removal of the sutures. As these patients are usually morbidly obese, it can be difficult to get the patient on an examination table, and so the removal of the sutures is sometimes done with the patient in a wheelchair or a sitting position. Placing the knots on the upper flap therefore makes access easier for removal of the sutures. Packing is then done with a Kerlix gauze soaked in saline and wrung out (Fig. 5.35). The packing is changed twice daily, and the sutures are removed starting at 2 weeks. This technique has been used successfully both for patients before bariatric surgery and in patients requiring hysterectomy or bowel surgery.

OPTIMIZING OUTCOMES

- Mark the lateral extent of the hanging pannus so there will be no dog ears.
- Consider either a midline excision or a lateral excision for patients with a lot of mid–upper abdominal laxity.
- The risk of seroma formation is increased in this population—use four drains.
- Resect the mons if redundant.

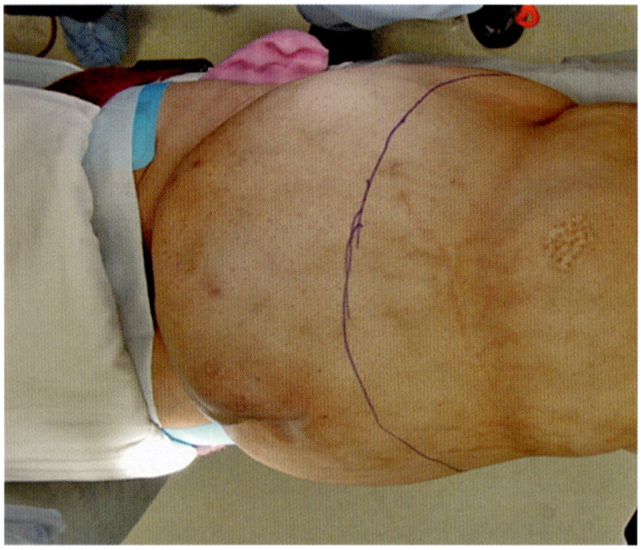

Figure 5.32 Massive pannus, the patient supine on the operating room table.

SUMMARY OF SURGICAL TECHNIQUE
(Figs 5.30–5.35)

1. Mark lateral extent of incision with patient in standing position.
2. Pannus prepared and draped.
3. Sterile draping of Hoyer crane or shoulder suspension device over table.
4. Large Adair clamps applied along extent of pannus.
5. Sterile rope passed through clamps and tied to crane.
6. Resection started at lateral aspects, and once the fascia is reached the dissection is carried to the midline simultaneously from each side.
7. As the pannus is resected, the crane is elevated and the pannus is raised off the patient.
8. Mattress sutures of a large nylon are placed every 4–6 inches.
9. Loosely pack in between the mattress sutures with Kerlix wet-to-dry.

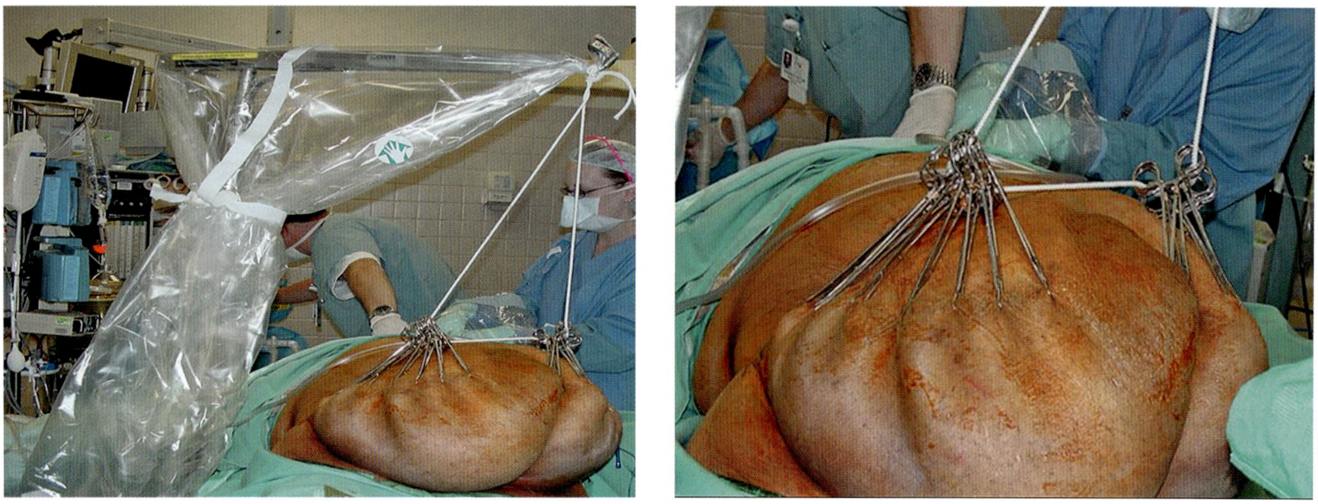

Figure 5.33 Elevation of a massive pannus with a shoulder suspension device.

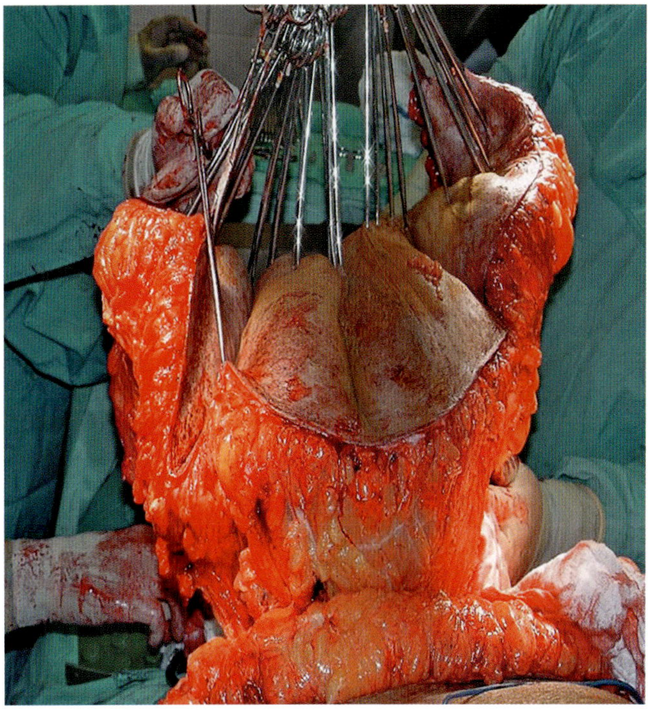

Figure 5.34 Resected pannus.

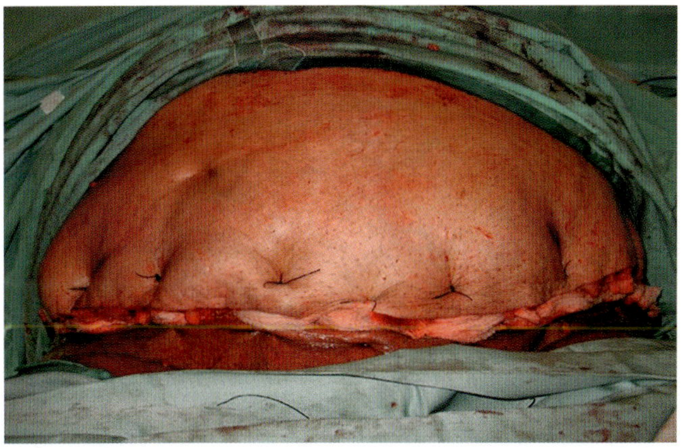

Figure 5.35 Pannus closed with #2 nylon mattress stitch and packed with Kerlix.

Although this population of patients can be some of our happiest patients, there are some factors that need to be taken into consideration to maximize the outcome. One of the most important is the avoidance of dog ears. Marking the patient in the standing position to delineate the lateral extent of the overhanging pannus (Fig. 5.7) will minimize this problem. The lower abdominal incision is much longer in post–massive weight loss patients than in other patients presenting for an abdominoplasty.

It is also important to resect a portion of the mons if lax. A patient who has undergone a panniculectomy and has been left with a redundant mons is often disappointed. We generally resect the mons horizontally down at three fingerbreadths above the labial cleft.[18] Undermining the mons will lead to increased risk of lymphatic drainage and should be avoided. My decision on how much mons to resect is made on the operating table, as it can be difficult to elevate the area under the pannus while the patient is standing (Fig. 5.9).

Recurrent laxity is a problem in any patients after massive weight loss. No matter how tight the skin is pulled, it can be expected to relax over time, leading to some recurrence of the defect. The upper abdomen is an area where recurrent laxity can be particularly bothersome to the patient. Patients are more willing to trade contour for scars, and the possibility of a midline incision should be considered. In some patients, a lateral excision could also be used, especially as a continuation of a brachioplasty incision and especially in patients with laxity lateral to their breast area.

The risk of seromas is higher in this population. The fat appears different in these patients—it is clear that there are still too many fat cells present (although they appear depleted), from the appearance of the fat. Use of four drains is advised to adequately drain the area. Even then, some patients will develop a seroma (see *Complications and their management* section).

POSTOPERATIVE CARE

Avoidance of pulmonary embolus is of utmost importance. During the procedure, pneumatic stockings are used, and early mobilization in the postoperative period is key. Some surgeons advocated the use of low-molecular-weight heparin starting before or after the procedure, but there is not a clear consensus at this time. What is agreed on is the importance of early mobilization as quickly as possible. We have found that it is useful to insist that in order to eat, the patients must be out of bed in a chair.

A one-night stay in either an aftercare facility or a hospital may be recommended because the amount of fluid shifts due to the amount of tissue that is removed, as well as to monitor for a hematoma. Some surgeons base their decision on the BMI of the patient at the time of abdominoplasty. In one study, patients with a BMI up to 34 kg/m^2 were considered for outpatient abdominoplasty. Patients with a BMI of 35 kg/m^2 were kept overnight in the hospital. For borderline cases involving an obese patient, the decision was made after a qualified anesthesia provider was consulted.[19]

As the skin is very stretched and there is a large dead space in these patients, it can be difficult to assess the abdomen for a hematoma, particularly in the early phase of a fluid collection. The abdominal skin may never become taut, despite even a liter of blood being present. If clinical suspicions are high (low blood pressure, increased drainage, or sanguinous drainage), then an ultrasound can be helpful in confirming the diagnosis.

COMPLICATIONS AND THEIR MANAGEMENT

An interesting observation has been made regarding the risk of complications between non-obese, borderline, and obese patients undergoing abdominoplasty. A multifactorial analysis of variance showed that the preoperative weight at the time of abdominoplasty had a highly statistically significant effect on the incidence of complications, whereas previous bariatric surgery did not.[20] One group of patients seems to have the highest complication rate for any body-sculpting procedure: those who have had the greatest change in their BMI from prebariatric surgery to postbariatric surgery. Also, patients with a high BMI (over 35 kg/m^2) at the time of plastic surgery have an increased complication rate, with seromas being the most common problem.[6]

For the abdominal procedures, those at greatest risk of problems would include the group with a subset of those patients who carried their weight in the abdominal area. These patients, who can be described as having the apple pattern or male pattern of fat distribution, have the greatest amount of residual abdominal fat and skin, and therefore would be at risk for the highest rate of complications. This stems from the large number of fat cells present in their abdominal areas. When the patients were heavy, they had too many fat cells (hyperplasia) and they were too large (hypertrophy). When the patients lose weight, they still have too many fat cells, although the cells are now shrunken. The skin and fat that are resected contain many shrunken fat cells, but the skin and fat left behind still contain more fat cells per area than in patients who have never been morbidly obese.

Fat cells are known to secrete many substances, such as leptin and inflammatory cytokines, that effect endothelial permeability. The secretion of these substances by this large population of fat cells may lead to the increased risk of seroma formation over the risk seen in patients undergoing abdominoplasty without massive weight loss. Ideally then, to minimize the risk of problems, one would choose to operate on the patient who has not lost a significant amount of weight and whose lost weight was not from their abdomen. Clearly, this is not the typical postbariatric patient, and therefore the risk of seroma formation must be dealt with. The use of four drains has already been discussed; this is important in adequately draining the space. Different surgeons manage the drains differently. Some surgeons routinely remove the drains at 2 weeks whether or not the drainage has decreased, and will then deal with the complication of seroma formation as it occurs. Others will remove the drains only when a certain drainage level (our criterion is 40 cc per day) has been reached. In either case, seroma formation can occur.

Serial aspiration is the most common method used to deal with seromas. Using a 14-gauge angiocatheter through the incision, many seromas can be dealt with by aspiration. The patient is then seen either weekly or biweekly for continued aspiration until the seroma has resolved. If the seroma cannot be aspirated in the office, then an ultrasound with drain placement may be required.

Various techniques have been suggested as methods to control seroma formation. Some surgeons use mattress-type sutures[21] to minimize the dead space and therefore reduce the available space for seroma formation. Others have used tissue sealants during the procedure. Surgeons have been using tissue sealants to minimize the occurrence of seromas during latissimus flap surgery[22] and have recently adapted its use to this area. The use of tissue sealants (most notably Tisseel, Baxter

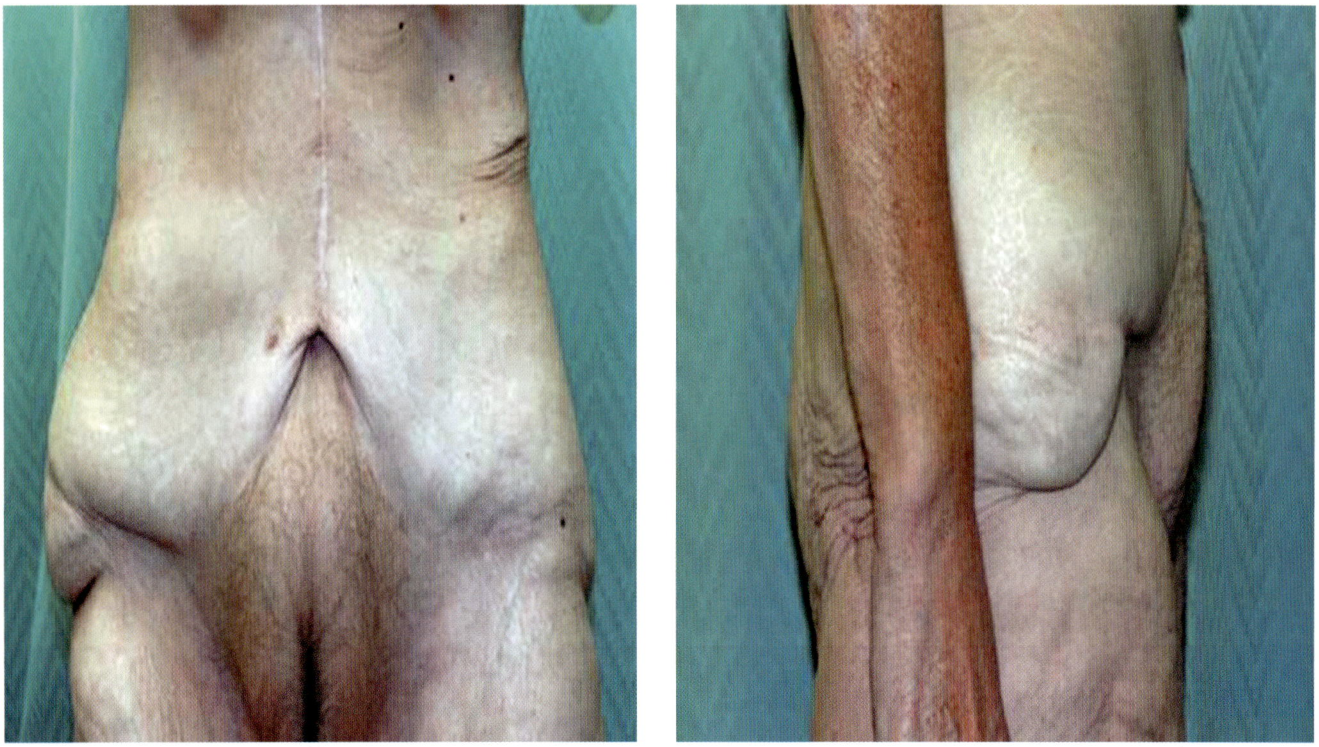

Figure 5.36 Result of T-juncture breakdown and secondary healing.

Corp., Deerfield, Illinois) for reducing the risk of seromas is an off-label use of the product. The use of Tisseel seems to reduce the number of seromas that occur and, when seromas do occur, their size is diminished.[23]

When drainage is persistent, some surgeons have been using doxycycline in the drains. Similarly to the use of doxycycline in thoracic surgery to decrease pleural effusions, the doxycycline is diluted (100 mg in 5 cc of saline) and injected into the drain. The drain is then left unclamped for 4 h and then suction is again applied. Some patients may complain of a temporary burning sensation, but most do not report any symptoms. The burning sensation, if felt, seems to be more common in patients who are less than 2 weeks out from their procedure. Anecdotal evidence shows that, for some patients, this method is effective in expediting the resolution of the seroma.

The most common site of wound breakdown is at the T juncture where the vertical and horizontal incisions come together. Debridement and packing will usually allow this area to heal, but patients may require a scar revision (Fig. 5.36).

Infections are not that common but, when they do occur, can be troublesome to manage. If a patient presents with an infection, it is important to recall which bariatric procedure the patient had undergone. Patients who have undergone a malabsorptive procedure, especially a duodenal switch, may not absorb adequate antibiotics and so may require intravenous therapy. We have handled this situation by admitting the patients, having a peripherally inserted central catheter line placed, and then continuing the intravenous antibiotics at home.

CONCLUSION

The post–massive weight loss patient is both challenging and rewarding. Although the surgery may be more difficult, in requiring different incisions or even a staged approach, the outcome may be life-changing for the patient. Careful planning and discussions with the patient, as well as some different intraoperative routines, can minimize the complications as well as undesirable outcomes.

REFERENCES

1. Kelly HA. Report of gynecological cases. John Hopkins Med J 1899; 10:197.
2. Kelly HA. Excision of the fat of the abdominal wall lipectomy. Surg Gynecol Obstet 1910; 10:299.
3. Thorek M. Plastic reconstruction of the female breast and abdomen. Am J Surg 1939; 43:268.
4. Matarasso A, Swift RW, Rankin M. Abdominoplasty and abdominal contour surgery: a national plastic surgery survey. Plast Reconstr Surg 2006; 117:1797–1808.
5. Aly AS, Cram AE, Heddens C. Truncal body contouring surgery in the massive weight loss patient. Clin Plast Surg 2004; 31:611–624.
6. Aly AS, Cram AE, Chao M, et al. Belt lipectomy for circumferential truncal excess: the University of Iowa experience. Plast Reconstr Surg 2003; 111(1):398–413.
7. Downey SE, Kelso R, Anthone G, et al. Review of technique for combined closed incisional repair and panniculectomy status post bariatric surgery. Surg Obes Relat Dis (in press).
8. Gmur RU, Banic A, Erni D. Is it safe to combine abdominoplasty with other dermolipectomy procedures to correct skin excess after weight loss? Ann Plast Surg 2003; 51(4):353–357.
9. Babcock W. The correction of the obese and relaxed abdominal wall with especial reference to the use of buried silver chain. Phila Obstet Soc 1916; May 4.
10. Savage RC. Abdominoplasty following gastrointestinal bypass surgery. Plast Reconstr Surg 1983; 71(4):500–507.
11. Rosenfield LK. Comprehensive abdominoplasty approaches using complementary techniques. In: Nahai F. The art of aesthetic surgery. St. Louis: Quality Medical Publishing; 2005.
12. Ward DJ, Wilson JSP. Abdominal reduction following jejunoileal bypass for morbid obesity. Br J Plast Surg 1989; 42:586–590.
13. Jensen PL, Sanger JR, Matloub HS, et al. Use of a portable floor crane as an aid to resection of the massive panniculus. Ann Plast Surg 1990; 25:234–235.
14. Acarturk TO, Wachtman G, Heil B, et al. Panniculectomy as an adjuvant to bariatric surgery. Ann Plast Surg 2004; 53(4):360–366.
15. Matory WE, O'Sullivan J, Fudem G, et al. Abdominal surgery in patients with severe morbid obesity. Plast Reconstr Surg 1994; 94(7):976–987.
16. Richard EF. A mechanical aid for abdominal panniculectomy. Br J Plast Surg 1965; 18:336–337.
17. Hopkins MP, Shriner AM, Parker MG, et al. Panniculectomy at the time of gynecologic surgery in morbidly obese patients. Am J Obstet Gynecol 2000; 182:1502–1505.
18. Matarasso A, Wallach S. Abdominal contour surgery: treating all aesthetic units, including the mons pubis. Aesthetic Surg J 2001; 21(2):111–119.
19. Williams TC, Hardaway M, Altuna B. Ambulatory abdominoplasty tailored to patients with an appropriate body mass index. Aesthetic Surg J 2005; March–April:132–137.
20. Vastine VL, Morgan RF, Williams GS, et al. Wound complications of abdominoplasty in obese patients. Ann Plast Surg 1999; 42(1):34–39.
21. Pollock H, Pollack T. Progressive tension sutures: a technique to reduce local complications in abdominoplasty. Plast Reconstr Surg 2000; 105(7):2583–2586.
22. Weinrach JC, Cronin ED, Smith BK, et al. Preventing seroma in the latissimus dorsi flap donor site with fibrin sealant. Ann Plast Surg 2004; 53(1):12–16.
23. Downey SE, Morales CL. The use of fibrin sealant in the prevention of seromas in the massive weight loss patient. Poster presentation at the Annual ASPS Meeting, September 2005, Chicago, Illinois.

ADDITIONAL READING

Al-Basti HB, El-Khatib HA, Taha A, et al. Intraabdominal pressure after full abdominoplasty in obese multiparous patients. Plast Reconstr Surg 2004; 113(7):2145–2150.

Baroudi R, Ferreira C. Seroma: how to avoid it and how to treat it. Aesthetic Surg J 1999; 18:439.

Belin RP, Stone NH, Fischer RP, et al. Improved technique of panniculectomy. Surgery 1966; 59(2):222–225.

Blomfield PI, Le T, Allen DG, et al. Panniculectomy: a useful technique for the obese patient undergoing gynecological surgery. Gynecol Oncol 1998; 70:80–86.

Bolton MA, Pruzinsky T, Cash TF, et al. Measuring outcomes in plastic surgery: body image and quality of life in abdominoplasty patients. Plast Reconstr Surg 2003; 112(2):619–625.

Carwell GR, Horton CE Sr. Circumferential torsoplasty. Ann Plast Surg 1997; 38(3):213–216.

Cosin JA, Powell JL, Donovan JT, et al. The safety and efficacy of extensive abdominal panniculectomy at the time of pelvic surgery. Gynecol Oncol 1994; 55:36–40.

Da Costa LF, Landecker A, Manta AM. Optimizing body contour in massive weight loss patients: the modified vertical abominoplasty. Plast Reconstr Surg 2004; 114(7):1917–1923.

Dardour JC, Vilain R. Alternatives to the classic abdominoplasty. Ann Plast Surg 1986; 17(3):247–258.

Daw JL, Mustoe TA. Use of a tourniquet in panniculus resection. Plast Reconstr Surg 1997; 99(7):2082–2084.

Desjardin A. Lipectomy for extreme obesity. Paris Chir 1911; 3:466.

El-Khatib HA, Bener A. Abdominal dermolipectomy in an abdomen with pre-existing scars: a different concept. Plast Reconstr Surg 2004; 114(4):992–997.

Goessl A, Redl H. Optimized thrombin dilution protocol for a slowly setting fibrin sealant in surgery. Eur Surg 2005; 37(1):43–51.

Grazer FM, Goldwyn RM. Abdominoplasty assessed by survey, with emphasis on complications. Plast Reconstr Surg 1997; 59(4):513–517.

Hagerty RF, Hawk JC Jr, Boniface K, et al. Resection of massive abdominal panniculus adiposus. South Med J 1974; 67(8):984–989.

Hensel JM, Lehman JA Jr, Tantri MP, et al. An outcomes analysis and satisfaction survey of 199 consecutive abdominoplasties. Ann Plast Surg 2001; 46(4):357–363.

Hester TR Jr, Baird W, Bostwick J III, et al. Abdominoplasty combined with other major surgical procedures: safe or sorry? Plast Reconstr Surg 1989; 83(6):997–1004.

Hunstad JP. Body contouring in the obese patient. Clin Plast Surg 1996; 23(4):647–670.

Kamper MJ, Galloway DV, Ashley F. Abdominal panniculectomy after massive weight loss. Plast Reconstr Surg 1972; 50(5):441–446.

Krueger JK, Rohrich RJ. Clearing the smoke. Scientific rationale for tobacco abstention with plastic surgery. Plast Reconstr Surg 2001; 108(4):1063–1073.

Kulber DA, Bacilious N, Peters ED, et al. The use of fibrin sealant in the prevention of seromas. Plast Reconstr Surg 1997; 99(3):842–849.

Lockwood T. High-lateral-tension abdominoplasty with superficial fascial system suspension. Plast Reconstr Surg 1995; 96(3):603–615.

Lockwood T. Lower body lift with superficial fascial system suspension. Plast Reconstr Surg 1993; 92(6):1112–1122.

Lockwood T. Superficial fascial system (SFS) of the trunk and extremities: a new concept. Plast Reconstr Surg 1991; 87:1009–1018.

Lockwood T. Transverse flank-thigh-buttock lift with superficial fascial suspension. Plast Reconstr Surg 1991; 87(6):1019–1027.

Lockwood TE. Lower-body lift. Aesthetic Surg J 2001; 21:335.

Matarasso A. Abdominoplasty. In: Achauer BM, Eriksson E, Guyuron B, et al, eds. Plastic surgery: indications, operations and outcomes, vol 5. Aesthetic surgery. St. Louis: Mosby; 2000:2783–2821.

Matarasso A. Liposuction as an adjunct to a full abdominoplasty revisted. Plast Reconstr Surg 2000; 106(5):1197–1202.

Matarasso A. The male abdominoplasty. Clin Plast Surg 2004; 31(4):555–569.

McCabe WP, Kelly AP Jr, Frame B. Panniculectomy following intestinal bypass. Br J Plast Surg 1974; 27:346–351.

McGraw LH. Surgical rehabilitation after massive weight reduction: case report. Annual Meeting of the American Society for Aesthetic Plastic Surgery, March 12, 1973, California.

Meyerowitz BR, Gruber RP, Laub DR. Massive abdominal panniculectomy. JAMA 1973; 225(4):408–409.

Micha JP, Rettenmaier MA, Francis L, et al. 'Medically necessary' panniculectomy to facilitate gynecologic cancer surgery in morbidly obese patients. Gynecol Oncol 1998; 69:237–242.

Oguz AT, Wachtman G, Heil B, et al. Panniculectomy as an adjuvant to bariatric surgery. Ann Plast Surg 2004; 53(4):360–366.

Petty P, Manson PN, Black R, et al. Panniculus morbidus. Ann Plast Surg 1992; 28(5):442–452.

Powell JL, Kasparek DK, Connor GP. Panniculectomy to facilitate gynecologic surgery in morbidly obese women. Obstet Gynecol 1999; 94(4):528–531.

Rubin JP, Nguyen V, Schwentker A. Perioperative management of the post-gastric-bypass patient presenting for body contour surgery. Clin Plast Surg 2004; 31:601–610.

Soundararajan V, Hart NB, Royston CMS. Abdominoplasty following vertical banded gastroplasty for morbid obesity. Br J Plast Surg 1995; 48:423–427.

Stanhope CR, Winburn KA, Silberman MB. Indicated noncosmetic panniculectomy in gynecologic surgery. J Pelvic Surg 2002; 8:197–201.

Van Geertruyden JP, Vandeweyer E, de Fontaine S, et al. Circumferential torsoplasty. Br J Plast Surg 1999; 52(8):623–628.

Van Uchelen JH, Werker PM, Kon M. Complications of abdominoplasty in 86 patients. Plast Reconstr Surg 2001; 107(7):1869–1873.

Young SC, Freiberg A. A critical look at abdominal lipectomy following morbid obesity surgery. Aesthetic Plast Surg 1991; 15:81–84.

Zook EG. Abdominoplasty following gastrointestinal bypass surgery. Plast Reconstr Surg 1983; 4:508–509.

Zook EG. Massive weight loss patient. Clin Plast Surg 1975; 2(3):457.

APPROACH TO THE LOWER BODY AFTER WEIGHT LOSS

6

Joseph F. Capella

Key Points

- A careful analysis of patient morphology is critical to proper treatment of the massive weight loss patient.
- Classification of patients by BMI assists with patient education and provides an algorithm for treatment.
- Careful preoperative evaluation and preparation are essential in the postbariatric population.
- The use of bony landmarks with preoperative patient marking helps control scar placement and scar perceptibility.
- Appropriate staging in postbariatric body-contouring procedures minimizes complications and maximizes the aesthetic and functional outcome.

The abdomen, thighs, and buttocks or lower body are often the areas of greatest concern to patients following massive weight loss. The well-described stigmata of the postpartum syndrome include redundant skin along the anterior abdominal wall, striae gravidarum, relaxed abdominal wall fascia, and diastasis recti. Massive weight loss leads to similar changes of the abdomen; however, other regions of the torso and the remainder of the body are affected as well.

The typical appearance of the massive weight loss patient derives from a combination of factors, including a gender-dependent body morphology and a change or changes in BMI that then lead to skin and soft tissue excess and poor skin tone.[1]

- Overweight women tend to have large deposits of fat at the hips, circumferentially along the thighs, lower abdomen, and mons pubis, and the axilla and flanks to a lesser degree, creating a gynecoid or 'pear-shaped' body habitus (Fig. 6.1a–c).
- Morbidly obese men have an android or central distribution of fat. Much of their adiposity is confined to the abdomen, axilla and flanks, and hips and medial thighs (Fig. 6.1d–f). In addition, the hip roll in men is slightly more cephalad, generally at the level of the iliac crest as opposed to below the iliac crest in women.

As a result of the characteristic location of fat deposition in both men and women, the contour deformities of morbidly obese individuals following massive weight loss are also quite typical.

- Women tend to have excess skin along the anterior abdominal wall, flank, and hip regions, as well as cellulite and excess skin along the thighs and buttocks. The buttocks and pubic areas are often ptotic and redundant (Fig. 6.1a–c).
- Men have similar changes to the abdominal, flank, hip, medial thigh, and pubic regions; however, the anterior, posterior, and lateral thighs and buttocks are affected to a lesser degree and are usually without cellulite (Fig. 6.1d–f).

The lower body contour stigmata of massive weight loss for both men and women is the consequence of the skin and soft tissues failing to retract completely following the metabolism of fat, either through bariatric surgery or following lifestyle changes. The excess skin and soft tissues descend inferomedially from the characteristic areas of fat deposition. The fat deposits of the axilla and flank produce rolls along the upper and mid back and flank. The hip fat deposit produces a roll just below the top of the iliac crest in men and often on to the proximal lateral thigh in women. The collapse of redundant tissues from the lower abdomen, mons pubis, and buttocks in both men and women contributes directly to the excess tissues along the medial thighs, as does the redundant tissues from the fat deposits of the medial thigh itself. The descent of redundant tissues from the fat deposits circumferentially along the thighs in women creates the potential for skin folds throughout the thighs. The circumferential deposition of fat along the thighs in women results not only in a vertical excess of tissues, but a circumferential or horizontal excess as well.

In addition to issues of skin and soft tissue excess, the postbariatric patient is different from the traditional body-contouring patient with regard to skin quality. Obese individuals have usually been overweight since childhood and nearly always since adolescence.[2] The average age for bariatric procedures is 37 years.[3] In the years prior to gastric reduction procedures, obese individuals have typically gained and lost weight numerous times in attempts to lose weight through

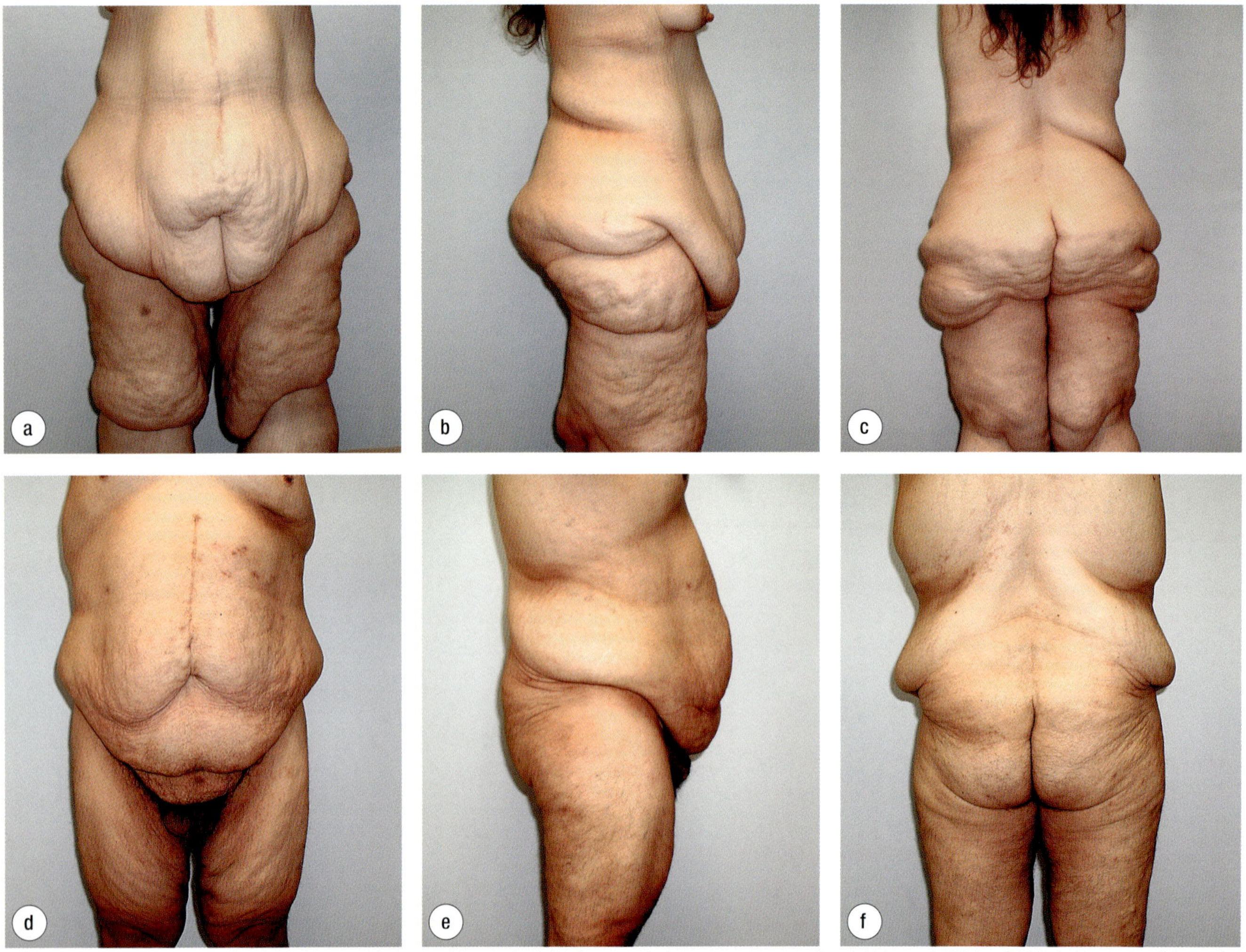

Figure 6.1 Type 3 patients. (**a–c**) A 40-year-old woman 40 months following gastric bypass surgery and weight loss of 269 lbs (122 kg). Current weight and BMI: 254 lbs (115 kg) and 41 kg/m^2, respectively. Highest weight and BMI: 522 lbs (237 kg), 84 kg/m^2. (**d-f**) A 39-year-old man 16 months following gastric bypass surgery and weight loss of 209 lbs (95 kg). Current weight and BMI: 229 lbs (104 kg) and 37 kg/m^2, respectively. Highest weight and BMI: 439 lbs (199 kg), 71 kg/m^2.

dieting or behavioral modification. The prolonged period of skin under tension and the frequent history of 'yo-yo' dieting lead to poor skin tone following massive weight loss. Striae and cellulite are common throughout the torso, particularly in women. The extreme body contour deformities that distinguish the routine patient from the massive weight loss patient have led to the development of operative techniques specific to these individuals.

The ideal lower body–contouring procedure for the massive weight loss patient should effectively address all or as many of the characteristic stigmata as possible in a safe, efficient, and consistent manner. Various techniques have been described to treat the lower body postbariatric condition; these include body lift, belt lipectomy, lower body lift, and circumferential torsoplasty.[1,4–6] While having different names, each in this group involves a simultaneous abdominoplasty, and thigh and buttock lift. The goal of all these procedures is to reverse or derotate the inferomedial collapse of the skin and soft tissues of the lower body (Fig. 6.2). Aside from the obvious advantage of addressing the thighs and buttocks as well as the abdomen in one stage, a simultaneous circumferential procedure offers another very important advantage: a standing cone is not a concern. In any procedure that is limited by the length of a scar, some graduation in the amount of skin traction that can be applied must exist to prevent skin redundancy along the lateral extent of the scar. Circumferential procedures allow for much higher levels of tension to be applied without this concern. This is particularly important for the body lift where the distal thigh and upper abdomen are being addressed from the waistline.

The surge in bariatric procedures in the USA and abroad over the past 5 years has led to increasing patient requests for body-contouring procedures.[7] To treat the postbariatric condition, some plastic surgeons are implementing traditional

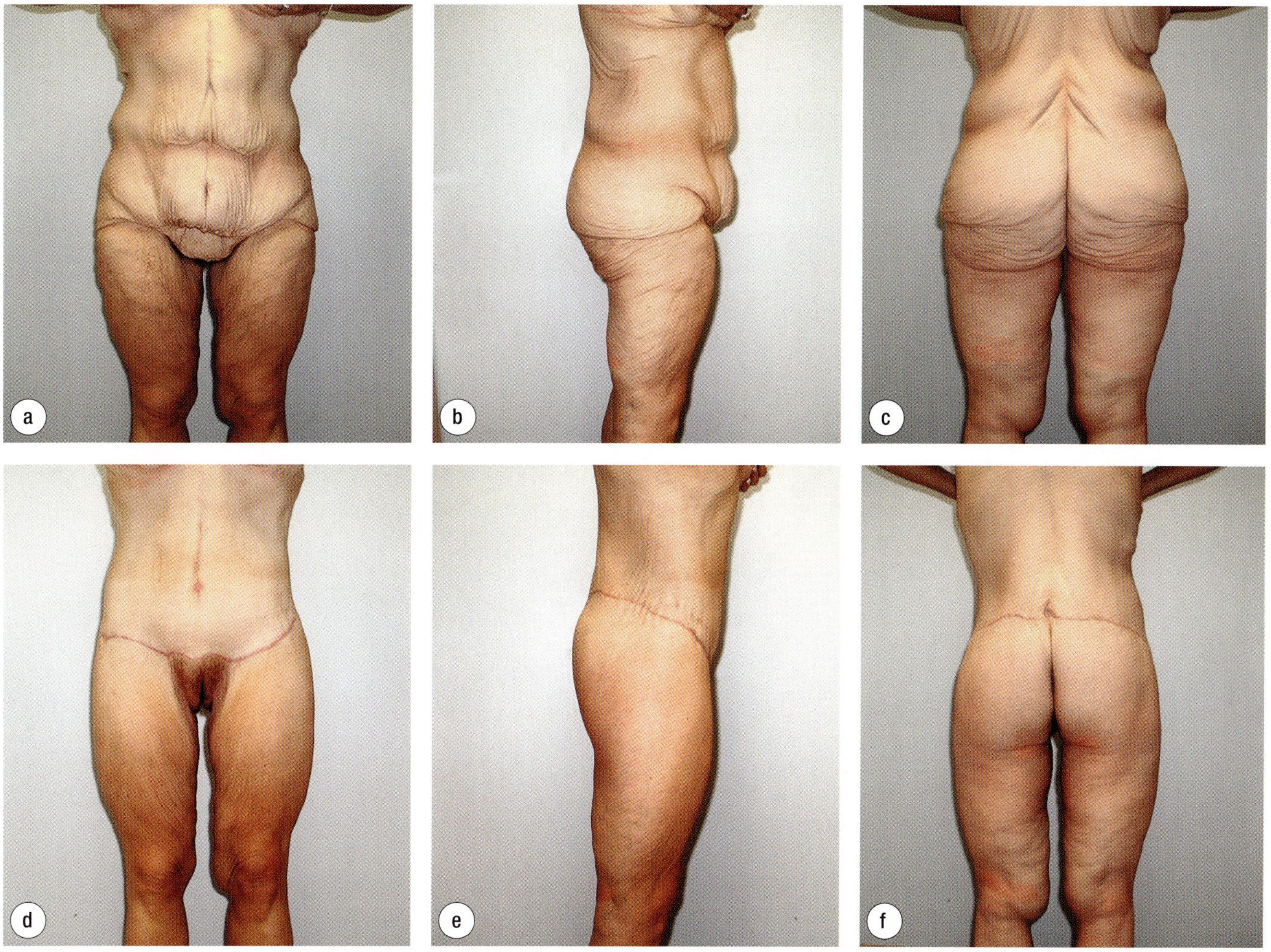

Figure 6.2 (**a–c**) A type 2 46-year-old woman 18 months following gastric bypass surgery and weight loss of 225 lbs (102 kg). Current weight and BMI: 176 lbs (80 kg) and 28 kg/m^2, respectively. Highest weight and BMI: 401 lbs (182 kg), 65 kg/m^2. (**d–f**) Seven months following body lift.

procedures and others are performing the more aggressive circumferential approaches.[1,4–6,8–12] Attempts to treat the postbariatric patient with abdominoplasty and liposuction alone are likely to result in an unsatisfactory outcome (Fig. 6.3a–c). Likewise, extending an abdominoplasty to be circumferential without thigh and buttock undermining usually produces less than optimal results.

Many plastic surgeons have been reluctant to apply skin-tightening procedures to deformities of the thigh and buttock region because of poor scars, unreliable scar location, high complication rates, and the magnitude of these procedures.[13] Largely because of Lockwood's many important contributions to body contouring and the increase in demand for these procedures, plastic surgeons are approaching postbariatric body contouring with renewed enthusiasm and interest.[5,14–17] Lockwood, by developing the lower body lift version 1 and later 2, approached the abdomen, thighs, and buttocks as a unit, realizing that each of these areas of the body had to be effectively treated to produce the best overall outcome. Treating the abdomen, thighs, and buttocks as singular units would negate the powerful benefits of a circumferential procedure. Lockwood also established the importance of approximating the superficial fascial system (SFS) with permanent sutures to maintain soft tissue contour over the long term and to maximize scar quality.

At the start of my career, practicing both bariatric surgery and plastic surgery along with my father, a bariatric surgeon, the lower body contour concerns, both functional and aesthetic, of the massive weight loss patient became very apparent.

- Women typically would present with the primary complaints of excess skin along the lower abdomen, an excess hair-bearing pubic area, and excess skin along the medial thighs. Other complaints might include sagging buttocks, cellulite, and excess skin along the remainder of the thighs. Lipodystrophy could also be a concern at any of these areas but was most frequent regarding the mons pubis, lateral and medial thighs, and knee region.
- Men would present with similar complaints regarding the lower abdomen, mons pubis, and medial thighs. In addition, men often had complaints about lipodystrophy

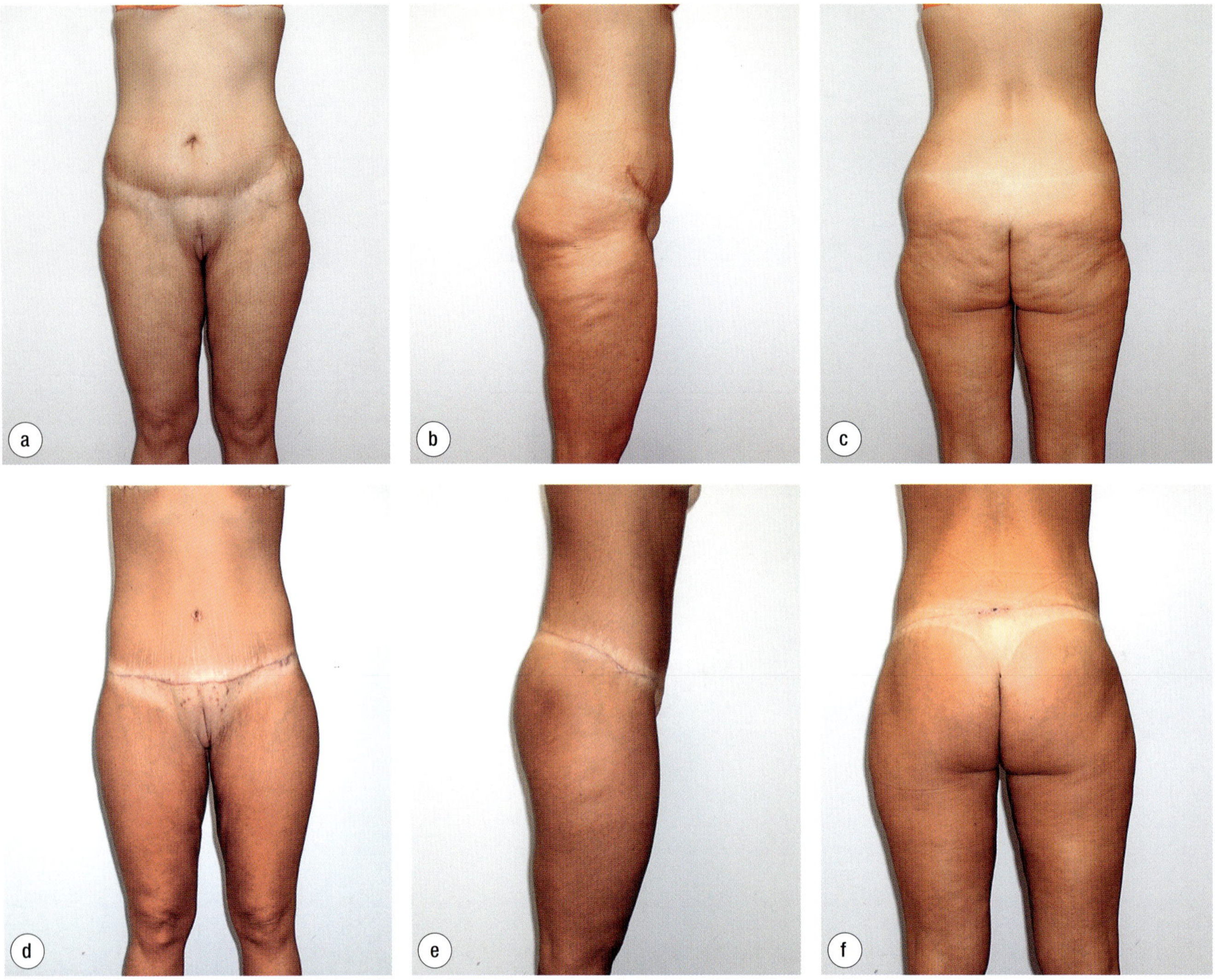

Figure 6.3 (**a–c**) A type 1 33-year-old woman 4 years following 163-lb (74 kg) weight loss from lifestyle changes and 2 years following abdominoplasty and liposuction. Current weight and BMI: 134 lbs (61 kg) and 21 kg/m^2, respectively. Highest weight and BMI: 298 lbs (135 kg), 47 kg/m^2. (**d–f**) Three months following body lift.

and excess skin along the hip region and less commonly the flank. Men, however, much less commonly complained about excess skin or lipodystrophy of the buttocks or anterior, lateral, and posterior thighs (Fig. 6.4).

Interestingly, the pattern of fat distribution among men appeared to vary very little. Therefore, their complaints were very similar. Women, on the other hand, had a much more varied presentation, with some having a typical gynecoid morphology and others a much more android appearance (Figs 6.1 and 6.5). Consequently, those with a more malelike fat distribution had complaints similar to those of men.

The functional concerns of both men and women usually included intertriginous dermatitis along the lower abdomen and on occasion the buttock cleft, periumbilical region, and medial thighs. We initially offered both men and women a circumferential or near-circumferential abdominoplasty. Undermining of the thighs and buttocks was not being performed. Liposuction would be applied to the abdomen, hips, and thighs when felt to be necessary. Men had satisfactory results with this technique, although the skin excess and lipodystrophy of the hips were never entirely corrected. The results with women, particularly those with a gynecoid morphology, were much less satisfactory, and liposuction had the potential of worsening the thigh skin and cellulite deformity.

Following the abdominoplasty, we then offered some patients a medial thigh lift with the approach limited to the thigh perineal crease. Following this procedure, the results also were frequently suboptimal. We began performing body lifts in March 2000. Our technique was based on Lockwood's description of the lower body lift, version 2, but differed in several ways, particularly with regard to our method of marking, choice for scar location, and intraoperative patient positioning. We have now performed over 319 body lifts since our first case in March 2000. Our technique for the body lift

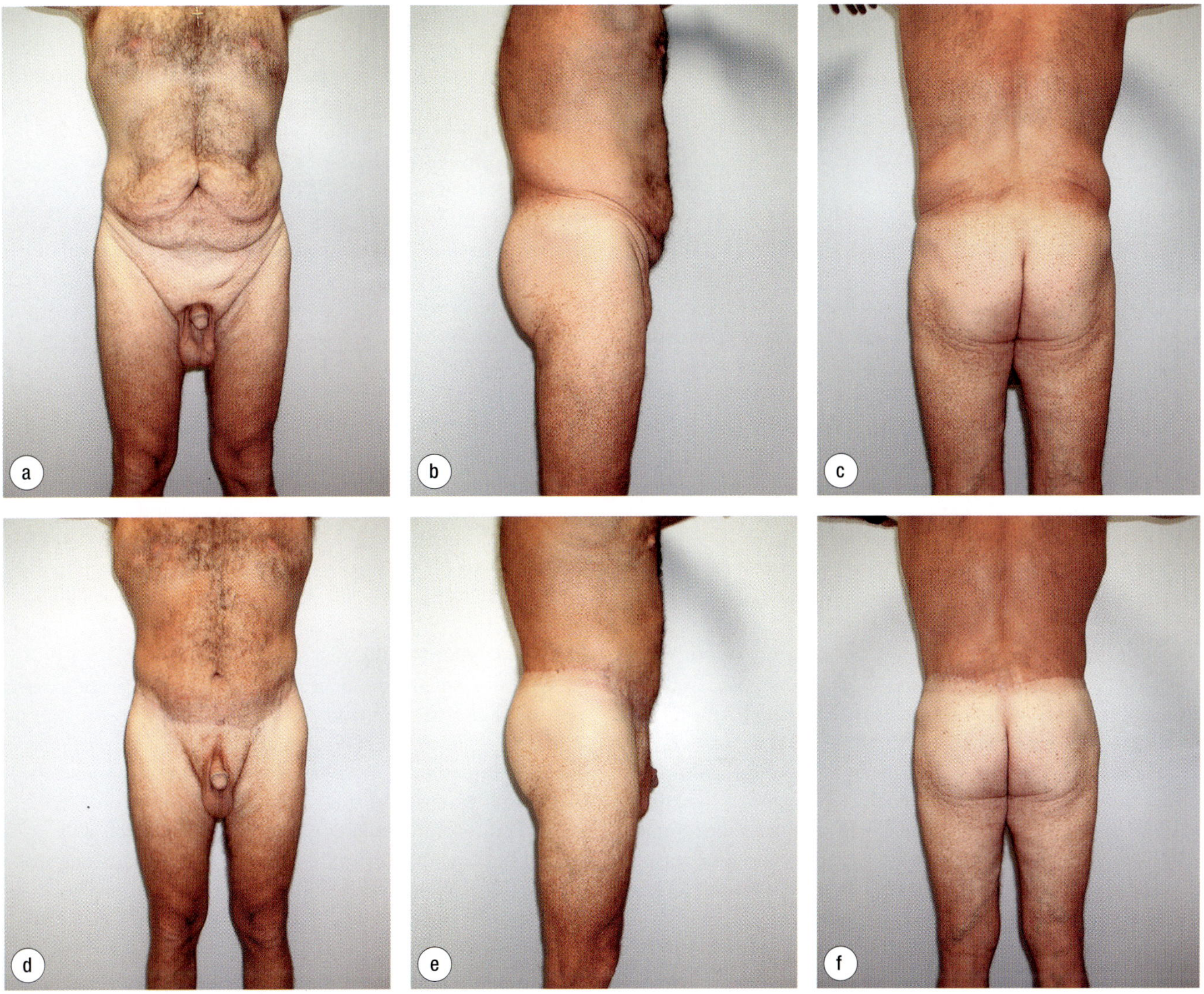

Figure 6.4 (**a–c**) A type 2 50-year-old man 1 year following gastric bypass surgery and weight loss of 150 lbs (68 kg). Current weight and BMI: 218 lbs (99 kg) and 29 kg/m^2, respectively. Highest weight and BMI: 368 lbs (167 kg), 48 kg/m^2. (**d–f**) One year following body lift.

has produced a substantial improvement over the circumferential abdominoplasty and has contributed to better results with secondary procedures such as a medial thigh lift. Our preference is now to perform a body lift or simultaneous abdominoplasty, thigh, and buttock lift on patients following massive weight loss when the appropriate indications are present and when patient selection criteria have been met.

PATIENT SELECTION AND PREPARATION

Proper patient selection and preparation prior to surgery are critical for maximizing the likelihood of a good outcome and minimizing complications following a body lift. Patients should have been at a stable weight for several months and ideally at their lowest weight prior to surgery (Table 6.1). Following gastric bypass surgery, this may range from 1 to 2 years, depending on prebariatric weight. For example, a 507 lb (230 kg) man following gastric bypass will take much longer to stabilize in weight than a 220 lb (100 kg) woman. Weight loss following gastric bypass surgery and other restrictive and malabsorptive procedures, such as biliopancreatic bypass, tends to be quite rapid during the first 8–12 postoperative months.[3,18] Weight loss following purely restrictive bariatric procedures, such as vertical banded gastroplasty and gastric banding, tends to be less and somewhat slower, with weight loss achieved over periods of as long as 3 years.[19,20]

The disadvantage of performing body-contouring procedures on patients with ongoing weight loss is the potential for early recurrence of tissue laxity. We avoid performing body lifts on individuals with a BMI of greater than 35 kg/m^2. Traction from the waistline in this population often has only a minimal effect on skin excess and cellulite along the lower buttocks and distal thighs. This heavier group of postbariatric patients typically

Table 6.1 Patient selection criteria

Feature	Criterion
Weight	Stable
BMI (kg/m^2)	<35
Age (years)	<55
Hemoglobin (g/dL)	≥12

has a large pannus present along the lower abdomen, extending to the hips and tapering over the buttocks. Difficulty with activities, severe intertriginous dermatitis, and back discomfort are usually their biggest complaints. We offer these patients a near circumferential abdominoplasty, a far less complex procedure. We do on occasion offer body lifts to this heavier group, particularly for patients less than 35 years of age, and usually men, but also women with a more central fat distribution.

We avoid performing body lifts on postbariatric patients greater than 55 years of age. Morbidly obese individuals who have sought bariatric surgery in the fifth and sixth decades of life have often developed degenerative arthritis, and in many instances have undergone joint replacement. We find the recovery from body lifts in patients with ongoing arthritis and following joint replacement to be difficult and protracted. We usually offer this group an abdominoplasty or an abdominoplasty to be followed in 6 months by a thigh and buttock lift.

Postbariatric patients, particularly menstruating women and those who have had malabsorptive procedures, i.e. gastric bypass and biliopancreatic bypass, are often anemic.[21] These anemias tend to be secondary to the poor absorption of both iron and folate. Patients considering a body lift are encouraged to take both an iron supplement and daily multivitamins. Severely anemic patients are referred to a hematologist. We prefer a baseline hemoglobin of 12 g/dL. All postbariatric surgery patients are encouraged to continue follow-up with their bariatric surgeon.

SURGICAL TECHNIQUE

The challenge of performing a consistently effective circumferential lower body-contouring procedure in the massive weight loss population relates directly to the properties inherent in this patient population and the objectives to be achieved. Common to the lower body of virtually all postbariatric patients is skin and soft tissue excess and a high degree of skin and soft tissue mobility. Attempting to affect change to the upper abdomen or distal thighs from the waistline, the usual location for circumferential procedures, requires a significant degree of traction. The combination of these patient properties with high levels of traction leads to the potential for inconsistent results with regard to scar location, scar quality, and overall outcome. Careful patient marking prior to a body lift is essential for an optimal outcome.

Circumferential body-contouring procedures have the common goal of minimizing scar perceptibility by placing the scar along the waistline. An analysis of where both men and women wear their pants, undergarments, bathing suits, bikinis, thongs, etc. reveals that the superior portion of most garments in the hip region lies at the level of the anterior superior iliac spine (ASIS) or approximately 6–7 cm below the superior edge of the iliac crest. Posteriorly, garments traverse horizontally along the lower back and above the buttocks, also at the level of the ASIS. Anteriorly, virtually all undergarments cover the interface between the hair-bearing pubic area and the hypogastrium (Fig. 6.6). Ideally, the scar for the body lift should be at the level of the ASIS along the hip and lower back, and gradually descend to the interface between the hair-bearing pubic area and hypogastrium anteriorly (Figs 6.6 and 6.7). An effective technique for marking the body lift should produce a scar that reliably lies along the waistline, despite the extreme tissue mobility of the massive weight loss patient and the high level of traction required to affect significant change from the waistline. To do so requires a marking technique that uses bony landmarks such as the ASIS to control scar placement.

Preoperative marking

1. With the patient standing, an area above the buttock cleft is marked first. This point (A), with downward traction to the skin, should be horizontal to the ASIS (Fig. 6.7). The ASIS is often difficult to palpate but is usually at a level approximately three fingerbreadths below the iliac crest (6–7 cm). With strong downward traction to the skin along the right anterior iliac region, a point (B) along the anterior axillary line should be marked that is horizontal to point A under downward traction (Fig. 6.7). A dotted line is drawn from A to B with downward traction over the right thigh and buttock. The dotted line with downward traction should be aligned with the patient's waistline.
2. Sitting in front of the patient, the surgeon identifies a symmetric point (C) along the left anterior axillary line. A dotted line is similarly drawn from C to A with downward traction to the left thigh and buttock. With downward traction to the right and left buttocks and thigh areas, a straight dotted line should result from point B on the right to point C on the left, passing through point A over the buttock cleft (Fig. 6.7). If the line is found to be straight, the dots are connected.
3. Point B′ is identified inferior to point B by the pinch technique. The two points, when approximated, eliminate cellulite along the anterior and lateral thigh. A similar procedure is performed on the left side and at the buttock cleft from point A. The redundant skin of the left and right buttocks is estimated with the pinch technique. Points B and B′ and C and C′ are called points of commitment, because the surgeon does not remeasure the distance between these points during surgery and commits to removing this skin. The remaining lower set of lines and point A′ are estimates only (Fig. 6.7).

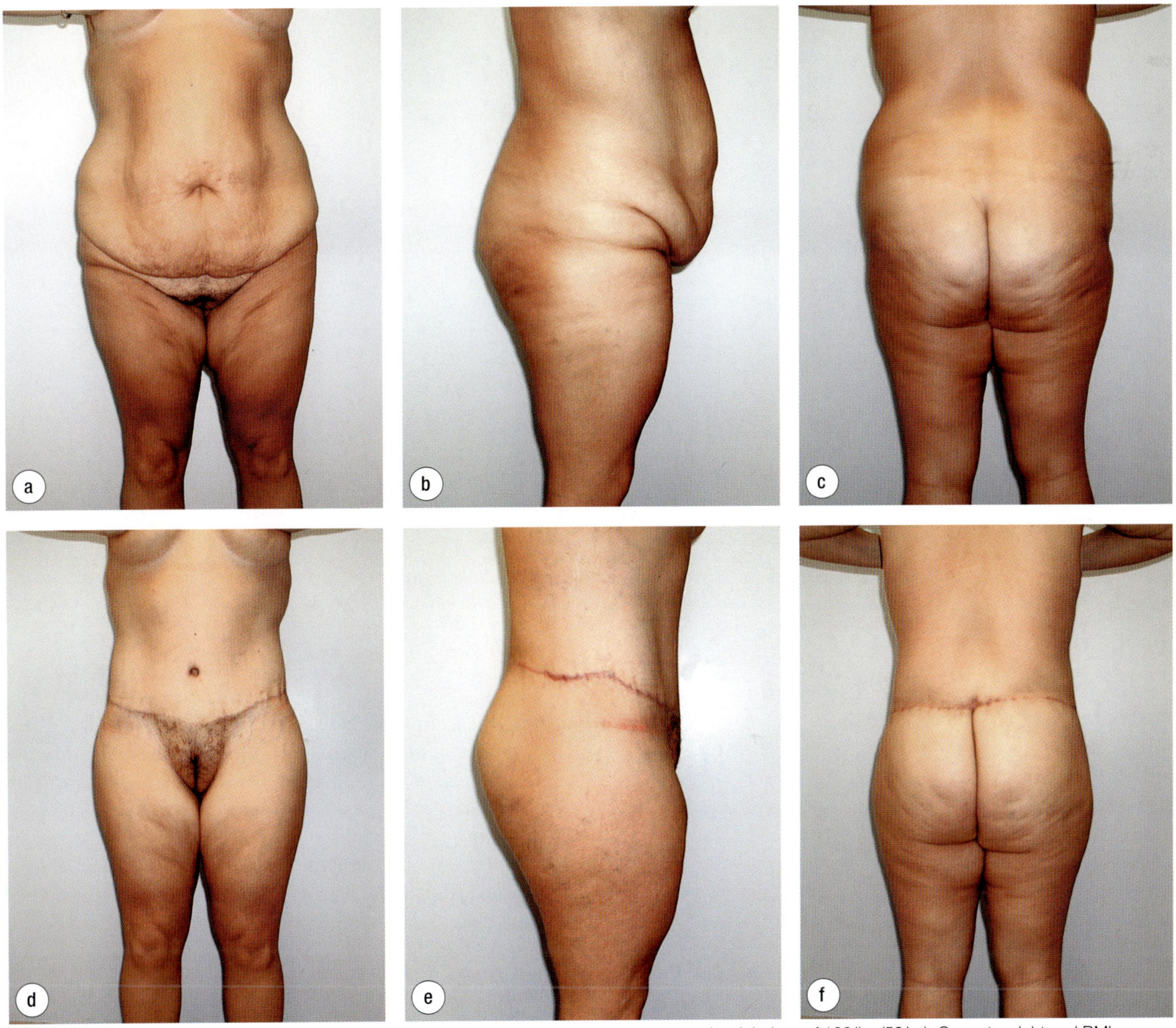

Figure 6.5 (**a–c**) A type 3 27-year-old woman 20 months following gastric bypass surgery and weight loss of 130 lbs (59 kg). Current weight and BMI: 216 lbs (98 kg) and 32 kg/m^2, respectively. Highest weight and BMI: 346 lbs (157 kg), 32 kg/m^2. (**d–f**) Seven months following body lift. Her body morphology is android.

4. The patient is then asked to lie supine and flat on the hospital bed. With firm, upward traction applied to the redundant skin along the anterior abdominal wall, a transverse line is drawn along the pubic region, D to D′. The line is placed approximately 6 cm superior to the vulvar anterior commissure or base of the penis. As described above, virtually every postbariatric patient has some degree of ptosis and redundancy of the mons pubis following massive weight loss. When marking the lower abdomen in this population, a normal spatial relationship must be restored between the top of the vulva, the top of the hair-bearing pubic area, and the umbilicus. An aesthetically pleasing distance from the top of the vulva to the top of the hair-bearing pubic area is approximately 6 cm. The umbilicus lies at approximately the level of the iliac crest. If the hair-bearing pubic area were not reduced in the postbariatric patient, an aesthetically pleasing lower abdomen could not be consistently achieved. With upward traction to the right lower quadrant of the anterior abdominal wall, a straight line is drawn from D to B′, and similarly between D′ and C′ with upward pressure to the left lower quadrant anterior abdominal wall. Traction along lower quadrants will permit correction of some or all of the excess skin along the anterior and medial thighs. In patients with moderate to severe degrees of skin excess, the lines from D to B′ and D to C′ will lie on the thighs when not on traction.
5. The patient is asked to stand, and any areas to be liposuctioned are marked at this time.

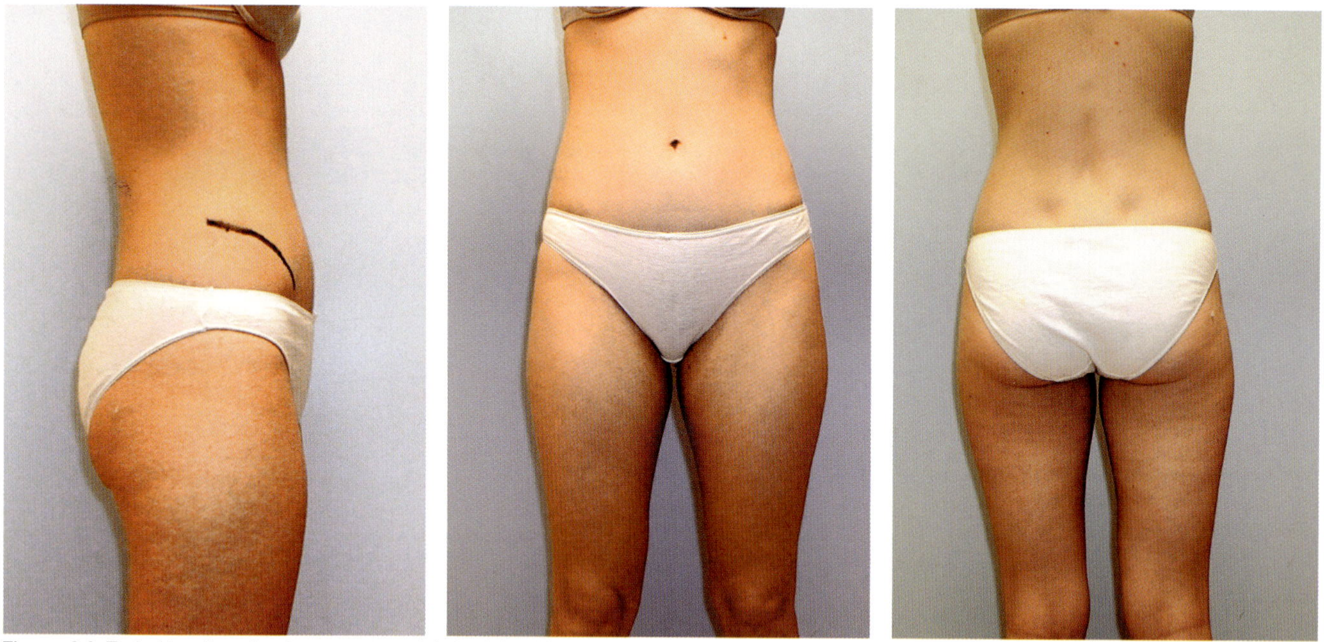

Figure 6.6 Typical location of undergarments and their relationship to bony landmarks. The dark line outlines the iliac crest. The upper portion of the garment lies at level of the anterior superior iliac spine.

Intraoperative surgical technique

In the operating room, the patient is prepared with povidone–iodine (Betadine) from the shoulders to the ankles while standing. The patient sits on a sterile draped operating table and is rotated into a supine and flat position. Sterile stockings and sterile sequential compression devices are placed. A drawsheet has been previously placed along the midportion of the table. Following general endotracheal anesthesia, a Foley catheter is placed, and a sterile sheet is stapled to the patient at the level of the inframammary fold and around either flank to nearly the midback. Drapes are placed from the operating table over either arm board. Finally, an ether drape is placed in the usual fashion over the chest area. Grounding pads are placed on each arm and secured with tape.

At the start of the surgical procedure, the skin along the lines A–B and A–C is scored superficially. A 1-cm vertical hatch mark is made above point A to demarcate the midline. The skin from B to B′ and from C to C′ and from C′ to B′ across the lower abdomen is superficially incised. If liposuction is to be performed to the thighs, it is done at this time. Tumescent fluid is infiltrated only into the tissues to be liposuctioned. Excessive tumescent fluid or tumescent fluid in tissues not to be liposuctioned can potentially distort tissues and prevent accurate tissue excision. In addition, the presence of tumescent fluid in tissues diffuses the energy of the cautery, decreasing its effectiveness.

The skin and soft tissues are then incised full thickness from C′ to B′ and down to the anterior abdominal wall fascia. The dissection is beveled inferiorly in the region of the mons pubis to directly excise fat in this area, particularly in the higher BMI patients. Direct excision is more efficient and accurate than liposuction in this area. The skin throughout the procedure is incised with a no. 10 blade while the subcutaneous tissues are divided and flaps elevated with cautery. The cautery is set to a high level. The anterior abdominal wall flap is elevated to the level of the umbilicus, which is preserved in the usual fashion. The skin and underlying subcutaneous tissue along the vertical lines C to C′ and B to B′ are divided to the underlying anterior abdominal wall fascia. Superior to the umbilicus, the dissection is kept primarily over the rectus abdominus muscles to the level of the xiphoid. Every effort is made to preserve intercostal perforators. For patients with more redundant fascia, wider dissection is necessary.

In nearly every massive weight loss patient, the anterior abdominal flap can be divided along the midline to the level of the umbilicus to allow better exposure of the xiphoid region. The back of the patient is elevated to approximately 35° to further demonstrate fascial laxity. To greatly assist in maintaining exposure of the epigastric fascia during plication, a Gomez retractor (Pilling Surgical, Horsham, Philadelphia) is placed to elevate the anterior abdominal wall flap (Fig. 6.9). The fascia to be plicated is marked as an ellipse from the pubic bone to the xiphoid. Two #1 Prolene looped sutures (Ethicon Inc., Sommerville, New Jersey) are used to plicate the redundant fascia from the pubic bone to the umbilicus. The two sutures are tied to each other in the midportion of the hypogastric region and buried. The technique avoids the possibility of suture extrusion near incisions or of palpating knots. Two more Prolene sutures are used to plicate the fascia from the umbilicus to the xiphoid. As the redundant fascia in the epigastric region is plicated, additional undermining of the flap may be performed to allow for appropriate contouring.

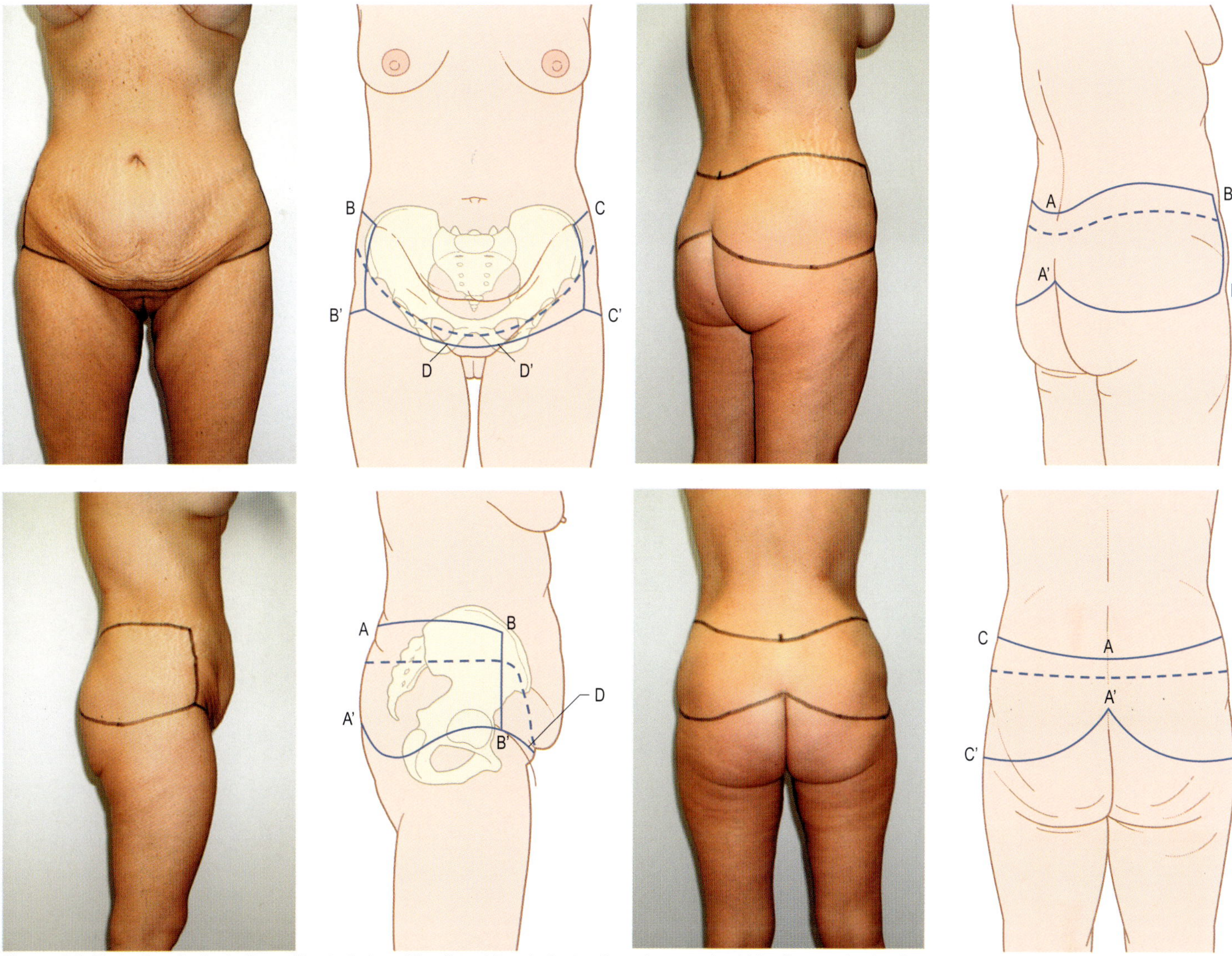

Figure 6.7 Illustrations for body lift marking technique. The dotted lines indicate where the scar should lie. See text for details.

The patient is then turned to the left lateral decubital position with assistance from the anesthesiologist behind the ether drape and the use of the drawsheet. With the patient then in the left lateral decubital position, the waist of the patient is flexed to approximately 30° and the knees to 45°. The skin from point B to A and approximately 10 cm beyond A toward C is incised full thickness. Incising the skin beyond the midline greatly facilitates undermining in the buttock cleft area and allows for an accurate determination of excess tissue in this region. The skin and subcutaneous tissues are elevated over the right hip, thigh, and buttock at a level superficial to the fascia overlying the musculature.

The entire deep fat compartment of the hip roll region is removed with this technique, except for some of the fat immediately posterior to the iliac crest. Enough fat should be left behind in this area to avoid an unnatural-appearing depression postoperatively. This is particularly important for higher BMI individuals. In men, a portion of the deep fat compartment of the hip may lie above the line of incision but can be removed along with the flap as it is pulled inferiorly (Fig. 6.10). Liposuction had been performed to the hips in the first 50 cases. We found that direct excision of fat was more efficient and precise. Continuous undermining is performed caudally to a level approximately four fingerbreadths in width inferior to the line from B′ to A′. In the thigh region, continuous undermining is performed to the level of the greater trochanter.

In some women, a 45-cm Lockwood underminer (Byron Medical, Tucson, Arizona) is passed to the knee over the anterior and lateral thigh just superficial to the thigh muscle fascia. The underminer is used on women who demonstrate excess skin and cellulite along the mid and distal one-thirds of the thigh. The waist is flexed to 90° to approximate a sitting position (Fig. 6.9). The right lower extremity is abducted to 30° with use of the Gomez retractor (Pilling Surgical). An abduction pillow maintains the knees approximately 30 cm apart. The right leg is hung by a sterile towel from the Gomez retractor

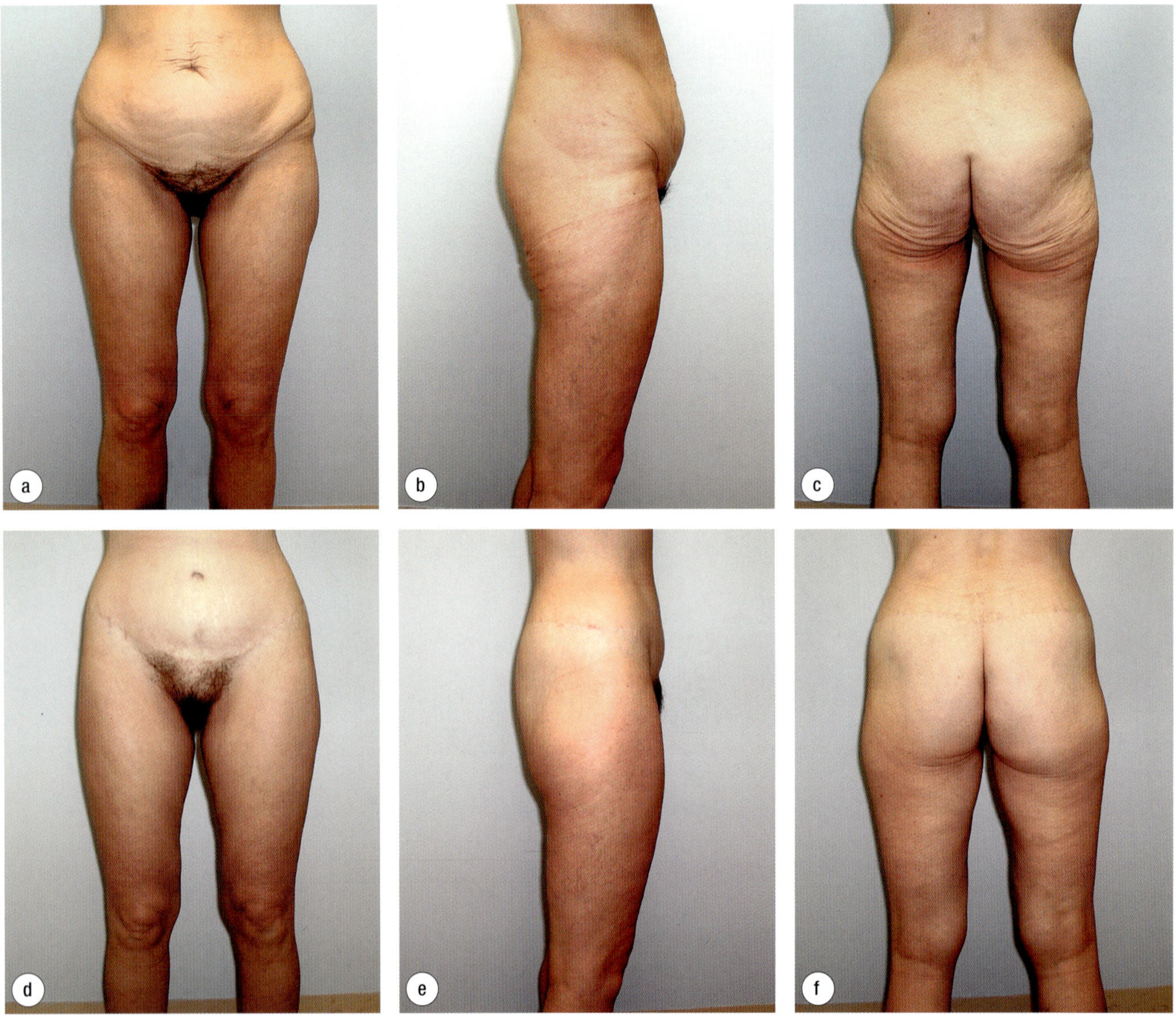

Figure 6.8 (**a–c**) A type 1 46-year-old woman 15 months following gastric bypass surgery and weight loss of 139 lbs (63 kg). Current weight and BMI: 141 lbs (64 kg) and 21 kg/m^2, respectively. Highest weight and BMI: 278 lbs (126 kg), 42 kg/m^2. (**d–f**) Two years following body lift.

(Pilling Surgical). An Adair clamp is placed between points B and B′, the previously marked points of commitment.

A Pitanguy (Padgett Instruments, Kansas City, Missouri) large flap demarcator is used to mark the excess skin along the buttock cleft region. Proper use of the Pitanguy skin marker requires that the clamp be placed in the same plane as the tissues to be measured. If the clamp is off this plane, the amount of tissue to be excised may be overestimated. In measuring with this technique, the amount of traction applied to the flap to be measured is critical. The technique involves securing the Pitanguy marker with an Adair clamp to the flap that has not been undermined, and advancing the marker toward the flap to be measured. The non-undermined flap edge usually glides several centimeters before it becomes stable. At this point, the undermined flap is manually advanced into the Pitanguy clamp for measurement. The flap should be advanced toward the clamp until the flap cannot be mobilized any further with moderate tension. The tension on the flap is then diminished to allow the flap to retract approximately 1–2 cm. The flap is marked at that point. The several extra centimeters are important for providing adequate tissue for an optimal closure (Figs 6.11 and 6.12).

The excess skin is incised, and the point A and a newly established A′ are approximated with an Adair clamp. With light traction to the right buttock and thigh flap in a cephalic direction, the Pitanguy clamp is used to mark excess skin along these flaps. The excess tissue is removed by incising the skin and beveling the subcutaneous tissues caudally. A 10-mm fully perforated flat drain (Zimmer Corp., Dover, Ohio) is placed through a small incision along the lateral aspect of the

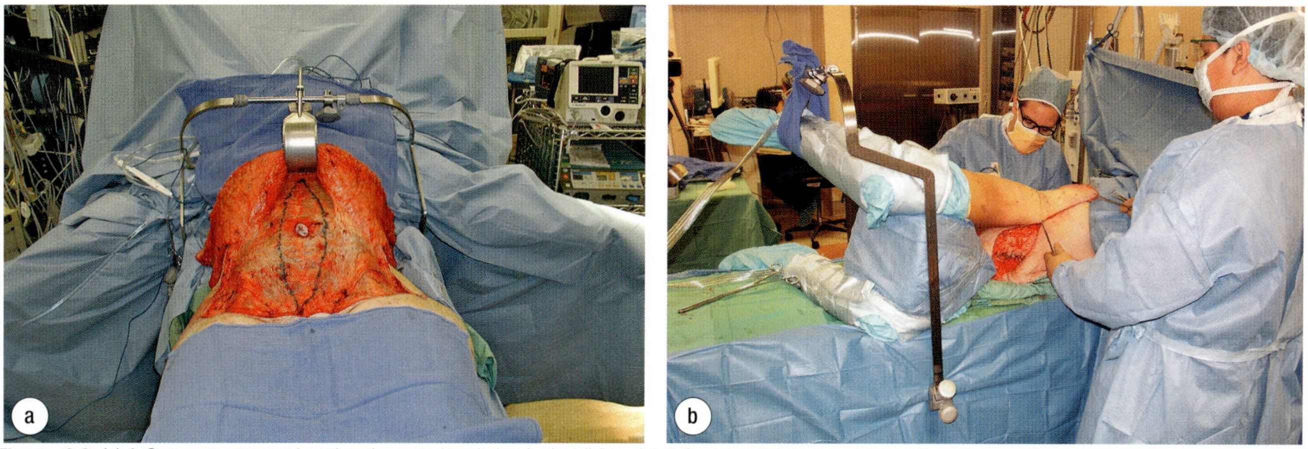

Figure 6.9 (**a**) A Gomez retractor elevating the anterior abdominal wall flap. (**b**) A Gomez retractor assisting with patient positioning.

right side of the pubic area and passed over to the buttock region. The drain is secured in the usual fashion. Adair clamps are used to approximate the upper and lower tissue edges of the right buttock and thigh flaps. Then #1 braided nylon (Ethicon Inc.) stitches are used to approximate the SFS and deep dermis. 2-0 Monocryl and 3-0 (Ethicon Inc.) stitches are placed at the level of the dermis (Fig. 6.12).

The skin is redundant along the closure line and appears as a ridge (Fig. 6.12). This minimizes tension along the incision during the early months of scar maturation. The patient is turned to the right lateral decubital position and a similar procedure performed to the left thigh and buttock. While rotating the patient, Adair clamps are placed at points B–B′ and A–A′ to prevent disruption.

Once in the supine and flat position, the back of the patient is elevated to 35°. Limited undermining of the flap in the epigastric region often leads to flap redundancy and an epigastric roll (Fig. 6.13). For patients with minimal or no lipodystrophy in the epigastric area, this can be addressed by discontinuous undermining either digitally or with Mayo scissors opened perpendicularly to the plain of dissection. For some patients, additional undermining may be necessary to eliminate the roll. Every effort is made to preserve intercostal perforators. For patients with an epigastric roll and lipodystrophy in this area, the Pitanguy clamp is used to mark the excess skin at the central portion of the flap. The flap is incised to this point and secured to the lower tissue edge with an Adair clamp. Excess flap is then marked on either side of the central portion of flap under slightly more tension than was applied along the midline.

Without resecting excess tissue at this time, the flap is then secured to the lower tissue edges with additional clamps along the right and left lower quadrants. The patient is returned to a supine and flat position. Liposuction is then performed to the epigastric portion of the flap until a roll is no longer present. Following liposuction, the patient's back is once again elevated to 35°. Typically, additional tissue can be marked for excision with the Pitanguy skin marker. Following excision of the excess tissue from the anterior abdominal wall flap, the flap is secured to the lower tissue edge with the patient in a supine and flat position. A new position for the umbilicus is marked, and a 1-cm shield-type incision is made. The opening should be made approximately 0.5 cm superior to the corresponding umbilical position on the anterior abdominal wall, to account for the additional retraction that occurs with the SFS and deep dermal approximation at the time of closure.

The umbilical stalk is secured to the abdominal fascia and dermis of the flap with 3-0 Vicryl (Ethicon Inc.) sutures. Four additional flat, fully perforated drains are placed through stab wounds in the pubic region. Two of the drains are placed into each thigh recess and two drains on to the abdominal wall fascia. The drains serving the abdominal wall exit the mons pubis medially, and the drains leading to each thigh exit the mons between the drains from each buttock and the abdominal wall.

Placing the drains via the mons pubis and in a certain order serves several purposes.

- Exiting the drains via the mons pubis allows patients to lie comfortably on their back and sides, the preferred positions for post–body lift patients.
- The scars from the drains are less perceptible in the hair-bearing pubic region.
- Not placing the drains along the incision avoids the potential for disruption of the closure.
- Placing the drains in a specific order and location allows the individual removing the drain to know from which area the drain is being removed.

This information can be helpful in preventing seroma formation. The back of the patient is raised to 40°, and the abdominal wall flap is secured to the lower tissue edge as was described for the thigh and buttocks. Interrupted 3-0 Prolene sutures are placed at the umbilicus following approximation with the previously placed Vicryl sutures. Sterile dressings are held in place by a loose binder. The patient is transferred to a hospital bed in a beach chair position following extubation.

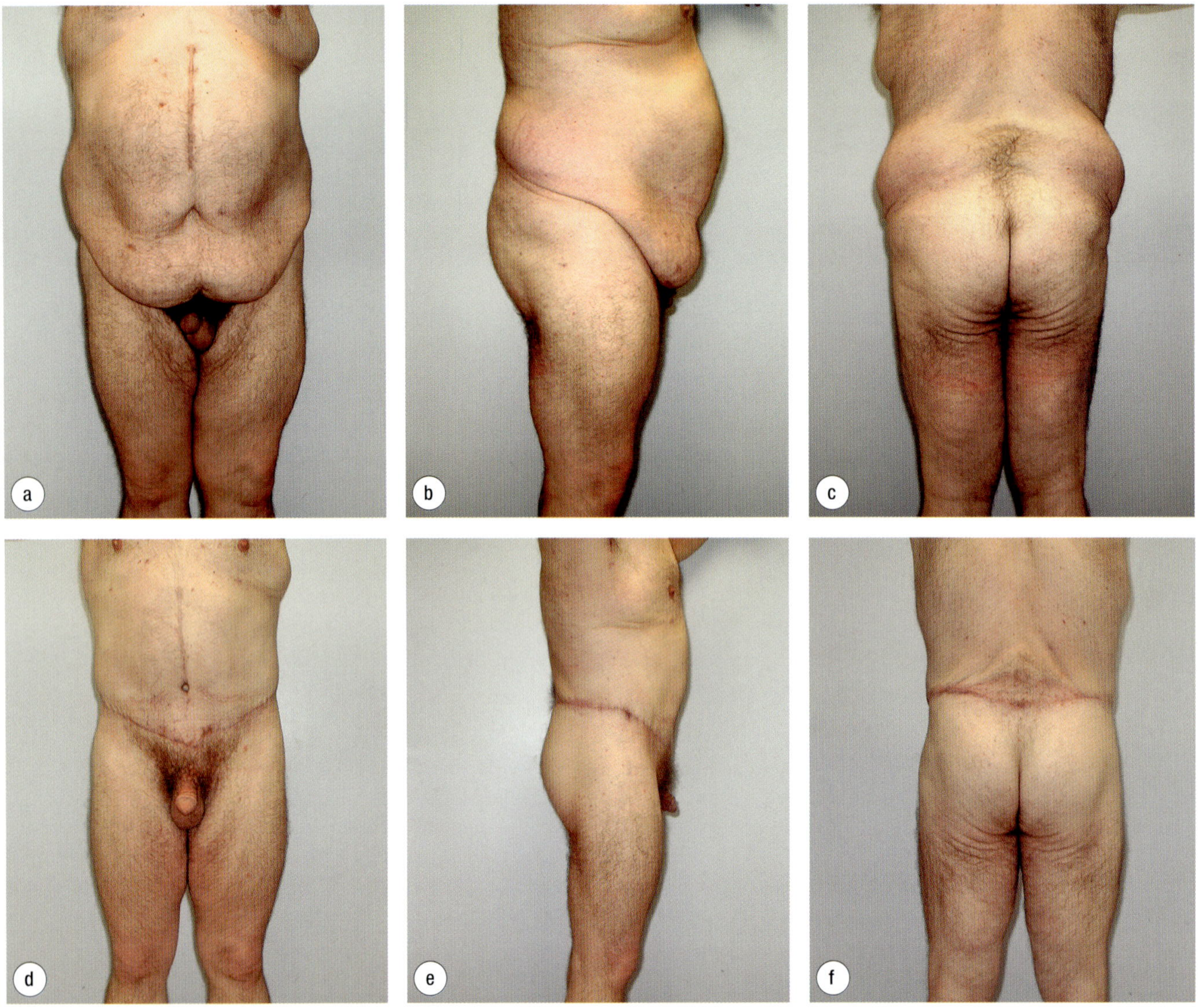

Figure 6.10 (a–c) A type 3 55-year-old man 2 years following gastric bypass surgery and weight loss of 152 lbs (69 kg). Current weight and BMI: 240 lbs (109 kg) and 35 kg/m^2, respectively. Highest weight and BMI: 392 lbs (178 kg), 58 kg/m^2. (d–f) Seven months following body lift. Hip roll was treated by direct excision.

OPTIMIZING OUTCOMES

Patient classification

Achieving the best results requires a careful assessment and an individual approach to each patient. We have found classifying patients into groups depending on BMI prior to the body lift to be very helpful in this regard. The reasons for classifying patients are several.

- Classifying patients helps us to better educate patients on the likelihood of complications.
- It provides patients with an idea of the expected outcome from the aesthetic and functional points of view.
- From the plastic surgeon's point of view, classifying patients helps to create a plan for management whether for selection or as an algorithm for treatment.

We classify patients into three groups (Table 6.2). Normal BMI is between 19 and 25 kg/m^2 (Table 6.3). We consider our type 1 patients to be, in effect, normal weight. Typically with removal of excess skin and soft tissue following a body lift, these patients drop to a BMI of below 25 kg/m^2 if they are not already at the time of the body lift (Figs 6.8 and 6.18). Type 2 patients usually remain overweight, and type 3 patients stabilize in the obese category (Fig. 6.25). The approach to each class of patients differs somewhat, particularly with regard to the management of lipodystrophy and the sequence of procedures.

Type 1 patient treatment (BMI < 28 kg/m^2)

Patients with a BMI less than 28 kg/m^2 following massive weight loss are the most likely to achieve an ideal body contour and usually have minimal lipodystrophy. Our approach

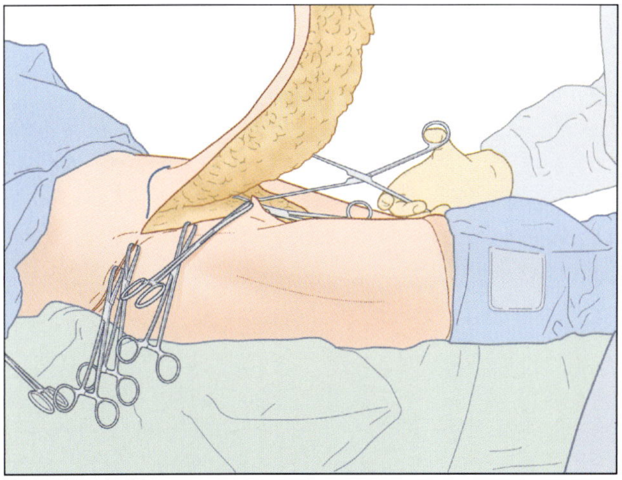

Figure 6.11 The appropriate use of the Pitanguy.

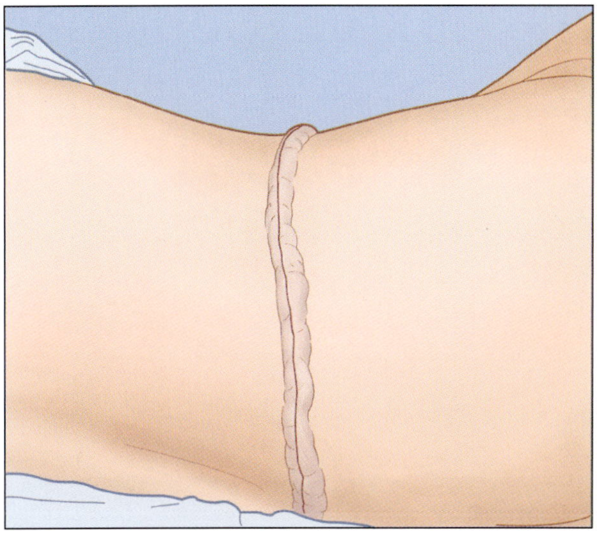

Figure 6.12 Creating skin redundancy: its appearance in the operating room.

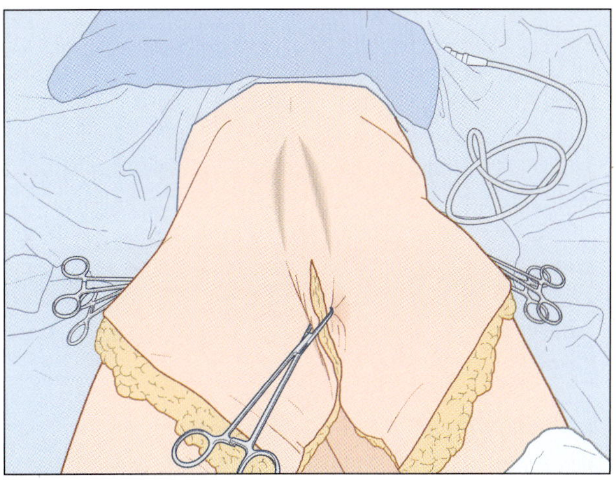

Figure 6.13 The appearance of roll.

Table 6.2 Patient classification by BMI

Type	BMI (kg/m^2)
1	<28
2	28–32
3	>32

Table 6.3 BMI and obesity

BMI (kg/m^2)	Classification
19–24.9	Normal weight
25–29.9	Overweight
30–34.9	Obese
35–39.9	Severely obese
40–49.9	Morbidly obese
50–59.9	Superobese

to the lower body in this class of patients, both men and women, is to offer a body lift first (Table 6.4) Women in this group may have remaining lipodystrophy along the abdomen, hips, and thighs. Liposuction immediately prior to undermining and resecting excess tissue not only serves to address lipodystrophy but also facilitates the mobilization of tissues with the body lift.

Liposuction plays less of a role in men in this group. Men with a BMI of less than 28 kg/m^2 following massive weight loss typically have little if any lipodystrophy and, if they do, it is unusually limited to the medial thighs. BMI as an indicator of fat content is very accurate except in muscular men. Men typically have a higher percentage of muscle mass as compared with overall body weight than women do. Men with a BMI of less than 28 kg/m^2 following massive weight loss, particularly if they are exercising regularly, may appear underweight but have a BMI that suggests a higher than normal weight. Men in this group often have excess skin at the medial thighs. Men or women with lipodystrophy at the medial thighs may benefit from liposuction to this area at the same time as the body lift. However, because the tension resulting from a body lift is less along the medial thighs, liposuction should only be performed to this area if a medial thighplasty is planned as a follow-up procedure. Otherwise, there is significant risk for skin contour irregularities that can only be corrected by a skin resection procedure. This concept applies to type 2 and type 3 patients as well (Fig. 6.17).

Three to six months following a body lift, the medial thighs of type 1 patients are reassessed. As discussed above, the tissue redundancy of the medial thighs is the result of both the inferomedial collapse of the excess tissues of the lower abdomen, mons pubis, thighs, and buttocks and the incomplete retraction of the skin and soft tissues of the thighs following

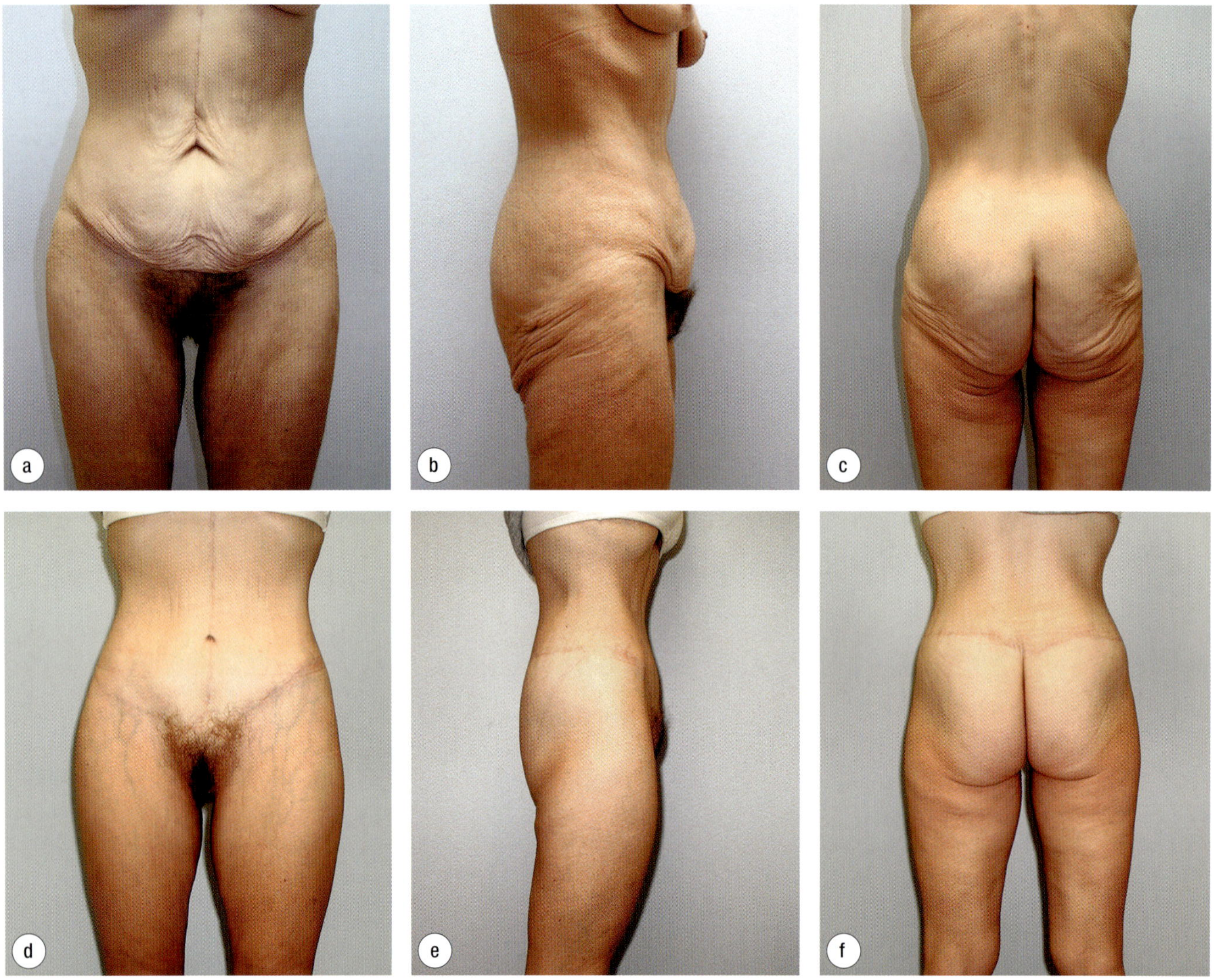

Figure 6.14 (**a–c**) A type 1 36-year-old woman 23 months following gastric bypass surgery and weight loss of 161 lbs (73 kg). Current weight and BMI: 121 lbs (55 kg) and 20 kg/m^2, respectively. Highest weight and BMI: 282 lbs (128 kg), 47 kg/m^2. (**d–f**) Eighteen months following body lift.

massive weight loss. Therefore, the postbariatric thigh deformity is both a vertical and horizontal problem. The body lift very effectively addresses the vertical component of the medial thigh deformity by the upward and outward rotation of these tissues. The body lift, however, only minimally addresses the horizontal or circumferential thigh deformity by drawing the narrower skin envelope of the distal thigh to the larger proximal thigh.

For many type 1 patients, particularly those less than 35 years of age and who have had a BMI change of less than 25 kg/m^2 following massive weight loss, the body lift may eliminate the need for a formal medial thigh lift (Figs 6.14 and 6.15). Those who are candidates for a medial thigh lift tend to be older and/or have had a large BMI change (> 25–30 kg/m^2) following massive weight loss, and women with a more gynecoid fat distribution (Figs 6.2 and 6.18–6.20).

The appropriate procedure for a medial thighplasty depends on the remaining thigh deformity following a body lift. In some cases, individuals with excess skin and soft tissue along the proximal medial thigh may be effectively treated with a medial thighplasty limited to the thigh perineal crease (Fig. 6.21). The addition of a longitudinal component in this group will nevertheless usually produce a better aesthetic result with regard to thigh contour and with regard to preventing scar migration from the genitofemoral crease. Patients with a deformity extending to the midthigh or beyond will need a longitudinal component added to their thighplasty. These individuals typically have a significant degree of a horizontal deformity or circumferential tissue excess that must be addressed. The excess in addition often leads to a saddlebag deformity that cannot be completely corrected by a well-performed body lift (Fig. 6.18).

Type 2 patient treatment (BMI 28–32 kg/m^2)

Type 2 patients represent more of a challenge. Lipodystrophy typically is of a much greater concern, particularly for women.

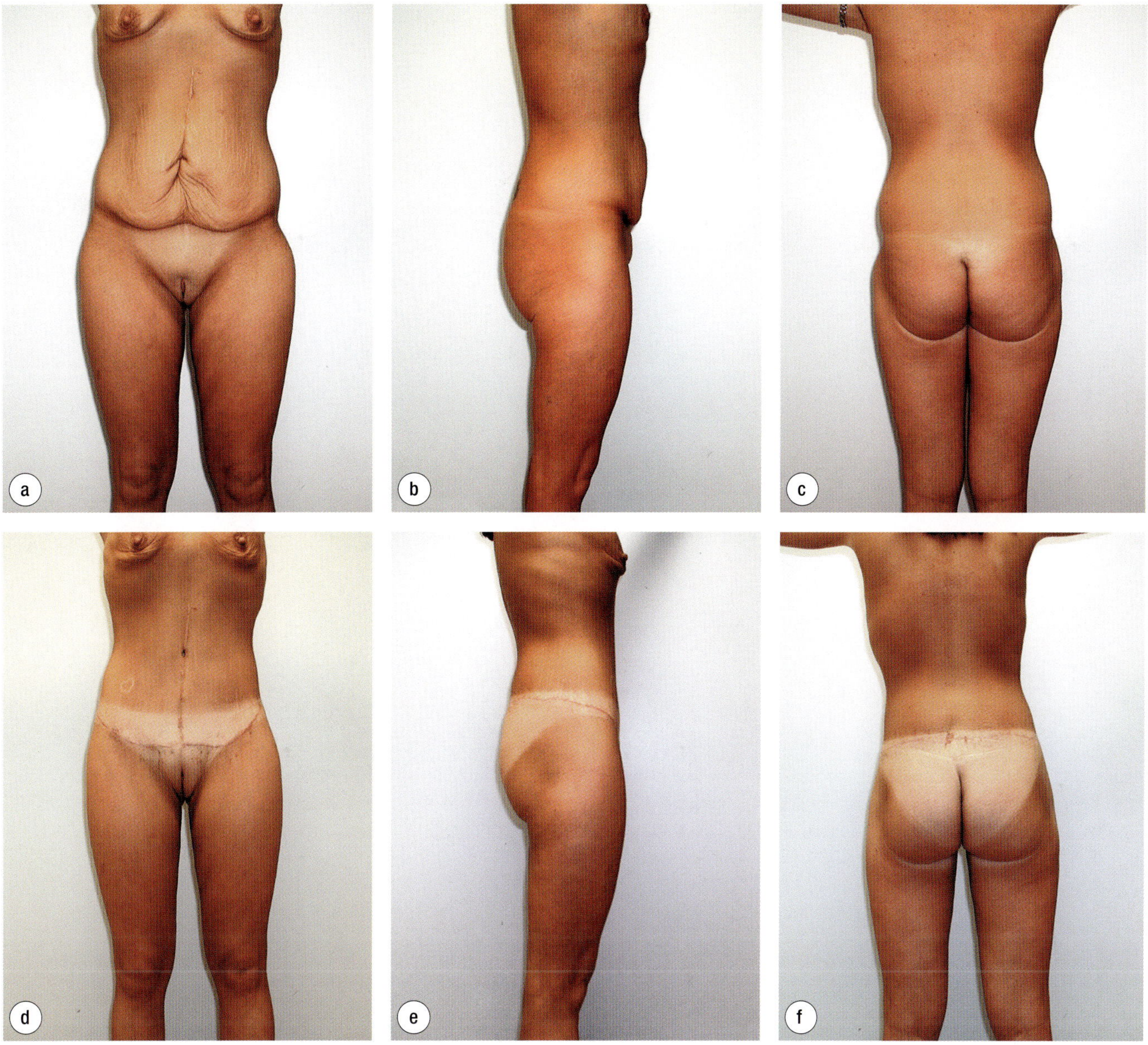

Figure 6.15 (**a–c**) A type 1 20-year-old woman 21 months following gastric bypass surgery and weight loss of 121 lbs (55 kg). Current weight and BMI: 134 lbs (61 kg) and 22 kg/m^2, respectively. Highest weight and BMI: 256 lbs (116 kg), 41 kg/m^2. (**d–f**) Seven months following body lift.

Achieving an ideal body contour is less likely for this group. These individuals have a BMI of between 28 and 32 kg/m^2, and are therefore either overweight or obese by definition. Following a body lift, they are unlikely to reach a normal BMI and usually stabilize between 25 and 30 kg/m^2. Liposuction usually plays an important role in thigh management in this group of patients, particularly among women, as does direct excision of fat at the hip region.

In general, women in this group, particularly those with a more gynecoid body habitus, are offered a body lift first with extensive circumferential thigh liposuction (Figs 6.16 and 6.22). Liposuction of the thighs at the time of the body lift addresses lipodystrophy and decreases overall thigh volume, allowing for more tissues to be excised vertically. Greater tissue excess may exist circumferentially at the thighs following the body lift and thigh liposuction alone; however, a much more effective thighplasty can then be performed as a second stage.

Men and women with a more android body habitus are offered a body lift as well; however, liposuction is usually limited to the medial thighs. Once again, liposuction to this area should only be performed if a medial thighplasty is planned. Direct excision of fat from the hip roll area is important for most type 2 men and women (Figs 6.4 and 6.23). As with the type 1 patients, a medial thigh lift may be necessary following a body lift. The same approach regarding timing and management is used for this heavier group of patients. Repeat liposuction of the thighs is often performed as part of a thighplasty.

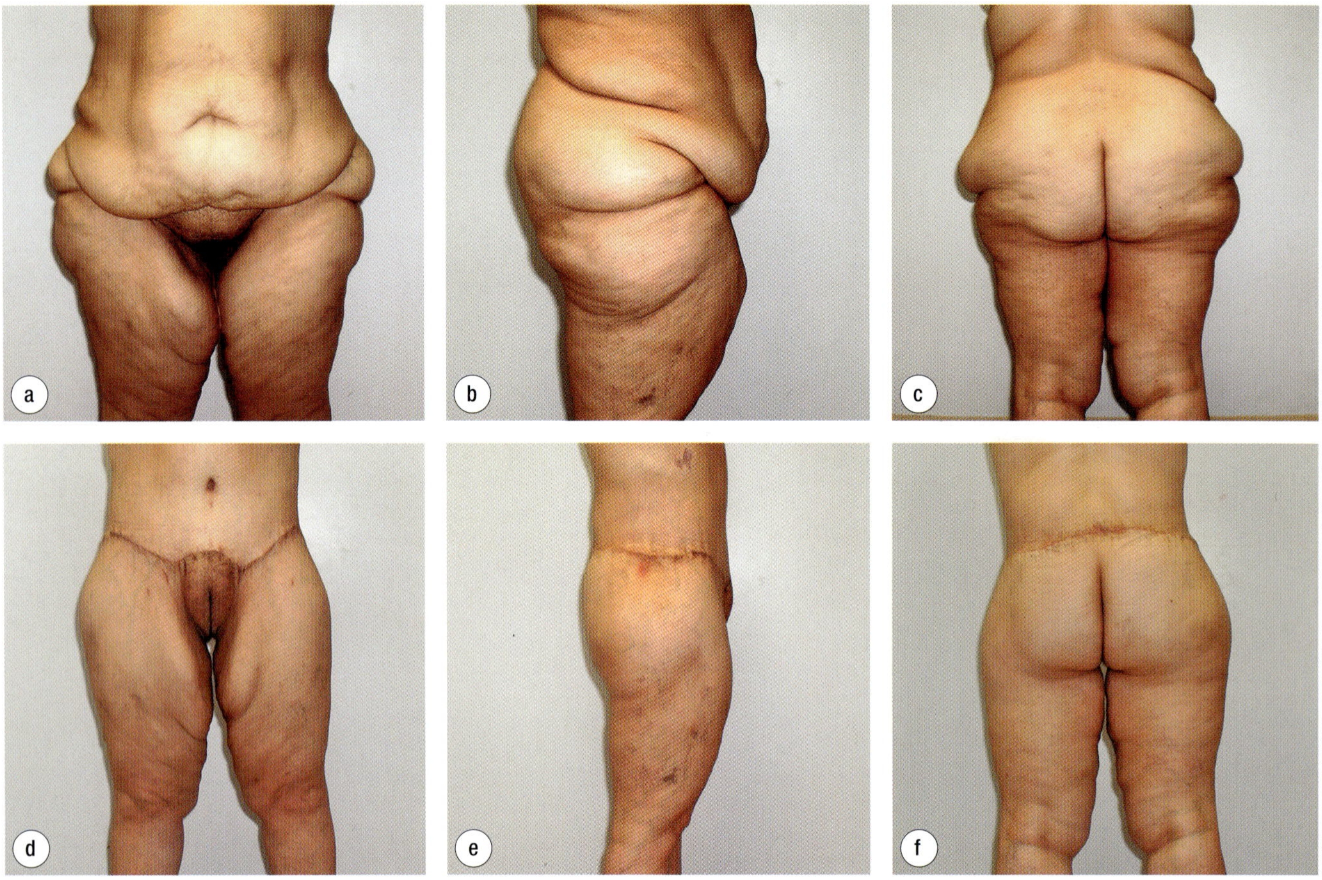

Figure 6.16 **(a–c)** A type 2 41-year-old woman 17 months following gastric bypass surgery and weight loss of 79 lbs (36 kg). Current weight and BMI: 165 lbs (75 kg) and 31 kg/m^2, respectively. Highest weight and BMI: 245 lbs (111 kg), 46 kg/m^2. **(d–f)** Seven months following body lift. The patient is scheduled for a medial thighplasty with a longitudinal component.

Type 3 patient treatment (BMI > 32 kg/m^2)

Type 3 patients, those with a BMI of greater than 32 kg/m^2, are the most challenging. They are the least likely to achieve an ideal body contour. Individuals in this category are obese, and are unlikely to fall into the overweight category (BMI 25–30 kg/m^2) following plastic surgery. Careful patient selection and staging is particularly important in this group of patients to minimize complications and maximize outcome (Table 6.4).

Our customary approach to these individuals is as follows. Within the type 3 category, we separate patients into those with BMI of less than 35 kg/m^2 and greater than 35 kg/m^2.

- For men with a BMI of less than 35 kg/m^2 and age less than 55, we offer a body lift first with possible liposuction of the medial thighs (Figs 6.20 and 6.24).
- Men older than 55 years and/or with a BMI greater than 35 kg/m^2 are considered for an abdominoplasty to be followed in 3–6 months by a simultaneous thigh and buttock lift as an alternative to the body lift.
- Women with a BMI of less than 35 kg/m^2, an android or central distribution of fat, and age less than 55 are offered a body lift (Fig. 6.25) with possible thigh liposuction.
- Women older than 55 years or with a gynecoid body habitus or a BMI of above 35 kg/m^2 should be considered for an abdominoplasty with thigh liposuction to be followed in 3–6 months by a simultaneous thigh and buttock lift (Fig. 6.1). Women of this weight and with a gynecoid body habitus typically have a degree of thigh lipodystrophy that would make a primary thigh-lifting procedure minimally effective in terms of correcting any distal thigh deformity. Large-volume thigh liposuction at the time of a body lift may significantly increase the morbidity of the procedure, and tissue edema may not permit an accurate assessment of tissue excess.

As with the other two categories of patients, type 3 men and women are evaluated for a medial thighplasty 3–6 months following their final procedure.

Variables affecting aesthetic outcome

An assessment of lower body contour following a body lift demonstrates that the technique produces very consistent results when patients of the same sex and similar age, body habitus, BMI, and maximum BMI are compared. For both

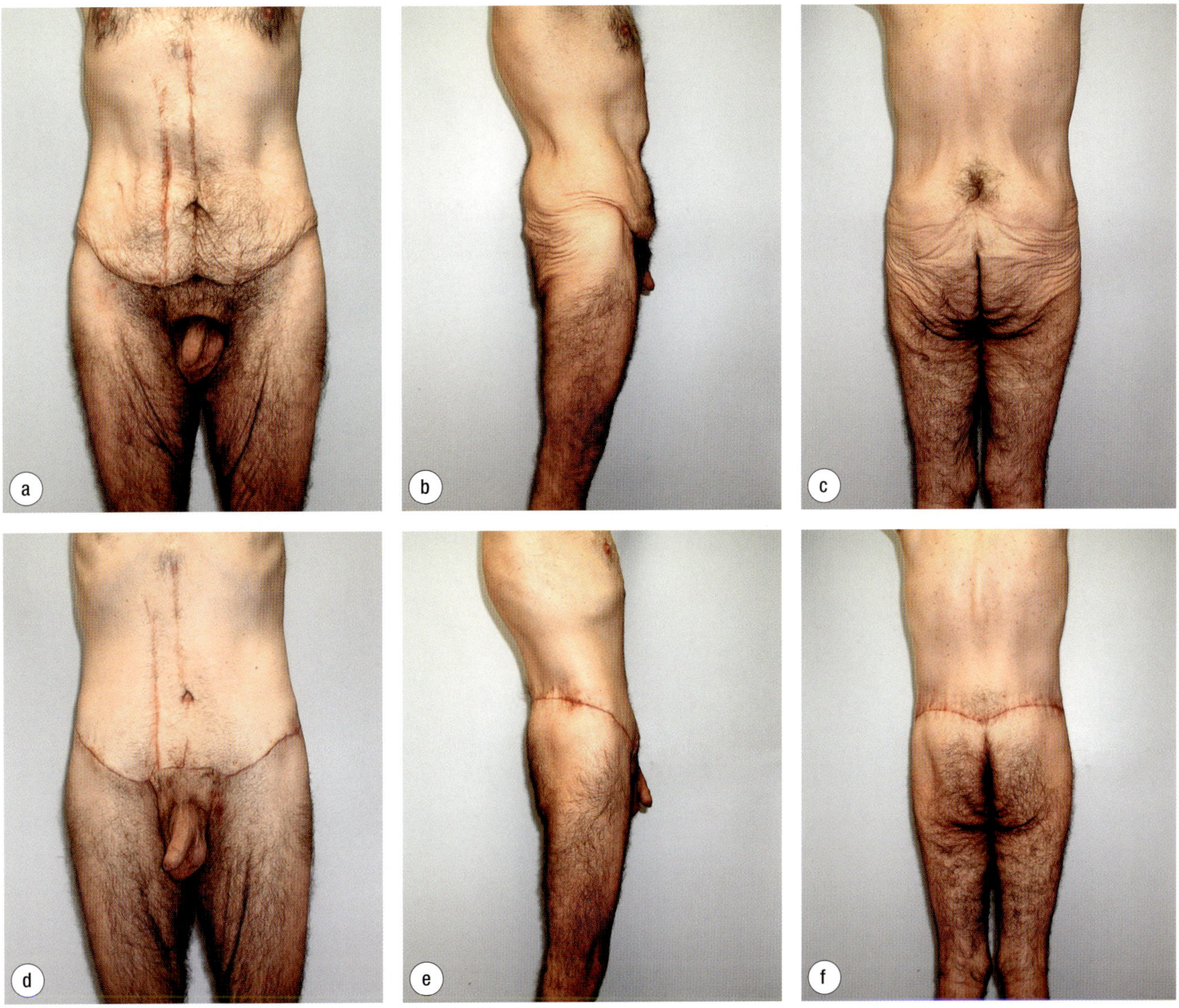

Figure 6.17 (**a–c**) A type 1 46-year-old man 14 months following gastric bypass surgery and weight loss of 179 lbs (81 kg). Current weight and BMI: 168 lbs (76 kg) and 23 kg/m^2, respectively. Highest weight and BMI: 346 lbs (157 kg), 48 kg/m^2. (**d–f**) Seven months following body lift.

men and women, higher BMI at the time of the body lift and higher maximum BMI prior to massive weight loss correlate with a lower aesthetic outcome. Age and body habitus affect men and women differently, however.

Advancing age and gynecoid body habitus in women correlate with a lower aesthetic outcome, particularly with regard to remaining skin and cellulite along the distal thighs. In female postbariatric patients with a gynecoid body habitus, a significant part of their thigh deformity is the result of a circumferential excess of tissues. The skin of the thighs, particularly in older patients, fails to retract completely to accommodate the smaller volume of the lower extremity. The forces of traction from the body lift originate from the waistline. As the body contour deformity of the massive weight loss patient extends farther from the waistline, the effect of the procedures diminishes. The body lift corrects the thigh and buttock deformity of the massive weight loss patient primarily by upward traction and the removal of tissues in this vector. However, the body lift only minimally addresses the circumferential excess of tissues that may be present at the thighs. As a result, older women and women with a more gynecoid body habitus are more likely to have excess skin and cellulite along the distal thighs following a body lift.

Men, on the other hand, may be spared entirely of cellulite along the thighs, with most their excess skin limited to the medial thighs. This appears to be true for older men as well. The deformities of massive weight loss in men are nearly always centered near and around the waistline, i.e. lower abdomen, hips, and proximal medial thighs. This is a direct result of the central or android distribution of fat in men. Consequently, the body lift is consistently effective across a wide range of BMIs and age groups in men.

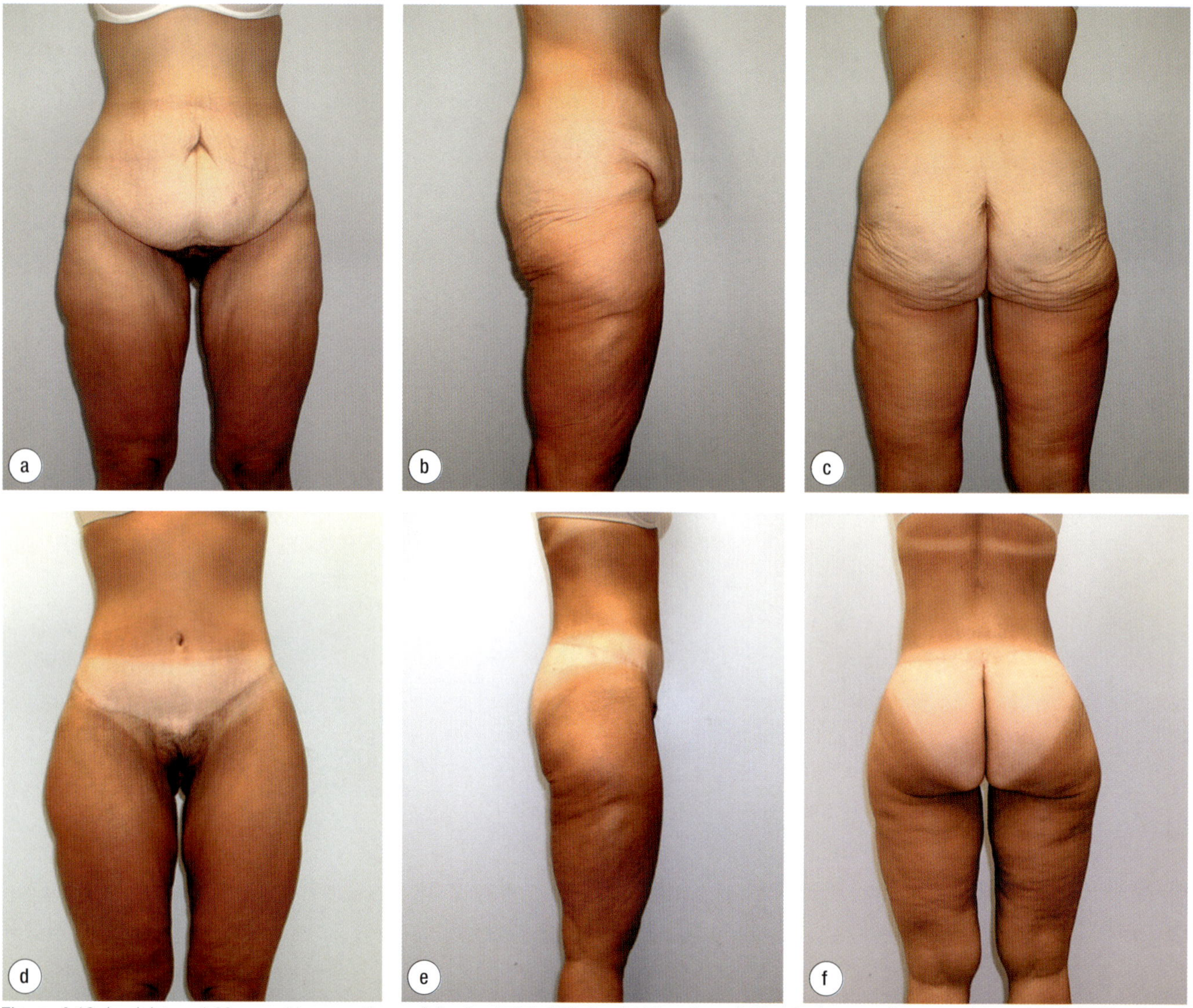

Figure 6.18 **(a–c)** A type 1 39-year-old woman 2 years following 174-lb (79 kg) weight loss through lifestyle changes. Current weight and BMI: 179 lbs (81 kg) and 26 kg/m^2, respectively. Highest weight and BMI: 353 lbs (160 kg), 51 kg/m^2. **(d–f)** Fourteen months following body lift. The patient has a gynecoid body habitus and is scheduled for a medial thighplasty with a longitudinal component.

The fat distribution in women is much more variable, with the most common being gynecoid. As would be expected, high-BMI women who have a more central fat distribution or android body habitus can expect better results from the body lift than women with a more gynecoid body morphology.

Scar quality

To affect change along the distal thighs and upper abdomen from the waistline requires significant tension. A properly performed body lift, therefore, creates the potential for wide and possibly unaesthestic scars. During the early part of our body lift series, the SFS was approximated with a braided nylon suture. The dermis was then approximated as a separate layer with absorbable sutures. While the soft tissue contour of this group of patients was good over the long term, the scar quality was variable. Some patients had wider and more hypertrophic scars than others (Fig. 6.23).

Following the recommendation of Dr. Lockwood (personal communication), we began incorporating a portion of the dermis with the SFS approximation (Fig. 6.12). This modification to our technique allowed us to create some degree of skin redundancy at the waistline closer for as long as 3 months, and in turn achieve consistent closure results with regard to scar quality. Our attempts to create skin redundancy at the waistline with approximation of the SFS alone, without the dermis, had been unsuccessful. With this change, we were in effect creating a low-tension skin closure with a body-contouring procedure incorporating a high level of traction.

From this observation, we were able to conclude that while SFS approximation is important for the maintenance of soft

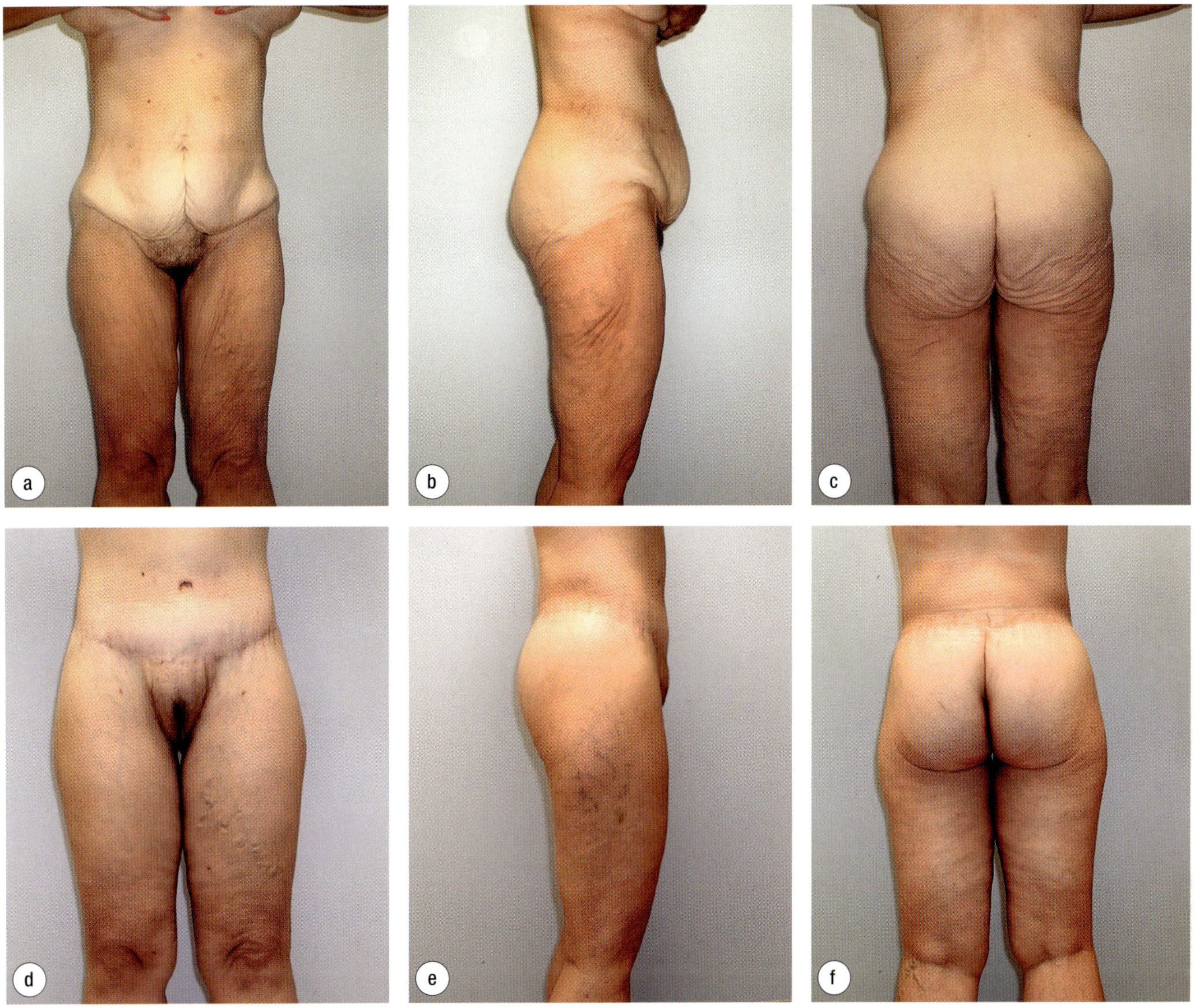

Figure 6.19 (**a–c**) A type 1 40-year-old woman 13 months following gastric bypass surgery and weight loss of 174 lbs (79 kg). Current weight and BMI: 187 lbs (85 kg) and 27 kg/m^2, respectively. Highest weight and BMI: 362 lbs (164 kg), 52 kg/m^2. (**d–f**) Four months following body lift and subsequent medial thighplasty with longitudinal component.

tissue contour, minimizing skin tension during the first several months of wound maturation is critical to producing consistently good scars with the body lift. The role of a nonabsorbable suture may be insignificant beyond 3–6 months, as it is unlikely that a scar would widen after that time. We are currently evaluating whether longer lasting absorbable sutures are able to maintain a redundant skin edge for a period of at least 3 months.

POSTOPERATIVE CARE

Patients are restricted to a hospital bed until the next day. Anticoagulants are not used perioperatively. Sequential compression devices are left in place. The following morning, the binder is loosened, and patients are assisted with ambulation after tolerating a sitting position. The Foley catheter and sequential compression devices are removed if the patient is ambulating well.

On postoperative day 2, the patient is usually discharged following a lower extremity venous Doppler study. Antibiotics are prescribed until all drains are removed. Oral narcotics and laxatives are prescribed as well. The first follow-up office visit is 1 week after surgery. At this visit, only drains with an output of less than 30 cc in the previous 24-h period are removed. At most, two drains are removed at each visit and preferably not from the same side. All drains are removed by 5 weeks, regardless of output. Patients are observed at 6 weeks, 3 months, 6 months, and annually thereafter.

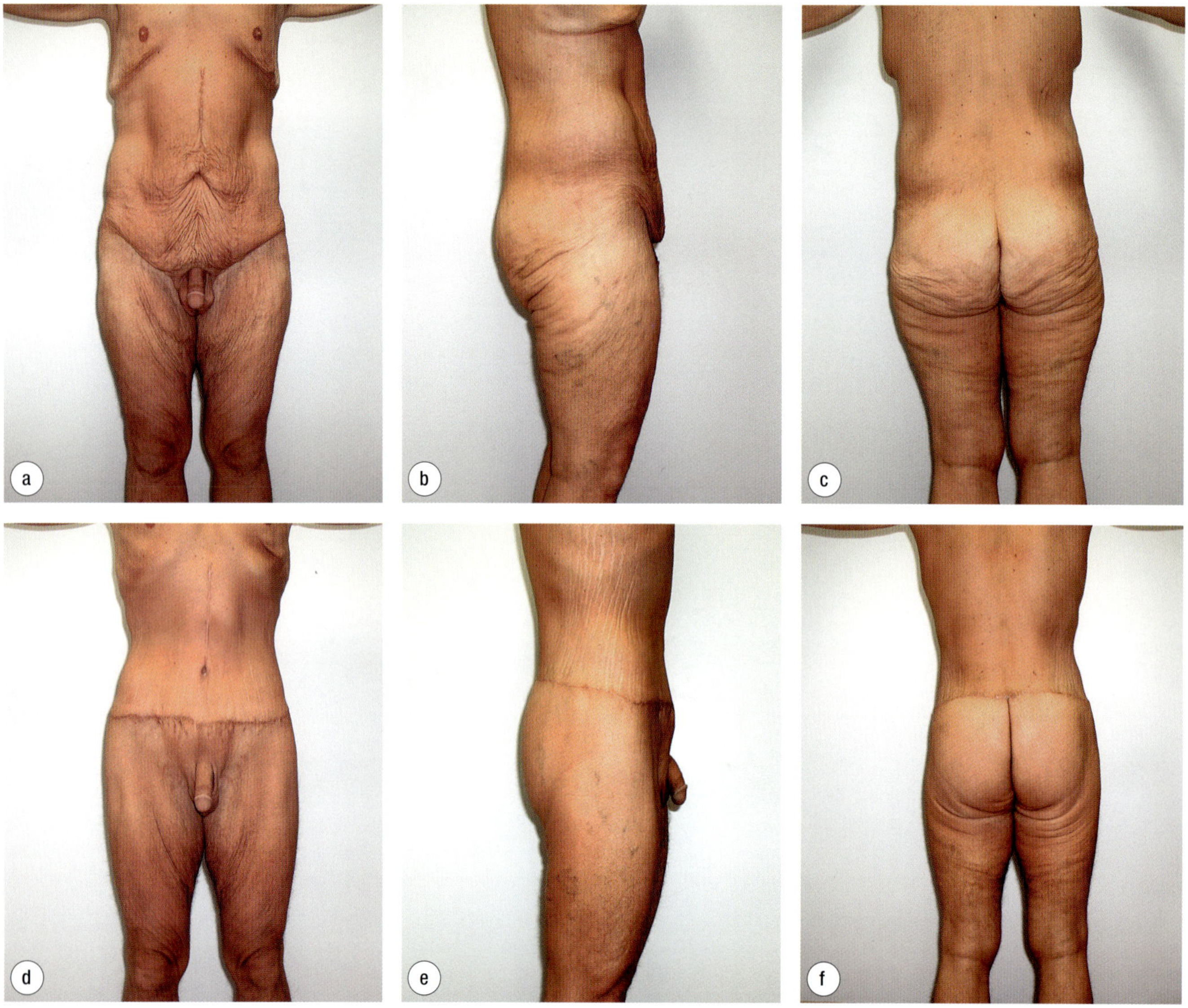

Figure 6.20 (**a–c**) A type 1 37-year-old man 2 years following gastric bypass surgery and weight loss of 295 lbs (134 kg). Current weight and BMI: 216 lbs (98 kg) and 27 kg/m^2, respectively. Highest weight and BMI: 511 lbs (232 kg), 66 kg/m^2. (**d–f**) Four months following body lift.

COMPLICATIONS: MANAGEMENT AND PREVENTION

Complications following the body lift are more frequent than with traditional body-contouring procedures such as abdominoplasty.[1,22,23] This finding is not surprising considering the much greater magnitude of this procedure and degree of deformity to be corrected in the massive weight loss population. Nevertheless, complications are generally well tolerated by this patient population because of the often dramatic functional and aesthetic benefits that come with these procedures.

The overall complication rate for 319 body lifts is 49% (Table 6.5). As with most surgical series, the frequency of complications has diminished over time. Statistical analysis of the data reveals the following.

- Patients with higher maximum BMIs prior to massive weight loss are at greater risk for complications following a body lift ($P < 0.01$). For example, an individual with a maximum BMI of 70 kg/m^2 prior to massive weight loss has a 15 times greater change of having complications following a body lify than somebody with a BMI of 40 kg/m^2.
- BMI at the time of the body lift was found to have a significant association with complications ($P < 0.05$).
- Patients with larger changes in BMI before and after weight loss were at greater risk for complications; however, the association was not found to be significant ($P < 0.06$).
- Patients with a history of smoking had more complications than non-smokers; however, the association with smoking was not found to be significant ($P < 0.13$).
- Men had more complications than women; however, the association with sex was not found to be significant ($P < 0.02$).

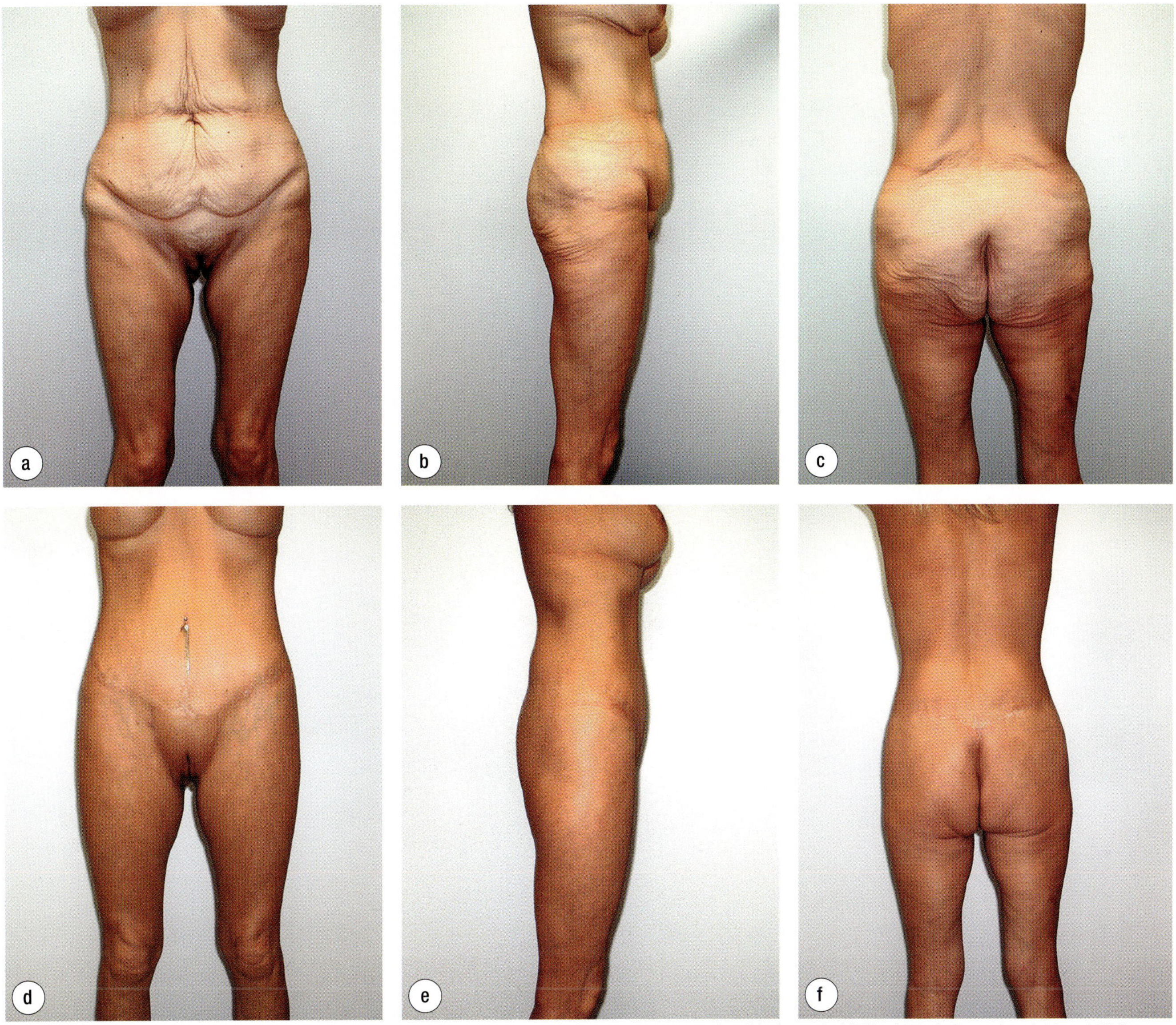

Figure 6.21 (**a–c**) A type 1 53-year-old woman 14 months following gastric bypass surgery and weight loss of 117 lbs (53 kg). Current weight and BMI: 137 lbs (62 kg) and 21 kg/m^2, respectively. Highest weight and BMI: 254 lbs (115 kg), 39 kg/m^2. (**d–f**) Twenty-four months following body lift and subsequent medial thighplasty with approach limited to the thigh perineal crease.

- Age at the tome of the body lift was also not found to be significantly correlated with complications.

Skin dehiscence

Skin dehiscence is our most frequent complication following a body lift (Table 6.5). This can be attributed to the facts that the procedure is circumferential, and that a high degree of traction is needed to produce an ideal outcome. Nevertheless, the frequency and severity of this complication has continued to diminish. Skin dehiscence in the vast majority of instances in our series has occurred at the buttock cleft and hips, the two areas of greatest tension following this procedure.

In the early part of the series, the skin to be removed at the buttock cleft was measured with the patient standing prior to surgery. During surgery, the waist was not completely flexed into a sitting position, and the previously marked skin to be removed appeared to be appropriate. When assuming a sitting position, patients place tremendous tension on this minimally mobile part of the lower back. In addition, the relatively greater period of time in bed in the early postoperative period may lead to some degree of ischemia over the sacrum and coccyx, likely contributing to poor healing in this area. Measuring the tissue to be removed intraoperatively, with the patient flexed into a sitting position, has greatly decreased the frequency and severity of this problem.

The hip had been another problem area for skin dehiscence in the early part of our series. Approximating the SFS along with a small dermal component with a permanent stitch, as suggested by Lockwood, allowed us to create some degree of tissue redundancy along the closure for several months. We

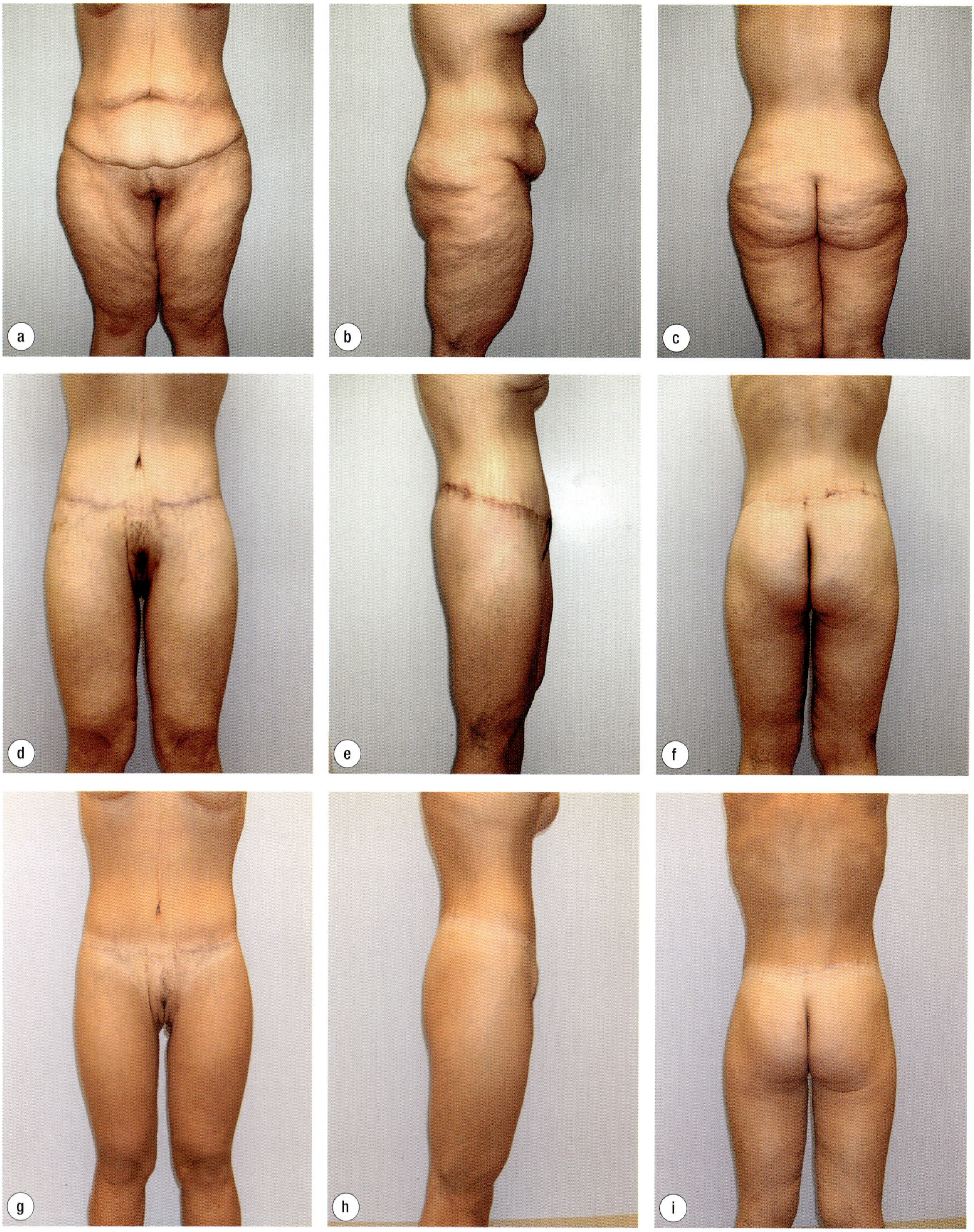

Figure 6.22 (**a–c**) A type 2 33-year-old woman 11 years following gastric bypass surgery and weight loss of 172 lbs (78 kg). Current weight and BMI: 179 lbs (81 kg) and 31 kg/m^2, respectively. Highest weight and BMI: 353 lbs (160 kg), 54 kg/m^2. (**d–f**) Five months following body lift and subsequent medial thighplasty with longitudinal component. (**g–i**) 24 months following body lift and 18 months following subsequent medial thighplasty with a longitudinal component.

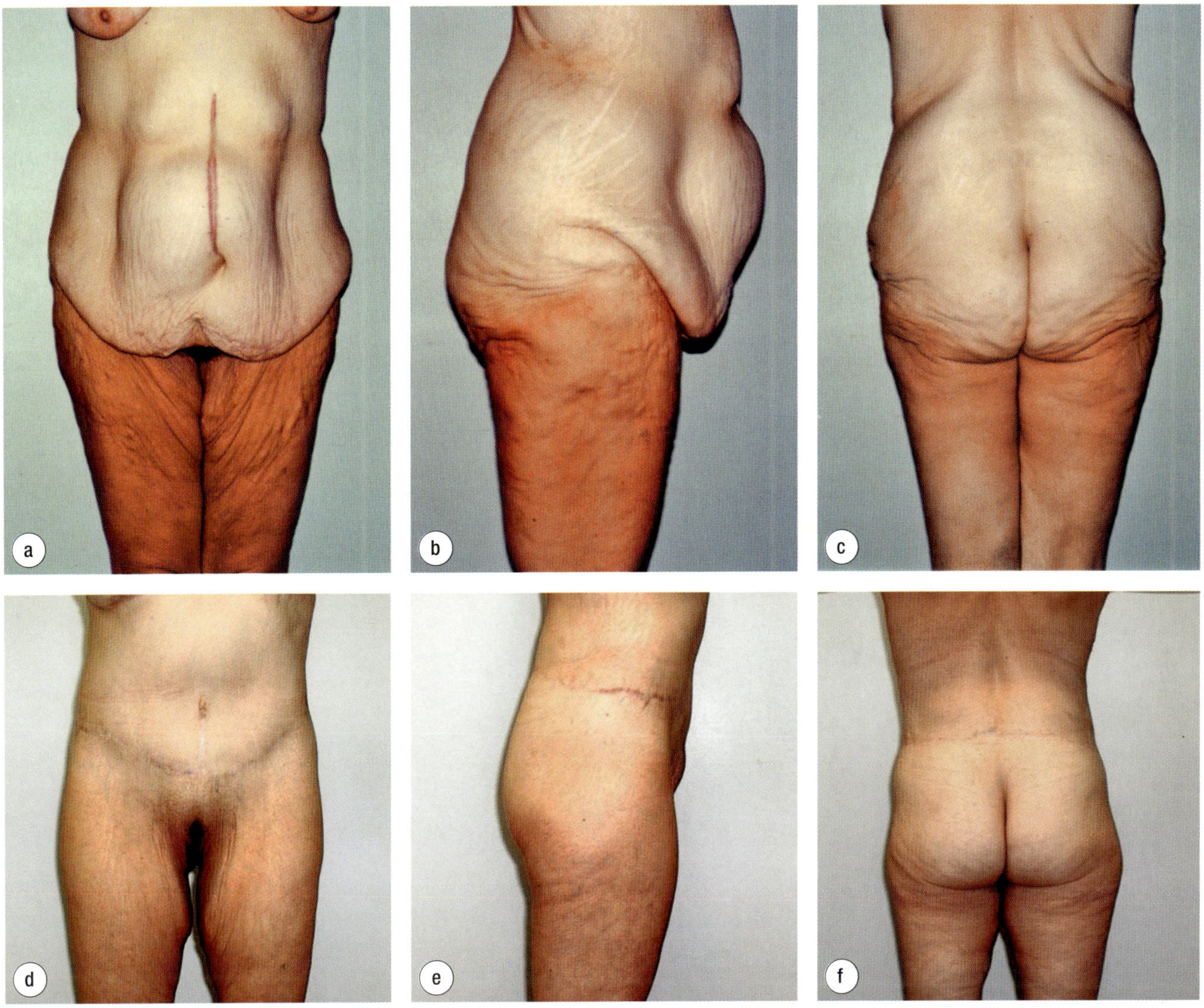

Figure 6.23 (**a–c**) A type 2 35-year-old woman 13 months following gastric bypass surgery and weight loss of 141 lbs (64 kg). Current weight and BMI: 183 lbs (83 kg) and 29 kg/m^2, respectively. Highest weight and BMI: 324 lbs (147 kg), 51 kg/m^2. (**d–f**) Forty-eight months following body lift and repair of ventral hernia. The lipodystrophy of the hip roll was treated by direct excision. The patient reports a history of smoking.

feel that this modification to our technique not only decreased the incidence of skin dehiscence but improved scar quality as well. The majority of skin dehiscences in our experience have been 1–2 cm in length and occurred more than 2 weeks following surgery. These dehiscences have been managed successfully with local wound care. Several of the dehiscences were managed surgically. In six cases, non-absorbable stitches were placed at the bedside on postoperative day 1 or 2 to approximate skin edges. In two other instances, patients fainted while showering for the first time, leading to a large wound dehiscence and an immediate return to the operating room.

The key elements to preventing skin dehiscence are:

- an effective and reliable preoperative marking technique,
- accurate intraoperative tissue measurement, and
- a closure technique that minimizes tension along the skin edges in the postoperative period.

Seroma

Seroma formation remains a frequent complication following body lifts in the postbariatric population. Extensive tissue undermining and the shearing of opposing subcutaneous tissue surfaces predispose patients to this complication. The reported incidence of seromas varies significantly in the literature, as does the approach to their prevention. Aly et al. report a rate of 37.5% and describe removing all drains by 2 weeks. Carwell and Horton and Van Geertruyden et al. describe seroma rates of 14 and 6.6%, respectively. On a series of 40 cases, Pascal and Le Louarn report having had no seromas and removing all drains by 3 days postoperatively. In our series of 319 cases, we have a seroma rate of 18.18%, with 23 days being the average for when the last drain is removed (Table 6.5). All seromas involved the thigh, and in some cases extended to either the buttocks or the anterior abdominal wall.

Table 6.4 Patient treatment

Type	Group	Treatment
1 (BMI $<28\,kg/m^2$)	Men and women	1. Body lift and thigh liposuction (possibly medial thighs for men, possibly circumferential for women). 2. Evaluate for possible medial thighplasty 3–6 months following body lift.
2 (28–32 kg/m^2)	Men and women	1. Body lift and thigh liposuction (possibly medial thighs for men, often circumferential for women). 2. Evaluate for possible medial thighplasty 3–6 months following body lift.
3 ($\geq 32\,kg/m^2$)	Men with BMI $<35\,kg/m^2$ and age <55 years	Body lift and possible medial thigh liposuction.
	Men with BMI $>35\,kg/m^2$ or age >55 years	1. Consider abdominoplasty with second-stage thigh and buttock lift. 2. Evaluate for possible medial thighplasty 3–6 months following body lift or second-stage thigh and buttock lift.
	Women with BMI $<35\,kg/m^2$, age <55 years, and android body habitus	Body lift and thigh liposuction.
	Women with BMI $>35\,kg/m^2$, age >55 years, or gynecoid body habitus	1. Consider abdominoplasty with thigh liposuction and second-stage thigh and buttock lift. 2. Evaluate for possible medial thighplasty 3–6 months following body lift or second-stage thigh and buttock lift.

Avoid medial thigh liposuction with body lift unless future medial thighplasty planned

The explanation for the pattern of seromas at the thigh most likely has to do with the motion of the greater trochanter with ambulation and this being the most dependent area of continuous undermining. As described earlier, in our technique the drains are placed through the mons pubis in a specific order and to a designated location. Our usual practice is to begin removing drains 1 week following surgery. Typically, the two drains serving the abdomen are removed first. The drains are removed only if they are draining less than 30 cc in a 24-h period. The following week, the drains servicing each thigh recess are removed, and at approximately 3 weeks the buttock drains are removed. The buttock drains treat the thigh recess as well. Any remaining drain is removed at 5 weeks, regardless of output. Knowing where each drain is placed eliminates the possibility of removing two drains from the same side of the body. Also, removing the drains in the order described always forms some degree of redundancy in treating any one area.

At each office visit, the drains are stripped to verify patency and proper function. We feel that this is very important, particularly in patients who may have had some oozing in the immediate postoperative period. Frequently, a drain that appears to be ready to be removed may in fact be obstructed by coagulated blood or fibrin. Our initial approach to seromas is to drain the collection by needle aspiration. If, however, the patient presents with any signs or symptoms of infection, or if the quality of the fluid suggests infection, the fluid is sent for analysis and a 10-mm fully perforated flat drain (Zimmer Corp.) is placed into the seroma cavity via the body lift scar. If the seroma is large, greater than 10 cm in diameter, and clinically sterile, the patient is also offered the possibility of having a drain placed in the cavity. For patients having to travel long distances for office visits, this is often the better choice. Seroma formation can be kept to a reasonably low level by keeping to a carefully prescribed drain protocol and meticulous drain care.

Skin necrosis

The most frequent sites for skin necrosis in our experience have been the suprapubic region and, less commonly, the hips and buttock cleft. Skin necrosis in body-contouring surgery is usually the result of poor tissue circulation, which can be influenced by variables such as tension, tobacco consumption, scars, liposuction, and in certain instances pressure from dressings and garments.[22,24,25] Necrosis along the suprapubic portion of the abdominal wall flap can be readily explained by the random and peripheral origin of its blood supply following an abdominoplasty. The necrosis along the hips and buttock cleft is usually marginal in presentation and may have more to do with the effect of tension on tissue perfusion. As described above, in an effort to preserve the blood supply to the hypogastric portion of the abdominal wall flap, we limit

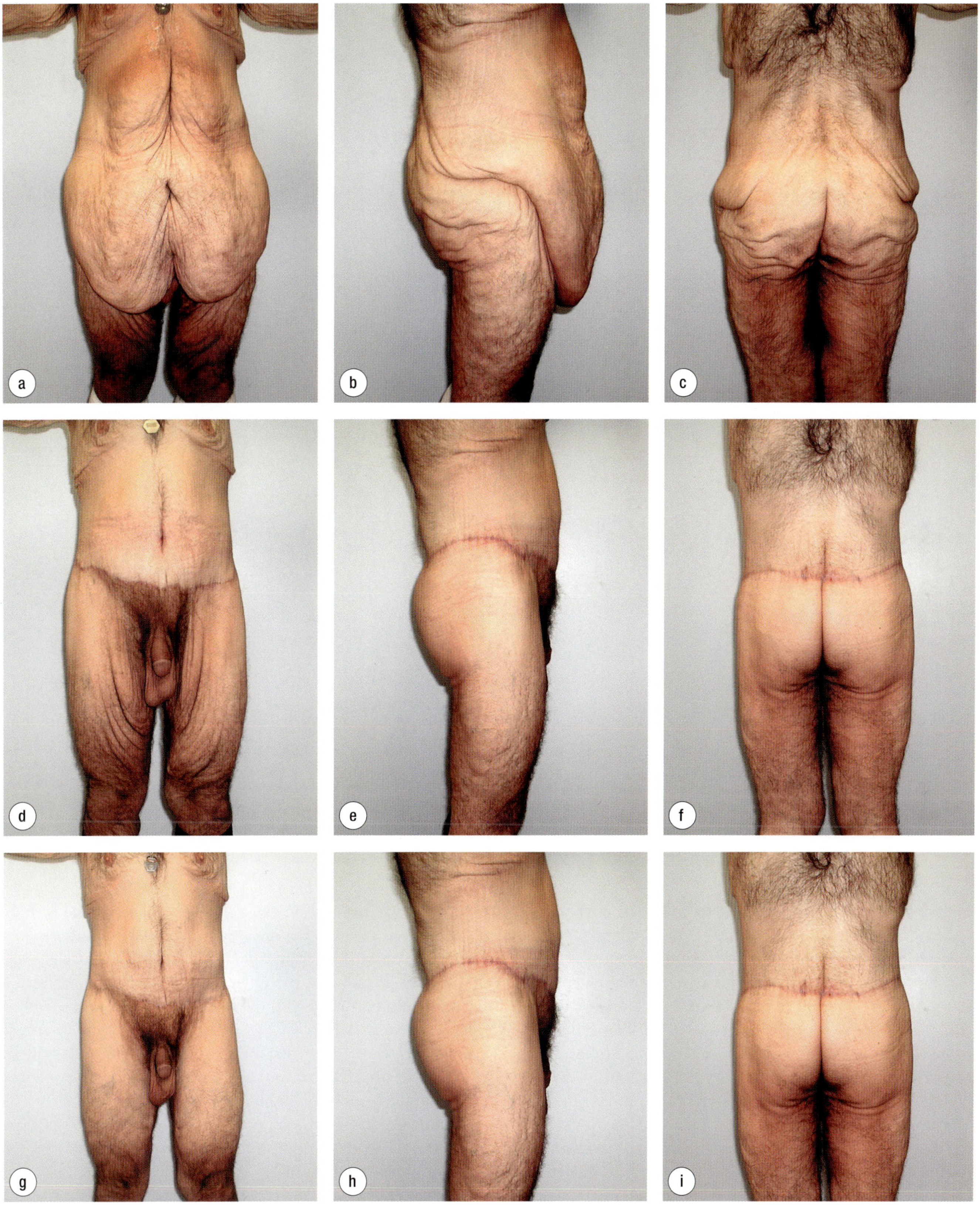

Figure 6.24 (**a–c**) A type 3 40-year-old man 21 months following gastric bypass surgery and weight loss of 165 lbs (75 kg). Current weight and BMI: 198 lbs (90 kg) and 32 kg/m^2, respectively. Highest weight and BMI: 366 lbs (166 kg), 59 kg/m^2. (**d–f**) Seven months following body lift. (**g–i**) Three months following medial thighplasty with a longitudinal component.

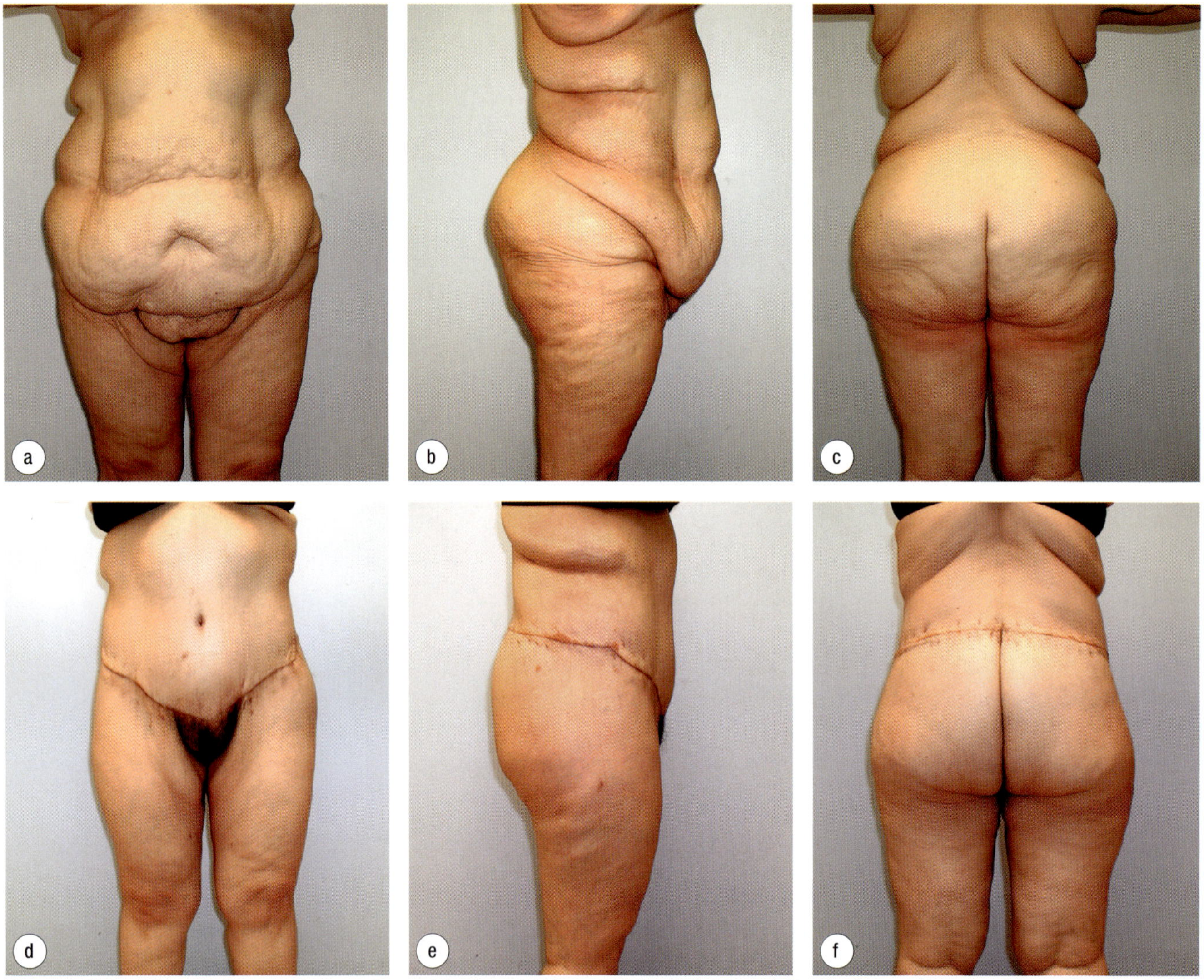

Figure 6.25 (**a–c**) A type 3 42-year-old woman 2 years following weight loss of 115 lbs (52 kg) through lifestyle changes. Current weight and BMI: 209 lbs (95 kg) and 36 kg/m^2, respectively. Highest weight and BMI: 324 lbs (147 kg), 54 kg/m^2. (**d–f**) Seven months following body lift.

undermining at the epigastrium as much as possible. This concept has been well described.[17] Tissue redundancy in the epigastrium may result from this technique.

Liposuction and/or discontinuous undermining can effectively treat this contour tissue. We prefer to directly excise any excess fat in the hypogastric portion of the flap. This is performed with curved Mayo scissors and is limited to the fat deep to Scarpa's fascia. The avoidance of liposuction to the infraumbilical portion of the flap has been advocated by others.[22] Our approach to the prevention of marginal skin necrosis at the hips is to apply only minimal tension to the thigh and buttock flap when measuring for excision. Because the thigh is abducted at the time the tissues are being measured, even minimal tension will result in significant tension along the lateral thigh when adducted.

Anecdotally, we have never seen an aesthetic or a functional benefit, in terms of preventing complications, from the use of abdominal or thigh garments. Early in our experience with the body lift, we had two instances where a netting used to hold dressings in place rolled into a cord, producing a tourniquet effect on the lower abdomen and subsequent skin necrosis. Therefore, because of the potential for garments to diminish circulation, particularly to the lower abdomen, we use only a loosely placed binder in the perioperative period to secure dressings. After 48 h, when the dressings are removed, patients are advised that they may remove the binder and, if they choose to continue to use it, it should be placed loosely.

Our necrosis rate is higher than rates reported by others (Table 6.5).[4,6,8,10] We can attribute this to the fact that 16.3% of our patients have a history of smoking. Tobacco consumption is a well-known appetite suppressant and, not surprisingly, smokers are overrepresented in our lowest BMI category of patients (Table 6.6). Although all our patients are advised to not consume tobacco during the perioperative period, we suspect that most smokers only diminish tobacco consumption during that time. We continue to operate on patients with a

Table 6.5 Patient outcome data

	No. of patients	Percentage	Length of stay (days)	Drain duration (days)	Complications (%)	Dehiscence (%)	Seroma (%)	Skin necrosis (%)	Infection (%)	Bleeding (%)	Deep vein thrombosis (%)	Pulmonary embolism (%)	Transfusions (%)
Total	319	100.00	2.75	23	48.90	29.78	18.18	9.40	4.39	1.88	1.88	1.25	15.36
Women	274	85.89	2.68	22	31.35	29.93	16.06	10.22	4.38	1.09	1.82	1.46	14.23
Men	45	14.11	3.22	27	53.33	28.89	31.11	4.44	4.44	6.67	2.22	0.00	22.22
Type 1	154	48.28	2.49	21	45.45	29.22	15.58	11.04	3.90	0.65	0.65	0.00	11.69
Type 2	96	30.09	2.82	25	45.83	29.17	18.75	6.25	3.13	2.08	3.13	2.08	17.71
Type 3	69	21.63	3.23	25	60.87	31.88	23.19	10.14	7.25	4.35	2.90	2.90	20.29
Non-smokers	267	83.70	2.78	24	46.07	28.09	16.48	8.24	5.24	2.25	2.25	1.50	17.23
Type 1	124	80.52	2.47	21	41.94	29.03	13.71	7.26	4.84	0.81	0.81	0.00	12.90
Type 2	83	86.46	2.92	25	43.37	26.51	18.07	7.23	3.61	2.41	3.61	2.41	19.28
Type 3	60	86.96	3.27	25	58.33	28.33	20.00	11.67	8.33	5.00	3.33	3.33	23.33
Smokers	52	16.30	2.62	21	63.46	38.46	26.92	15.38	0.00	0.00	0.00	0.00	5.77
Type 1	30	19.48	2.60	20	60.00	30.00	23.33	26.67	0.00	0.00	0.00	0.00	6.67
Type 2	13	13.54	2.23	23	61.54	46.15	23.08	0.00	0.00	0.00	0.00	0.00	7.69
Type 3	9	13.04	3.00	22	77.78	55.56	44.44	0.00	0.00	0.00	0.00	0.00	0.00

history of smoking after careful education and selection, because the functional and aesthetic benefits have far outweighed any sequelae from skin necrosis (Figs 6.23 and 6.26).

Upper abdominal scars, particularly those in the right and left subcostal region, represent a risk factor for skin necrosis along the lower abdomen. Our approach to patients with these scars is to proceed with the abdominoplasty portion of the operation, as described above, with careful attention to minimizing dissection in the epigastric region. The portion of the flap inferior to the scar is monitored carefully. If the lower portion of the flap appears viable, in nearly all instances, we have completed the procedure as usual with no adverse sequelae. If there is concern for the viability of the flap during the procedure, the ischemic area may be excised in a fashion similar to a fleur de lis procedure.

The majority of cases of skin necrosis in our series were 1 or 2 cm at greatest diameter, and in all instances were treated with sharp debridement and/or dressing changes. Patients are advised that scars from skin necrosis can be evaluated for revision at 1 year postoperatively. Skin necrosis can be minimized by:

- the judicious use of continuous dissection and liposuction in the epigastric region;
- the appropriate use of tension when marking for tissue excision; and
- the avoidance of garments that may affect circulation, particularly in the early postoperative period.

Individuals with a history of tobacco consumption may be eliminated entirely as candidates for a body lift or considered on a case-by-case basis after careful and detailed education.

Infection

Infections have been a relatively infrequent problem in our series (Table 6.5). We describe infections as cases where surgical intervention has been required to drain a collection or abscess. We have not had a case of cellulitis without a collection. The infections in our series all appear to be seromas that

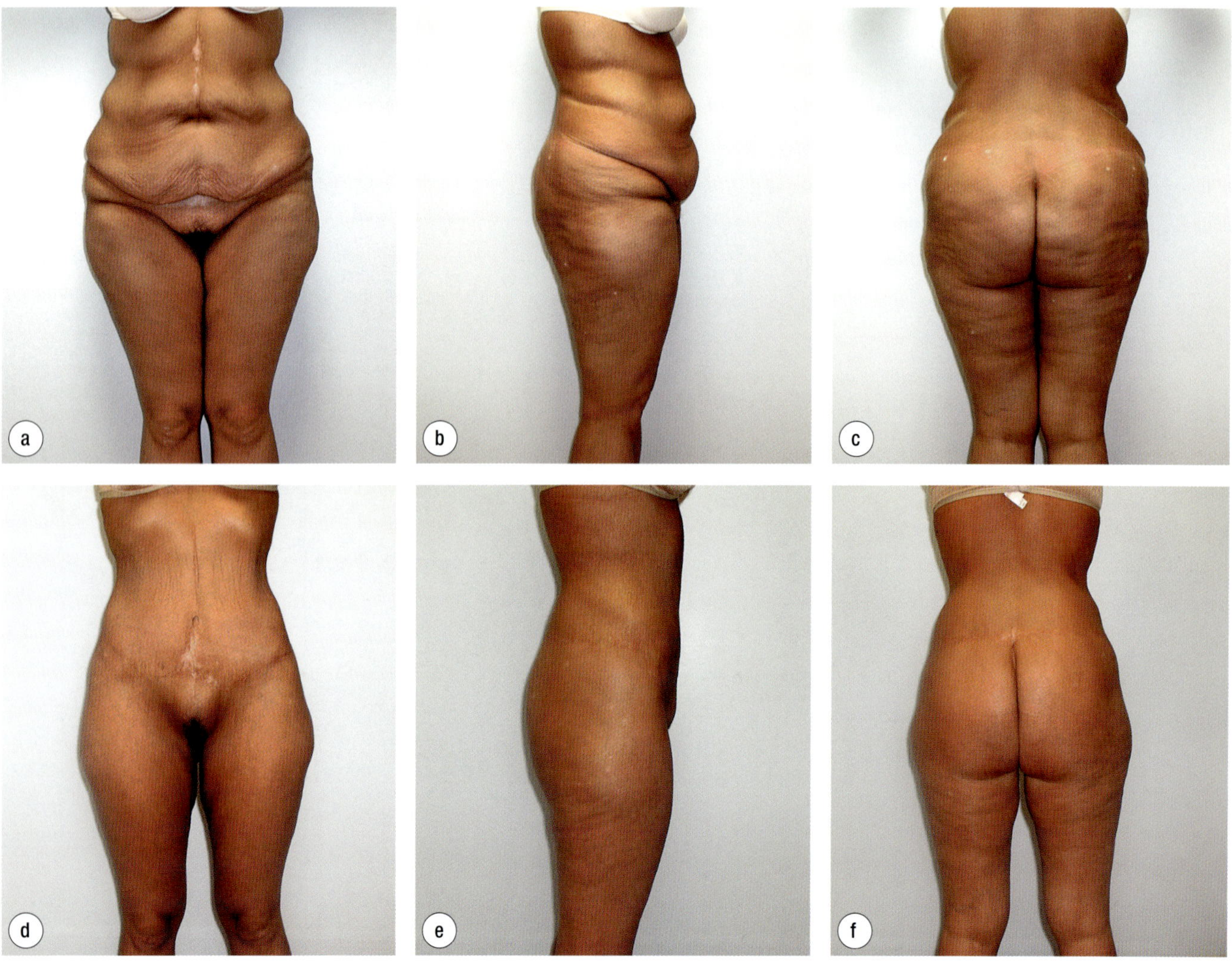

Figure 6.26 **(a–c)** A type 2 24-year-old woman 11 months following gastric bypass surgery and weight loss of 115 lbs (52 kg). Current weight and BMI: 170 lbs (77 kg) and 28 kg/m^2, respectively. Highest weight and BMI: 287 lbs (130 kg), 47 kg/m^2. **(d–f)** Thirty months following body lift. The patient reported a history of smoking and developed skin necrosis in the suprapubic region.

Table 6.6 Patient characteristics

	No. of patients	Percentage	Maximum BMI (kg/m^2)	Current BMI (kg/m^2)	BMI change (kg/m^2)	Smoking (%)	Diabetes (%)	Hypertension (%)
Total	319	100.00	50	29	21	16.30	3.45	8.15
Women	274	85.89	49	28	20	14.60	3.28	6.93
Men	45	14.11	57	32	25	8.89	4.44	11.11
Type 1	154	48.28	45	25	20	19.48	3.25	2.60
Type 2	96	30.09	50	30	20	13.54	4.17	13.54
Type 3	69	21.63	60	35	24	13.04	2.90	13.04
Non-smokers	267	83.70	50	29	21	0	3.75	8.24
Type 1	124	80.52	45	25	20	0	3.23	2.42
Type 2	83	86.46	50	30	20	0	4.82	14.46
Type 3	60	86.96	59	35	24	0	3.33	11.67
Smokers	52	16.30	48	28	20	100.00	1.92	7.69
Type 1	30	19.48	45	25	20	100.00	3.33	3.33
Type 2	13	13.54	49	29	20	100.00	0.00	7.69
Type 3	9	13.04	63	36	27	100.00	0.00	22.22

were either clinically evident or undiagnosed and that became infected. All patients were treated with open drainage or open drainage with replacement of a 10-mm fully perforated flat drain (Zimmer Corp.) in the collection cavity. The drainage was sent for analysis, and the patients were placed on either oral or intravenous antibiotics. No return to the operating room was required.

The pathogenesis of infected seromas is unclear. A possibility includes bacteria tracking from the skin on drains and infecting devitalized tissue, probably fat. Drains kept for long periods of time may create a risk factor for this problem. Our current protocol is to keep patients on antibiotics until the last drain is removed. This extended antibiotic regimen may predispose patients to infections with more resistant organisms. We are currently reassessing our protocol regarding this matter.

Hematoma/bleeding

Bleeding and blood loss during and following body lifts are a major concern. Many aspects of these procedures predispose patients to a risk for blood loss. To effectively treat the lower body contour deformity of the massive weight loss patient requires extensive tissue undermining, and with that the need to either ligate or cauterize a multitude of blood vessels. Meticulous hemostasis is critical throughout these procedures. We have found cautery set to a high level to be very helpful in this regard. Heavier patients, men, and those with larger BMI changes are at greater risk for significant blood loss. We avoid the routine use of anticoagulants in the perioperative period because of the concern for bleeding.

Menstruating women following malapsorptive bariatric procedures often present with significant degrees of anemia. All postbariatric patients are advised to take iron supplements when considering body-contouring surgery, and those with more severe cases of anemia are referred to a hematologist. We avoid having an already anemic patient bank autologous blood in the 1-month period prior to a body lift. Rather, we prefer to transfuse non-autologous blood if it becomes necessary. Our transfusion rate has decreased slightly over the course of the series.

Our hematoma rate has remained relatively low at 1.88% (Table 6.5). We defined a hematoma as a collection of blood that required surgery for evacuation. We presume that there may be other, smaller hematomas that go unnoticed and/or are evacuated by the drains themselves.

Deep vein thrombosis and pulmonary embolism

Deep vein thrombosis and pulmonary embolism represent the most serious risks for body lift patients. Several recognized risk factors for deep vein thrombosis are fundamental to these procedures.[26] The population of patients on average are overweight (Table 6.6), and the body lift is a lengthy procedure, routinely over 4 h. To complicate matters further, early ambulation can be difficult, and the early, routine use of anticoagulants may create a significant risk for bleeding.

Our approach to the avoidance of deep vein thrombosis is to provide the continual use of mechanical anticoagulation until the patient is ambulatory. Patients are kept on bed rest until the day following surgery. A lower extremity venous Doppler is then obtained on the day of discharge. Our deep vein thrombosis rate is 1.88%. We would expect this number to be significantly lower if all our patients were not routinely studied.

Pulmonary embolism remains relatively rare in our series. The management of this life-threatening complication in the post–body lift patient presents special challenges. Heparinization of the early postoperative patient may lead to significant bleeding. The timing and dosing of heparin must be evaluated carefully, as should the possible need for a vena caval filter.

SEQUENCE AND COMBINATIONS OF PROCEDURES

Massive weight loss individuals are often candidates for and are eager to have multiple procedures. Younger patients tend to present initially with more concerns about their torso and breasts, while older patients often have issue with their face and arms. The medial thighs and flanks can be of primary concern for both groups. Our preference regarding the torso is to perform a body lift first, as a single procedure. As we discussed before, the body lift may eliminate the need for a formal medial thigh lift in many patients, particularly those less than 35 years of age and who have had a BMI change of less than 20–25 kg/m^2 prior to the body lift. Furthermore, a more effective medial thigh lift can be performed in a patient following a body lift.

The body lift can often have a significant effect on the upper body, i.e. breasts, flanks, and back (Figs 6.20, 6.24 and 6.26). In men, it may eliminate the need for upper body-contouring surgery or reduce the magnitude of the procedure required. In women, while the body lift can positively impact the back and flanks, it can also cause significant downward migration of the inframammary fold. For this reason, ideally we prefer not to perform breast surgery prior to or concomitantly with a body lift. Following a body lift, other body-contouring procedures we commonly perform are combination brachioplasty and mammoplasty, thighplasty alone, or thighplasty with brachioplasty.

CONCLUSION

The lower body in the massive weight loss patient presents an extreme form of traditional aesthetic and functional body contour concerns. Routine body-contouring procedures usually produce only suboptimal results in this patient population. The body lift described above is an excellent alternative to treat the lower body deformity of the postbariatric patient. As with every technique, careful patient selection, education, and preparation are critical to minimizing complications and optimizing outcome.

REFERENCES

1. Capella JF, Oliak DA, Nemerofsky RB. Body lift: an account of 200 consecutive cases in the massive weight loss patient. Plast Reconstr Surg 2006; 117(2):414–430.
2. Capella JF, Capella RF. Bariatric surgery in adolescence. Is this the best time to operate? Obes Surg 2003; 13:826–832.
3. Capella JF, Capella RF. An assessment of vertical banded gastroplasty—Roux-en-Y gastric bypass for the treatment of morbid obesity. Am J Surg 2002; 183:117–123.
4. Aly AS, Cram AE, Chao M, et al. Belt lipectomy for circumferential truncal excess: the University of Iowa experience. Plast Reconstr Surg 2003; 111:398–413.
5. Lockwood TE. Lower-body lift. Aesthetic Surg J 2001; 21:355–370.
6. Van Geertruyden JP, Vandeweyer E, de Fontaine S, et al. Circumferential torsoplasty. Br J Plast Surg 1999; 52:623–628.
7. Mallory GN. American Society for Bariatric Surgery membership survey. Gainesville: ASBS; 2004.
8. Carwell GR, Horton CE. Circumferential torsoplasty. Ann Plast Surg 1997; 38:213–216.
9. Hurwitz DJ. Single-staged total body lift after massive weight loss. Ann Plast Surg 2004; 52:435–441.
10. Pascal JF, Le Louarn C. Remodeling body lift with high lateral tension. Aesthetic Plast Surg 2002; 26:223–230.
11. Hamra ST. Circumferential body lift. Aesthetic Surg J 1999; 19:244–251.
12. Morales Gracia HJ. Circular lipectomy with lateral thigh–buttock lift. Aesthetic Plast Surg 2003; 27(1):50–57.
13. Regnault P, Daniel R. Secondary thigh–buttock deformities after classical techniques: prevention and treatment. Clin Plast Surg 1984; 11:505–516.
14. Lockwood TE. Fascial anchoring technique in medial thigh lifts. Plast Reconstr Surg 1988; 82:299–304.
15. Lockwood T. Superficial fascial system (SFS) of the trunk and extremities: a new concept. Plast Reconstr Surg 1991; 87:1009–1027.
16. Lockwood T. Transverse flank–thigh–buttock lift with superficial fascial suspension. Plast Reconstr Surg 1993; 92:1112–1122.
17. Lockwood T. High-lateral-tension abdominoplasty with superficial fascial suspension. Plast Reconstr Surg 1995; 96:603–615.
18. Marceau S, Hould FS, Simard S, et al. Biliopancreatic diversion with duodenal switch. World J Surg 1998; 22:947–954.
19. Chapman AE, Kiroff G, Game P, et al. Laparoscopic adjustable gastric banding in the treatment of obesity: a systematic literature review. Surgery 2004; 135:326–351.
20. Capella JF, Capella RF. The weight reduction operation of choice: vertical banded gastroplasty or gastric bypass? Am J Surg 1996; 171:74–79.
21. Brolin RE. Metabolic deficiencies and supplements following bariatric operations. In: Martin L, ed. Obesity surgery. New York: McGraw-Hill; 2004:275–300.
22. Matarasso A. Liposuction as an adjunct to a full abdominoplasty. Plast Reconstr Surg 1995; 95:829–836.
23. Chaouat M, Levan P, Lalanne B, et al. Abdominal dermolipectomies: early postoperative complications and long-term unfavorable results. Plast Reconstr Surg 2000; 106:1614–1623.
24. El-khatib HA, Bener A. Abdominal dermolipectomy in an abdomen with pre-existing scars: a different concept. Plast Reconstr Surg 2004; 114:992–997.
25. Manassa EH, Hertl CH, Olbrisch R. Wound healing problems in smokers and nonsmokers after 132 abdominoplasties. Plast Reconstr Surg 2003; 111:2082–2087.
26. Geerts WH, Heit JA, Clagett GP, et al. Prevention of venous thromboembolism. Chest 2001; 119:132S–175S.

APPROACHES TO UPPER BODY ROLLS

7

J. Peter Rubin, Al S. Aly and Felmont F. Eaves III

Key Points

- An upper body lift is defined as correction of upper back or flank rolls by excision of tissue on the upper torso.
- Excision of upper back rolls can be accomplished with a transverse scar on the upper back or with bilateral lateral or oblique scars.
- Excision of upper back rolls may be combined with breast reshaping or gynecomastia correction.
- A circumferential approach or near-circumferential approach may be employed.

A subset of patients will present with significant rolls of skin along the upper back and lateral chest. This chapter describes technical approaches for correcting these deformities. There is little historical basis for these procedures; rather, they represent an early step in the evolution of approaches for contouring regions that have not traditionally been the focus of plastic surgeons.

DEFORMITIES OF THE UPPER TRUNK

As with any problem faced in plastic surgery, an accurate assessment of the deformity and how it is formed is needed. A surgical plan can then be devised based on this analysis. The thoracic region will often undergo dramatic changes during the process of massive weight gain and subsequent loss. The soft tissue envelope develops varying degrees of laxity in both the horizontal and the vertical directions. Zones of adherence, located over the sternum and spine, restrict movement of the overlying skin and act like hooks that tissues drape off, leading to both anterior and posterior inverted V deformities (see Fig. 7.1).

The lateral thoracic soft tissues descend inferiorly to varying degrees, causing a 'dropout' of the lateral inframammary crease. Some patients will experience no descent of the lateral inframammary crease, while others will drop significantly, manifesting this change into lateral breast rolls. The lateral breast rolls become upper back rolls as they traverse posteriorly. Although many patients will develop the full extent of deformities described here, there are others whose fat deposition pattern may lead to less severe deformities. If the lateral chest rolls dissipate in the region of the posterior axillary line, their correction may be incorporated into an extended mastopexy or gynecomastia correction. If the back rolls extend further, a decision must be made about the suitability of liposuction. Rolls with ptosis and poor skin tone will likely require excision for adequate treatment. Additionally, the position of the lateral inframammary crease is important. If it has dropped out laterally, then some form of an upper body lift will usually be required.

Three surgical approaches are demonstrated.

1. Transverse excision of back rolls combined with mastopexy and brachioplasty.
2. Transverse excision of back rolls combined with mastopexy.
3. Lateral excision of trunk tissue combined with mastopexy.

APPROACH 1: TRANSVERSE EXCISION OF BACK ROLLS COMBINED WITH MASTOPEXY AND BRACHIOPLASTY

Three goals are accomplished with this upper body lift approach.

1. Elimination of horizontal excess through an extension of the brachioplasty procedure on to the lateral chest wall.
2. Elimination of vertical excess by elevating the lateral inframammary crease to its correct position and excising lateral breast/upper back rolls.
3. Building the breast based on a repositioned inframammary crease.

Markings

The patient is marked in the sitting position (see Fig. 7.2).

The arms are marked utilizing a double-ellipse technique. The ellipses cross the axilla onto the lateral chest wall, with their widths and lengths of the lateral chest wall extension based on the amount of excess that the particular patient presents with. The outer ellipse of the double-ellipse technique is based on the estimation of the pinch of redundant tissue just inferior to the underlying musculoskeletal core. Because the pinch technique does not take into account the amount of

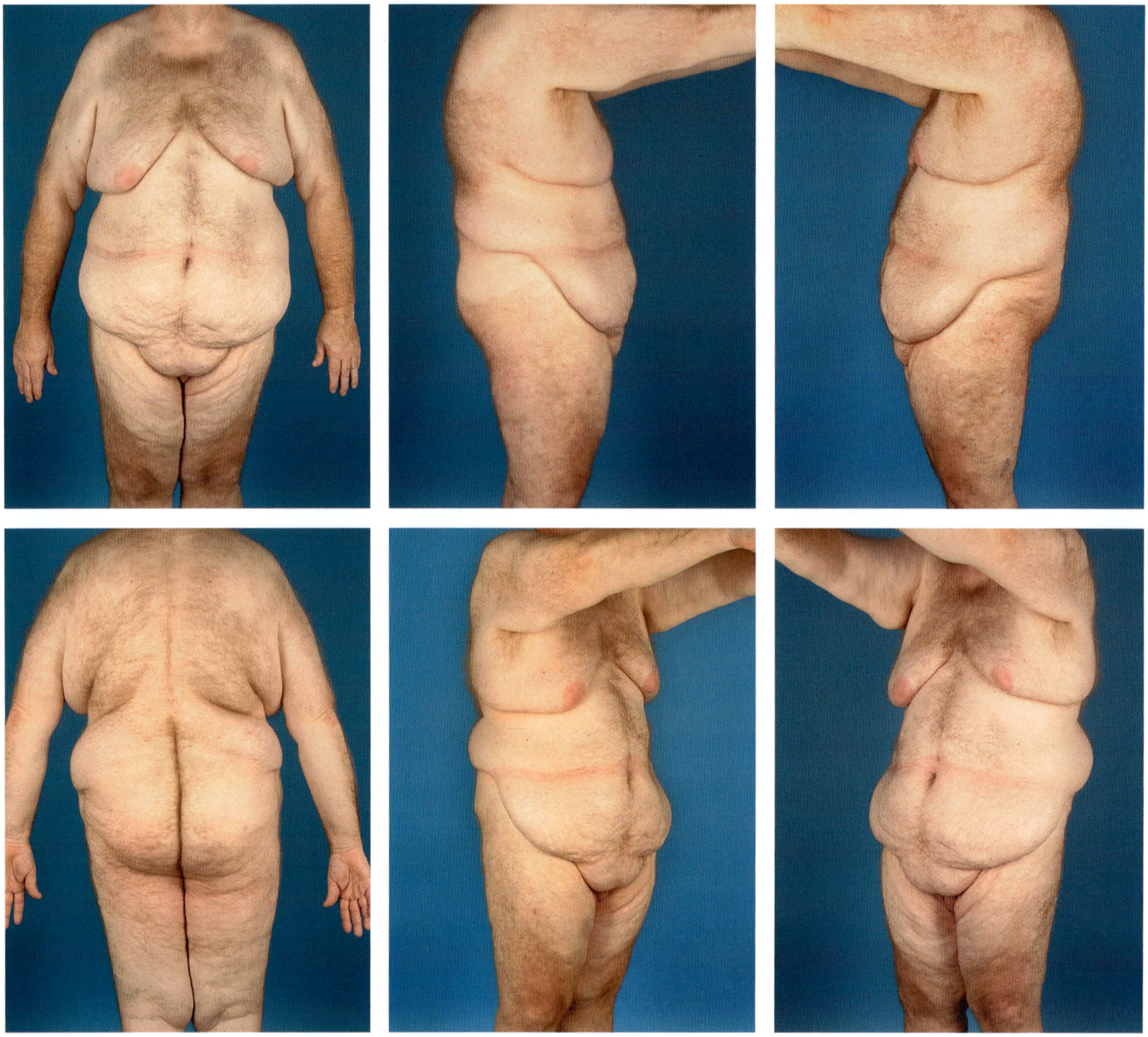

Figure 7.1 Note the inverted V deformities of the anterior and posterior chest caused by the zones of adherence overlying the sternum and spine and the 'dropout' of the lateral inframammary crease in this 48-year-old man who lost 200 lbs (91 kg) and dropped from a BMI of 54 kg/m^2 to 38 kg/m^2.

extra skin needed to fill the gap between the pinched fingers, a second inner ellipse is marked on the inside of the first one to allow appropriate closure.

Next, the lateral breast/upper back roll is pinched to delineate the amount that needs to be resected. This maneuver will demonstrate how far the lateral inframammary crease needs to be lifted to create an appropriate upward curve. Based on the pinch, an ellipse is marked with its medial edge located on the lateral edge of the breast, with the overall vector of the ellipse following the relaxed tension lines of the back. This ellipse may reach the level of the brachioplasty markings in the male, but most often it does in the female patient. The medial edge of the ellipse may reach the midline of the back in some patients.

Next, appropriate markings on the breast are made. A variety of procedures are required in the female patient, which include augmentation, augmentation/mastopexy, autoaugmentation/mastopexy, or reduction augmentation based on the particular patient's presenting anatomy and desires. In the male patient, a reduction of gynecomastia is usually required.

Surgical technique

The patient is placed in the lateral decubitus position to allow access to the arm, lateral chest wall, and back simultaneously. The brachioplasty aspect of the procedure is performed first. The inner ellipse is excised utilizing a segmental resection closure technique, where the procedure progresses from distal to proximal in segments that are excised and immediately closed

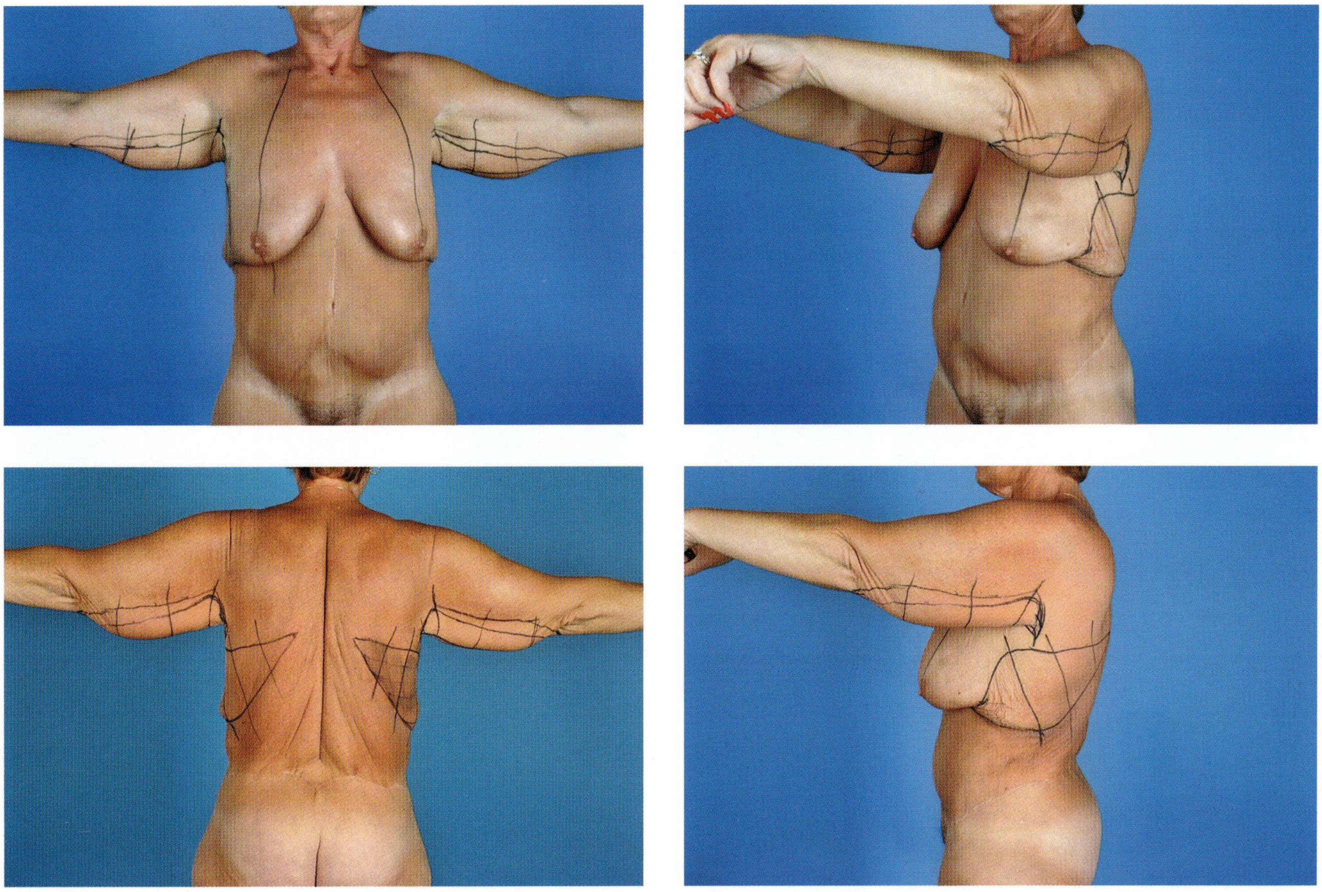

Figure 7.2 This 47-year-old woman had a 250 lb (113 kg) weight loss and dropped from a BMI of 70 kg/m^2 to 26.5 kg/m^2. She presented, after undergoing a belt lipectomy, complaining of all the typical sequelae of massive weight loss of the thoracic region. Note the lateral inframammary crease descent, which dictates the need for an upper body lift. The arms demonstrate the double-ellipse technique, which crosses the axilla on to the lateral chest wall. The lateral breast/upper back roll ellipse is marked along relaxed skin tension lines and reverses the inverted V deformity of the back. This particular patient was also marked for an augmentation/mastopexy.

to prevent intraoperative swelling from developing. At the axillary crease, a Z plasty is created to prevent contracture across the axilla.

Next, the lateral breast/upper back roll is excised, starting with incising the superior edge of the marked ellipse. An inferiorly based skin and fat flap is elevated at least as far down as the proposed inferior mark. The shoulder is then pushed inferiorly and the flap is pulled superiorly, and the excess is tailored from the flap.

The patient is then turned to the other lateral decubitus position and has the identical procedure performed on the opposite side. The patient is then placed in the supine position and whatever breast procedure is chosen is then undertaken.

Postoperative care

Patients are usually admitted overnight for an upper body lift. They are required to keep their arms elevated above heart level for at least 1 week and sometimes up to 3 weeks. Each side will have two drains: one draining the arm and the other draining the lateral/upper back pocket. Often they can be removed in 4–7 days once they reach 40 cc/day or less of drainage. Most patients are able to get back to normal activity in 2–4 weeks, depending on their lifestyle.

Results

Figure 7.3 shows the patient marked in Figure 7.2 before and 5 months after an upper body lift. Note the following.

- The elevation of the lateral inframammary crease to a higher, more appropriate position after surgery.
- The elimination of the lateral breast/upper back roll.
- The reduction in the upper arms.
- The lift and augmentation in the breasts.

In essence, an upper body lift is a complete rejuvenation of the entire thoracic unit, along with a reduction in upper arm excess.

Complications

Fortunately, complications are relatively infrequent when compared with other massive weight loss plastic surgery procedures such as body lifts. They include:

- infection,
- bleeding,
- seroma formation in the arms or back,

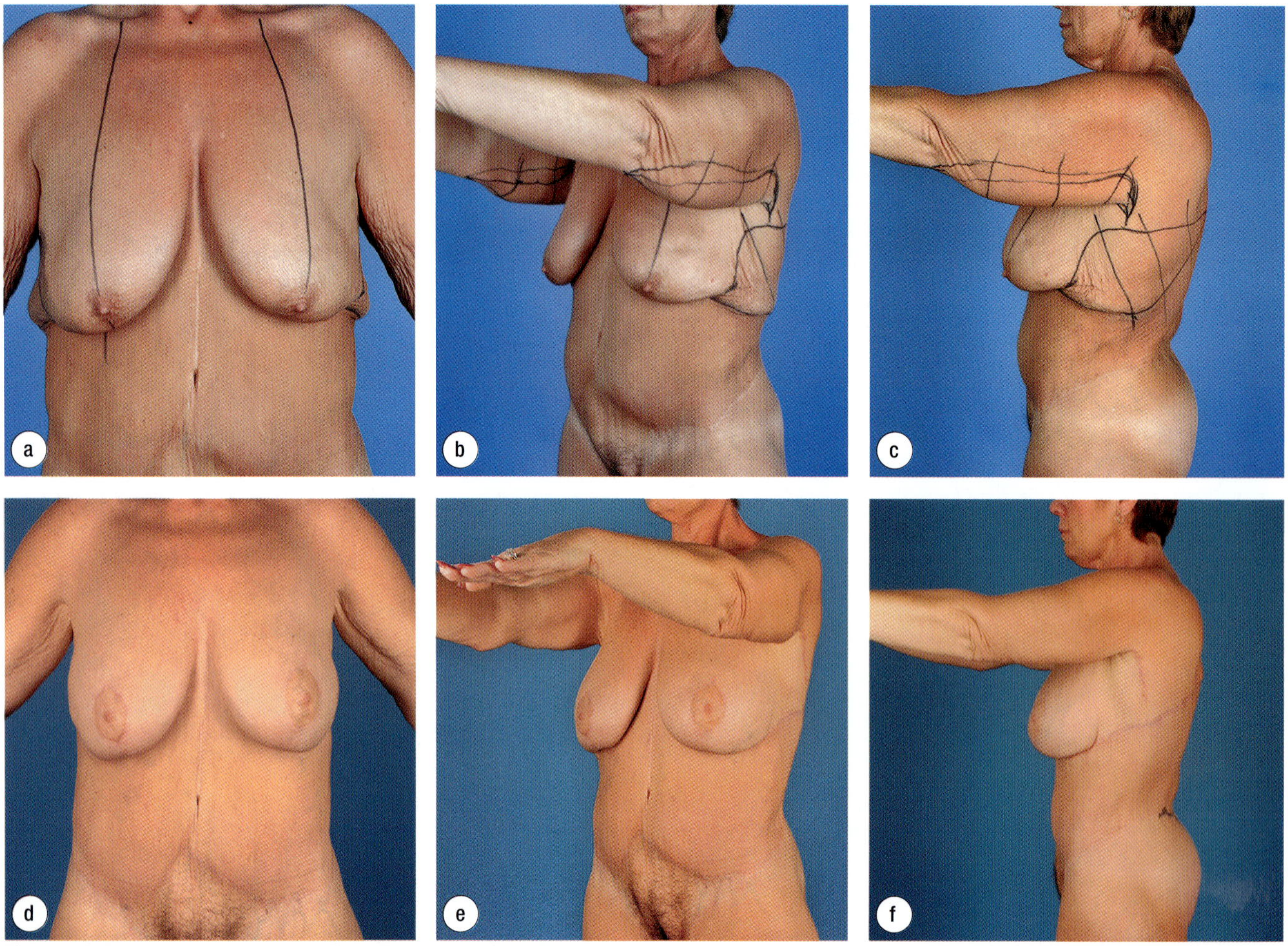

Figure 7.3 The same patient shown in Figure 7.2 is shown (**a–c, g,** and **h**) before and (**d–f, i,** and **j**) 5 months after an upper body lift. Although the results are still maturing, they demonstrate the needed elevation of the lateral inframammary crease, which creates a correct base on which the breast reconstruction can take place; the elimination of the lateral breast/upper back roll; and the improvement in the upper arms.

- asymmetry,
- persistent edema of the distal extremity,
- permanent lymphedema of the upper extremity,
- inability to close the arms,
- unattractive scarring of the arms, and
- nerve damage of the upper extremity.

APPROACH 2: TRANSVERSE EXCISION OF BACK ROLLS COMBINED WITH MASTOPEXY

This approach relies on a transverse posterior excision that merges with a mastopexy. Brachioplasty with extension onto the chest wall, when necessary, is performed as a staged procedure to avoid a confluence of scars.

Markings

A 49-year-old woman is shown in Figure 7.4 and demonstrates prominent back rolls and breast ptosis. The patient is marked in the standing position (Fig. 7.5). The patient is instructed to wear her brassiere, and the borders of the garment are marked (red lines). The intended transverse scar position is then marked within the borders of the brassiere (thin blue line). A superior anchor line (heavy blue line) is marked several centimeters above the intended scar line to allow for descent of the tissues under tension. Note that the anchor line is closer to the intended scar line at the midline (approximately 1 cm), where the tissues are not as mobile.

Next, a pinch test is employed to estimate the amount of skin that can be resected. Vertical reference lines can assist in maintaining symmetry of the marks. The inferior line of excision will be lifted to the anchor line once the tissue is resected. More tissue will be resected laterally than medially. The lateral border of the posterior pattern is generally set at the posterior axillary line and marked with a heavy vertical line.

Focus is then shifted to the mastopexy markings. These are commenced based on a Wise pattern. The lateral portion of the Wise pattern stops several centimeters from the marked border of the posterior resection.

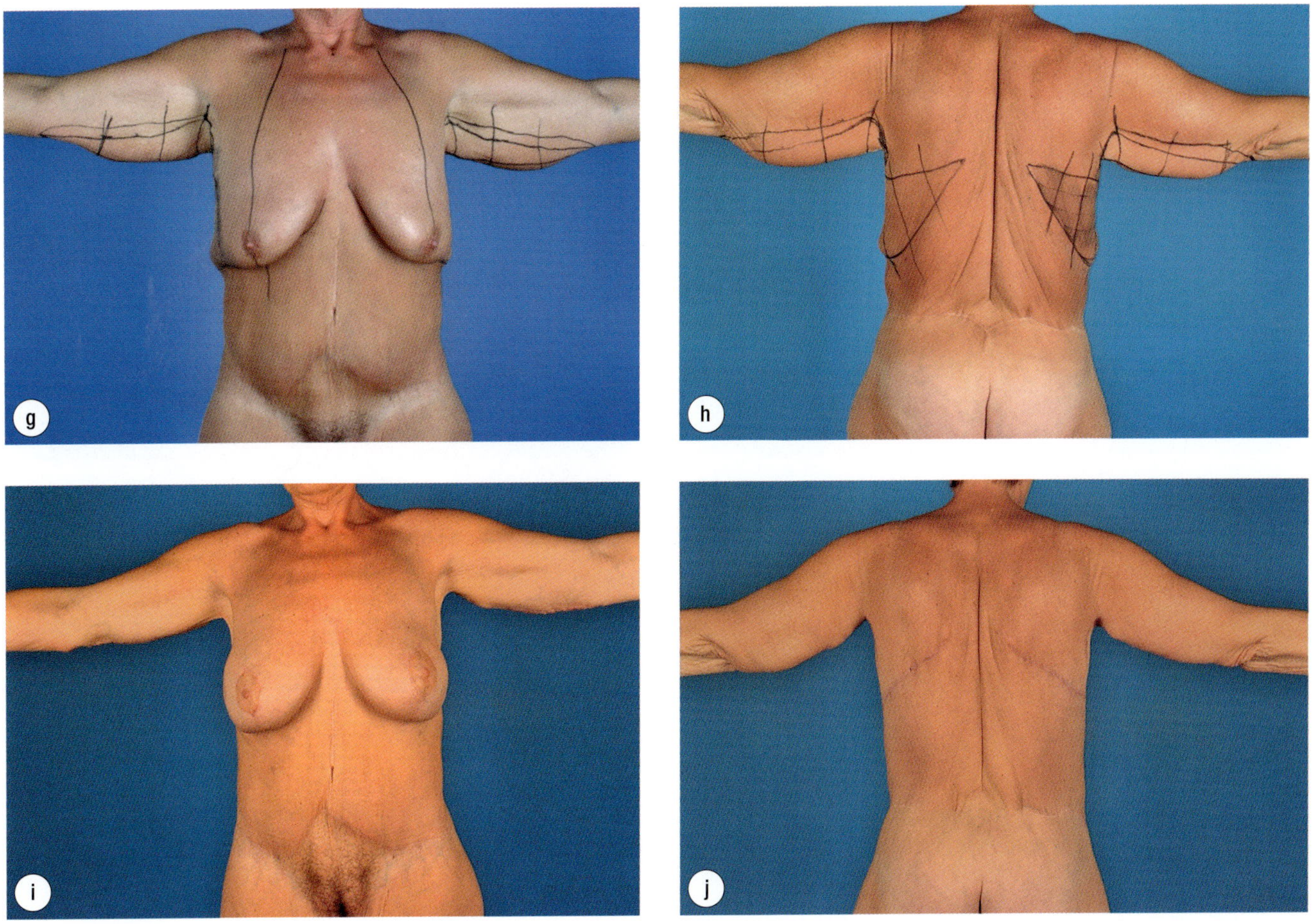

Figure 7.3 (*cont'd*)

Surgical technique

The patient is placed in the prone position after induction of general anesthesia, and then widely prepared and draped. The superior anchor line is incised along its entire length, and a flap undermined at the level of the deep fascia in a caudal direction. The inferior line of resection that was marked preoperatively serves as an estimate for the extent of undermining. Rather than commit to this inferior mark, a segmental resection is performed to precisely judge the amount of tissue to be removed. Multiple vertical incisions are made on the flap and the base of the incision secured to the anchor line with towel clips (Fig. 7.6). The vertical lines marking the borders of the posterior pattern, at the level of the posterior axillary line, are incised in a similar manner.

Once the margins of resection have been accurately set, the excision can be completed by marking between the towel clips. The wound is then closed with 0-braided absorbable interrupted sutures in the deep layer and 3-0 absorbable monofilament suture in the dermis. Because there is very little direct undermining outside the area of excision, drains are not routinely used on the back. A large 'dog ear' will be present at each lateral edge of the closure. This is simply closed with staples while the patient is in the prone position.

The patient is then turned to the supine position and reprepped for the mastopexy. A Wise pattern mastopexy is then performed. While the specific technique and pedicle design are not crucial, the dermal suspension method described in Chapter 4 is useful in this patient population. The breasts are closed with 3-0 absorbable monofilament sutures in the dermis and a single large Jackson–Pratt drain placed in each breast. Because the lateral Wise pattern marks stopped several centimeters anterior to the border of the posterior pattern, an intervening 'double dog ear' will be present on each flank. This small tissue flap is excised as a final step in the operation.

Postoperative care

A compressive dressing is kept in place for 5 days and the drains removed when output is less than 30 cc in 24 h. Oral antibiotics are prescribed while the drains are in place. Heavy lifting and vigorous exercise are avoided until 4 weeks postoperatively.

Results

Figure 7.7 shows preoperative and postoperative views at 3 months after surgery. Note the correction of breast ptosis, lateral chest rolls, and back rolls. The scar is hidden beneath the patient's brassiere.

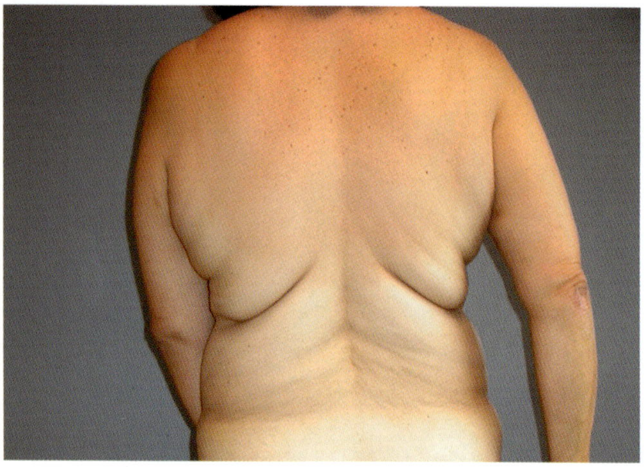

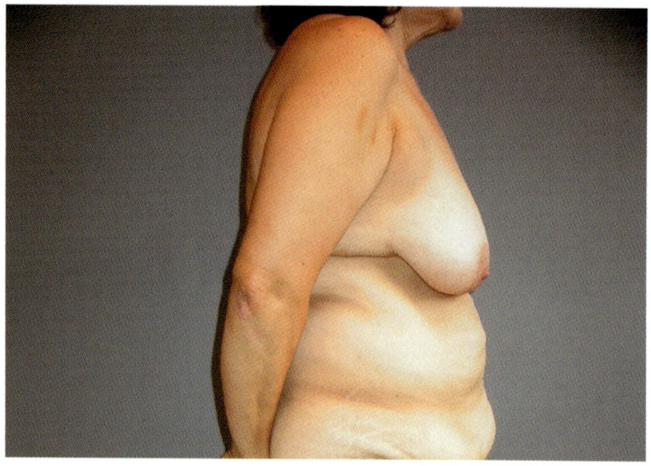

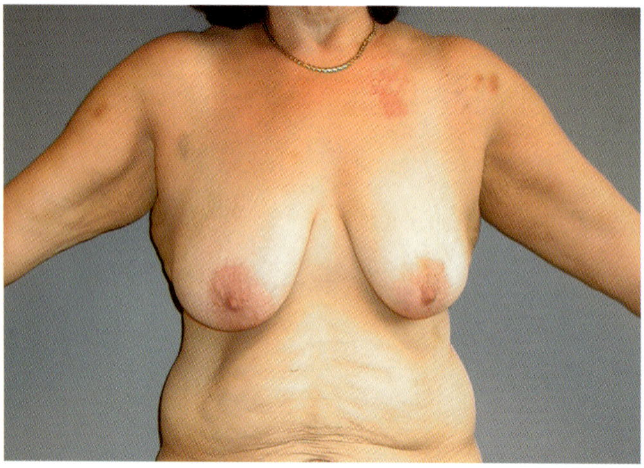

Figure 7.4 A 49-year-old woman after 110 lb (50 kg) weight loss who demonstrates significant back rolls and breast ptosis.

Complications

Complications have been minor with this procedure, consisting primarily of small wound dehiscences that healed with local wound care. Patients are advised of the risk of prominent scars from this procedure.

APPROACH 3: VERTICAL EXCISION OF BACK ROLLS WITH SCARS ALONG MIDAXILLARY LINE COMBINED WITH MASTOPEXY

This approach employs a bilateral flank excision and allows for elevation of generous faciocutaneous flaps that can be used for autologous breast augmentation.

Markings

The patient is marked in the standing position, utilizing a pinch test to determine the width of resection along the flank (Fig. 7.8). A key point is to have an assistant hold the tissues under tension on one side while the other side is marked. This helps prevent over-estimation of the resection and asymmetry between the two sides. The resection is marked in the style of a classic transposition flap, with the anterior margin extending into the dome of the axilla so the flap can be turned into the breast.

Surgical technique

The patient is placed in the supine position after induction of general anesthesia and widely prepped and draped. The anterior border of the flap is incised along its entire length and a flap undermined in a posterior direction at the level of the deep fascia. Care is taken to avoid injury to the long thoracic nerve. Once the flap is undermined and the posterior mark is double-checked to ensure closure of the wound, the posterior line is incised. The flap is then elevated and trimmed distally until adequate bleeding from the flap edge is noted. Introperative fluorescien may also be used to assess flap viability. The flap is deephelialized and a subglandular pocket dissected. The flap is then turned into this pocket and secured to the pectoralis fascia with absorbable O-braided suture (Fig. 7.9). The wound is then closed with O-braided absorbable interrupted sutures in the deep SFS layer and 3–0 absorbable monofilament suture in the dermis. Drains are placed prior to completing the closure (Fig. 7.10).

Postoperative care

A compressive dressing is kept in place for 5 days and the drains removed when output is less than 30 cc in 24 h. Oral antibiotics are prescribed while the drains are in place. Heavy lifting and vigorous exercise are avoided until 4 weeks postoperatively.

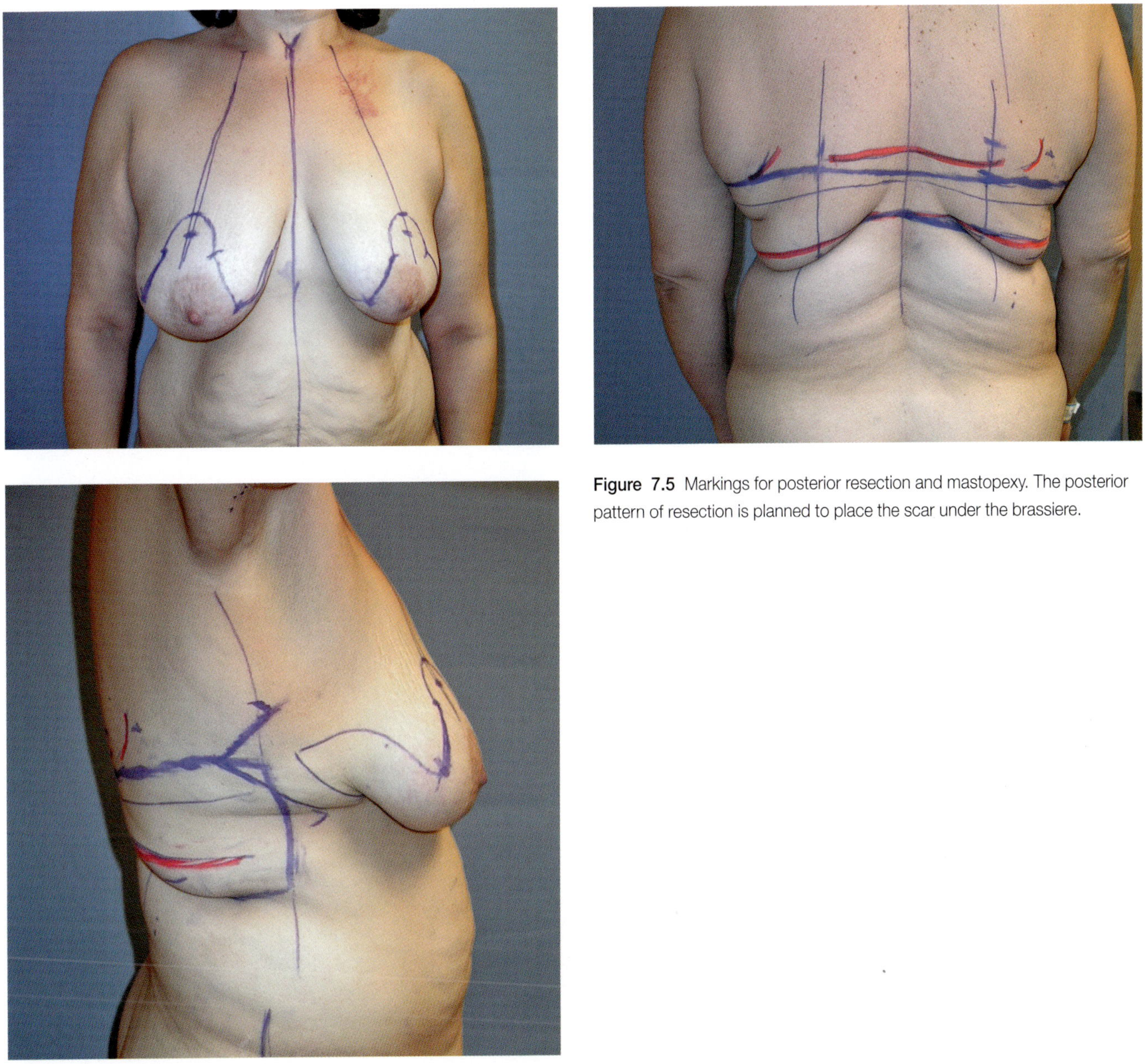

Figure 7.5 Markings for posterior resection and mastopexy. The posterior pattern of resection is planned to place the scar under the brassiere.

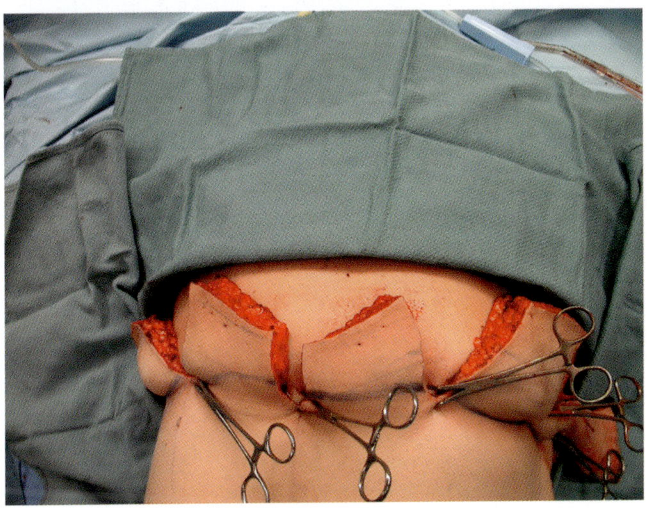

Figure 7.6 Segmental resection of posterior tissue avoids overresection and inability to close. The superior anchor line is excised first.

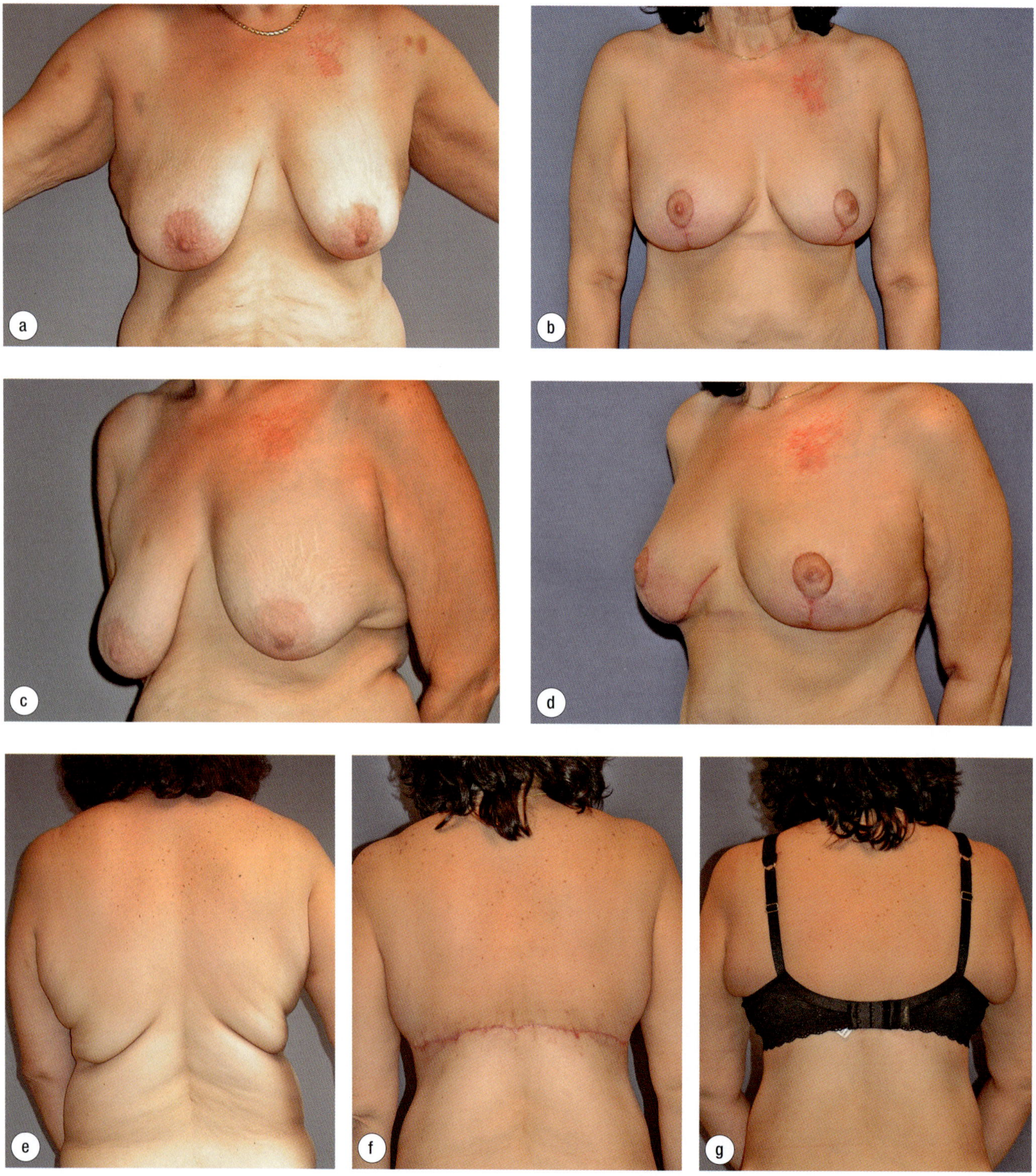

Figure 7.7 (**a, c,** and **e**) Preoperative views and (**b, d, f,** and **g**) postoperative views at 3 months after surgery.

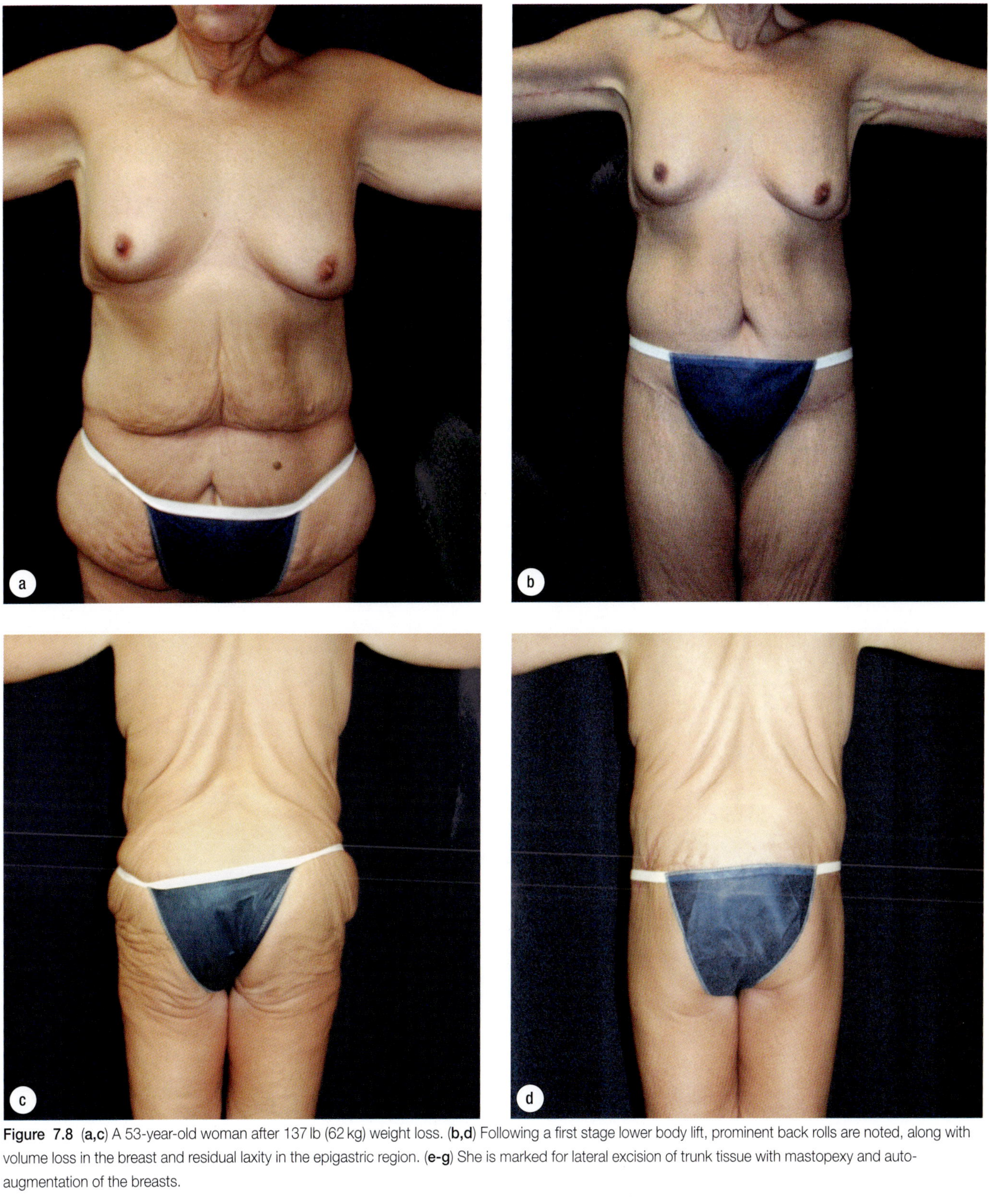

Figure 7.8 (**a,c**) A 53-year-old woman after 137 lb (62 kg) weight loss. (**b,d**) Following a first stage lower body lift, prominent back rolls are noted, along with volume loss in the breast and residual laxity in the epigastric region. (**e-g**) She is marked for lateral excision of trunk tissue with mastopexy and auto-augmentation of the breasts.

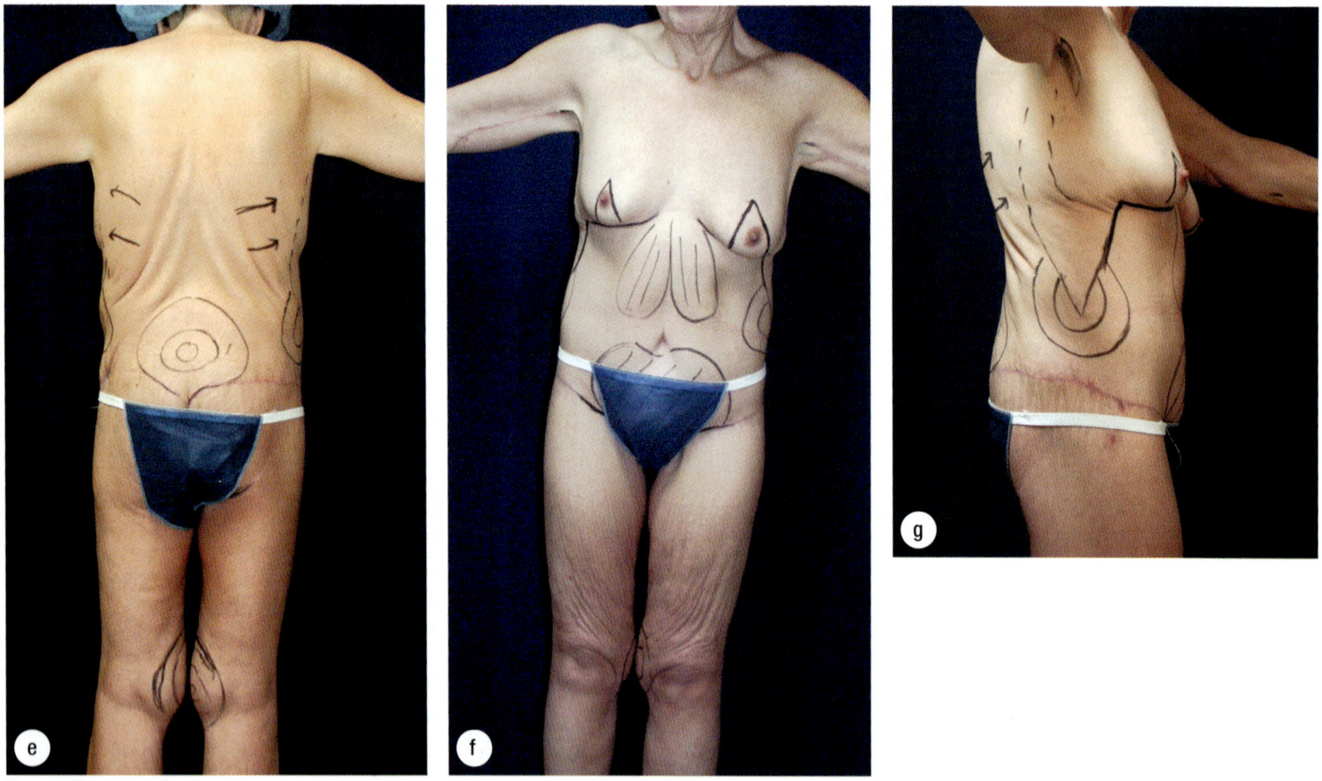

Figure 7.8 (*cont'd*)

Results

Figures 7.11 and 7.12 show preoperative and postoperative views at 6 months after surgery. Note the correction of breast ptosis, lateral chest rolls, and back rolls. While liposuction of the flap pivot point may be considered post-operatively to debulk the lateral prominence and prevent a 'boxy' appearance to the breasts, this has not been necessary in the cases performed to date.

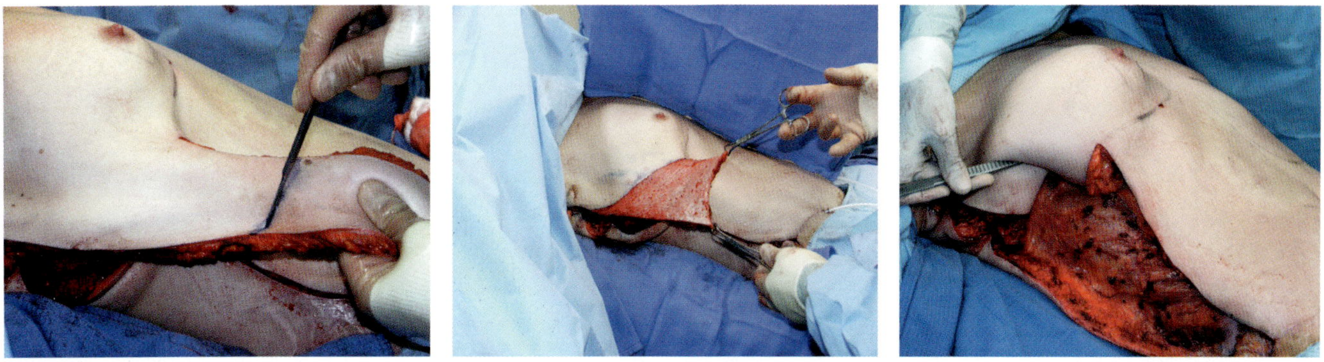

Figure 7.9 Intraoperative views showing elevation of tissue flap along flank, deepithelialization of flap, and transposition of flap into subglandular breast pocket.

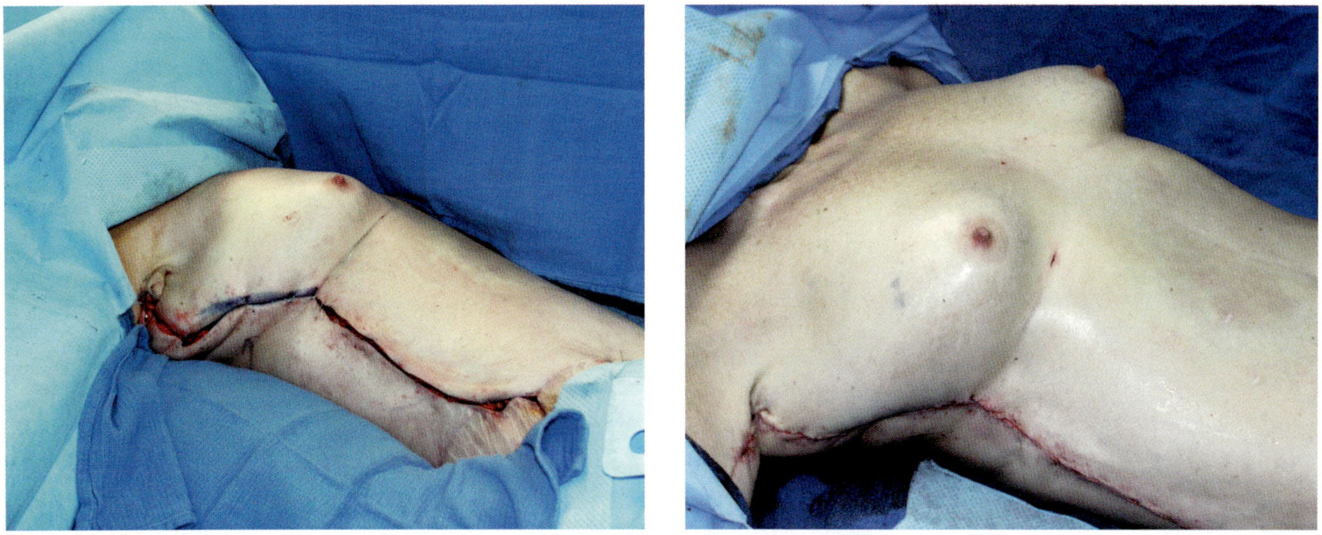

Figure 7.10 Intraoperative views demonstrating lateral scar and increased breast volume from autologous augmentation.

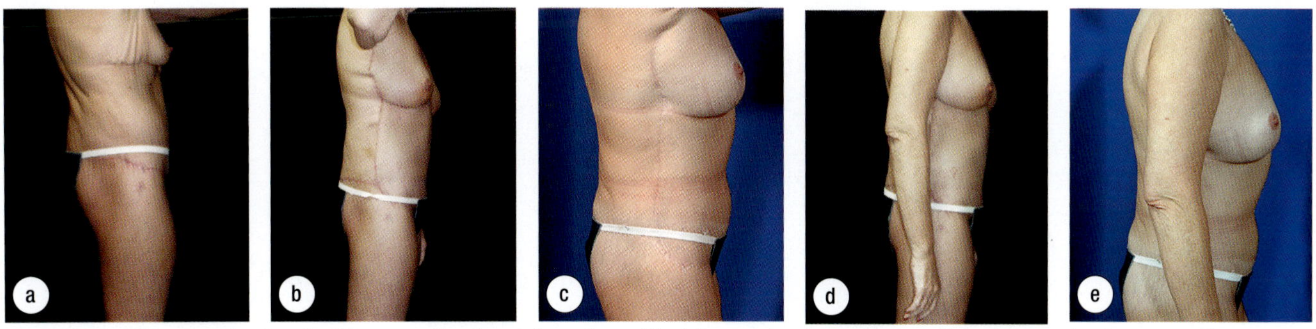

Figure 7.11 (**a**) Preoperative view. (**b,d**) Postoperative view at 2 months and (**c,e**) 2 years showing maturation of lateral scar and maintenance of breast shape.

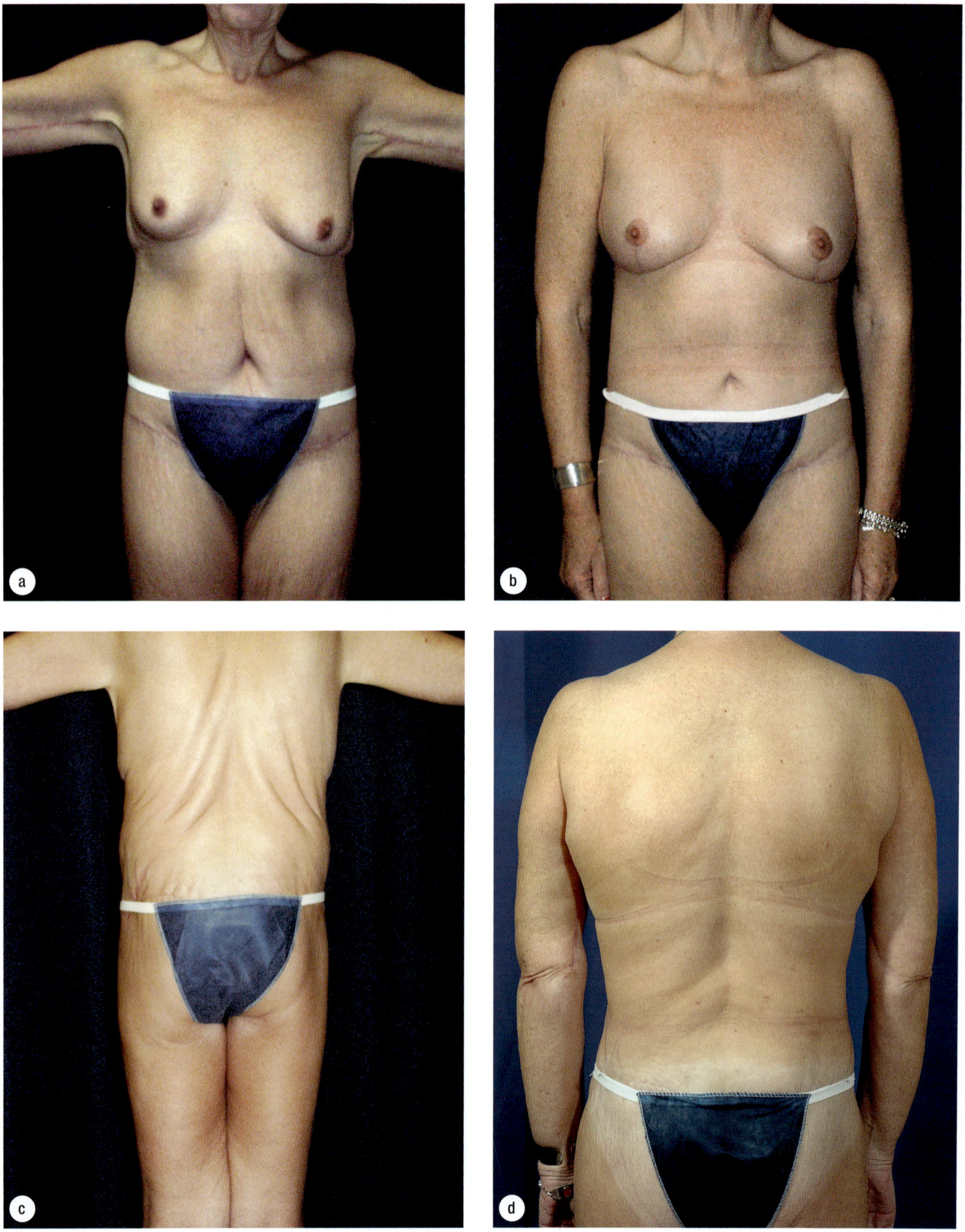

Figure 7.12 (**a,c**) Preoperative views and (**b,d**) postoperative views at 2 years.

APPROACH TO THE MEDIAL THIGH AFTER WEIGHT LOSS

8

Dennis J. Hurwitz

> **Key Points**
> - Single-stage integration of the medial lift and type incision into the lower body operative correction.
> - Accurate presurgical marking of a unique excision design using multiple positions.
> - Efficient use of prone and supine operative positions.
> - Excision of medial thigh skin from groin to knee improves the entire thigh contour.
> - Minor delayed wound healing in the upper medial thighs and seromas of the lower medial thighs are common.

Medial thighplasty is aesthetic reshaping of the thigh following removal of excess medial skin and fat. The new contour should be attractive, the scars inconspicuous, and complications minor. Medial thighplasty may be solely an upper thigh crescent excision adjacent to the labia majora (or scrotum),[1–4] extended with a wide band excision tapering at the knee for distal deformity,[3,5] or something in between. The extent of surgery depends on the deformity, patient expectations, and acceptance of trade-offs.

Recontouring thighs after massive weight loss is daunting for the following reasons.

- The deformity is considerable and complex.
- Thighs are large and exposed.
- The therapeutic index is narrow.
- A range of only several centimeters of skin resection is the difference between skin laxity and descended scars.
- Vertical extension scars are visible.
- Operative positioning and wound closure are awkward.
- Symmetry and optimal aesthetics are uncommon.
- Delayed healing, prolonged edema, and seromas are common.
- Distortion of the vulva and thrombophlebitis are concerns.

The L thighplasty integrates into the lower body lift and abdominoplasty to improve the vertical thighplasty, just as the brachioplasty integrates with the upper body lift.[5] The 'L' relates to the shape of the excision and resulting scar, with the long limb along the length of the medial thigh and the short limb between the thigh and the labia majora and mons pubis. The essential approach involves the following.

- Accurate presurgical marking of a unique excision design using multiple positions.
- Excision of medial thigh skin to improve the thigh contour.
- Single-stage integration of the medial lift into the lower body operative correction.
- Efficient use of prone and supine operative positions.

The thigh weight loss deformity varies by genetics, extent of loss, and residual obesity. For women who have lost most of their excess weight, there is a characteristic presentation (Fig. 8.1). Except for the lower lateral thigh, the skin is diffusely loose and flaccid. The medial thighs invariable sag most, with cascading transverse rolls. The anterior thighs have layered waves of skin. The upper lateral thighs slump into bulging saddlebags, abruptly stopping at the midthigh. The buttocks atrophy, with inferior accordion-like pleats of skin. Looseness of the upper posterior thigh is subtle. Inadequate weight loss leaves bulging thighs (Fig. 8.2).

Weight loss patients hate their thighs and hide them. Pungent odors emanate between the legs. Skin chafes under medial folds. Patients may avoid exposure during intimacy or avoid sexual activity altogether. Patients invariably welcome an upper medial thighplasty but may need encouragement to have the vertical excision extension. The surgeon should integrate medial thighplasty into complex operative planning.

Contrary to the opinion of some experts,[1,2,6–8] I favor upper medial thighplasty concomitant to lower body lift and abdominoplasty.[9–11] I believe these combined procedures are synergistic, capitalizing on the biomechanics of skin excess. For the most favorable cases without a vertical thigh extension, I offer single-stage total body lift surgery.[10]

PREOPERATIVE PREPARATION

Evaluation

The intrinsic medial thigh problem needs to be fully evaluated and then placed in the context of the remaining thigh and lower body deformity. During the examination, the lower body lift

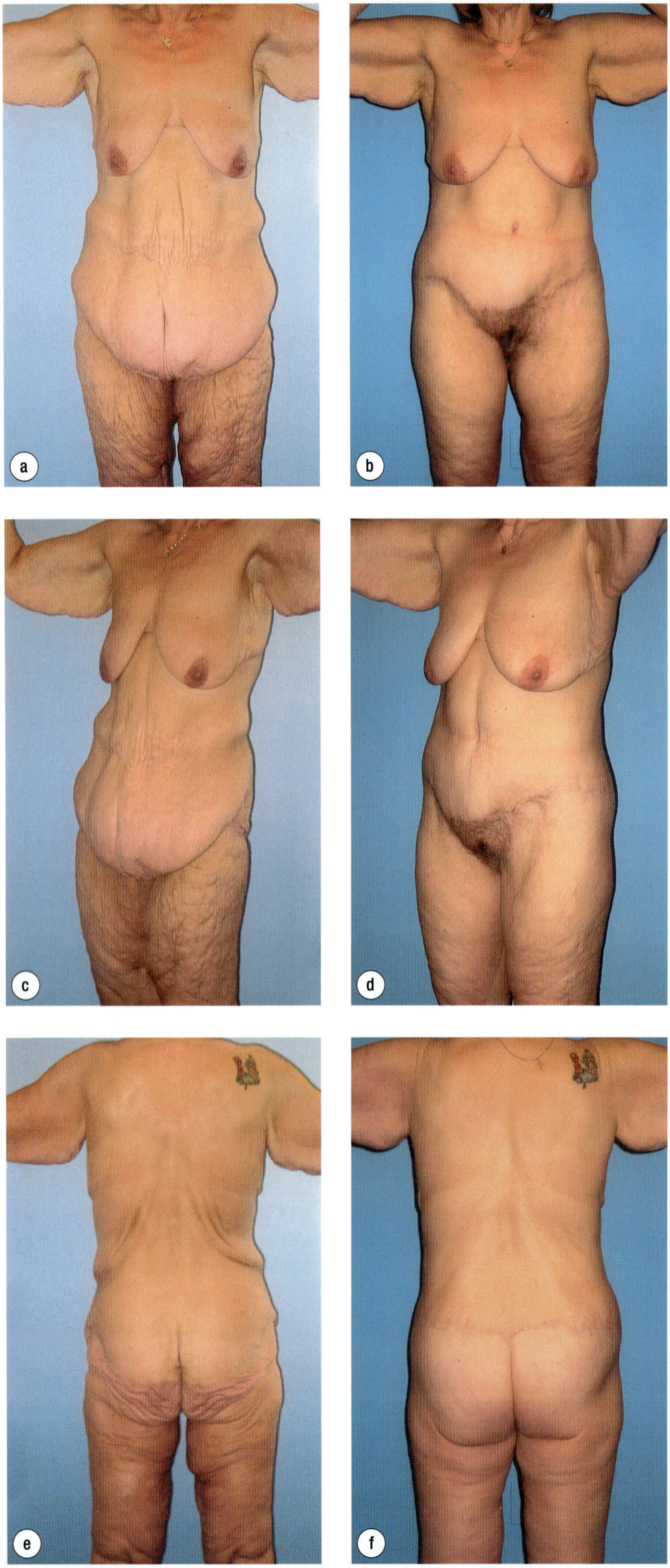

Figure 8.1 Multiple views of the thighs of a 49-year-old, 5' 7" (1.70 m), 157-lb (71 kg) woman (**a, c, e, g, i**) before and (**b, d, f, h, j**) 5 months after an L thighplasty with an abdominoplasty and lower body lift reported in the *Aesthetic Surgery Journal*.[5] She had lost 230 lbs (104 kg) subsequent to a gastric restrictive procedure and hated her thighs. Her rolls of redundant skin were worst medial, and least upper anterior and lower lateral thigh. The medial thighs had cascading transverse loose rolls of skin. The middle anterior thighs had stacked layers of skin like melted candle wax. Loose skin hung from the hips to the midlateral thigh. The buttocks had inferior accordion-like pleats. Except for the distal thigh, the postoperative views show these deformities corrected by a single complex 10-h operation, as described. The scars are level, symmetric, and narrow. There are long but inconspicuous scars running down the medial posterior thighs, between the labia and thigh, and in a beltlike manner around the lower torso. The buttock curvature is full due to the adipose flap reconstruction. There is some residual looseness below the buttocks and about the knees, which will be corrected secondarily.

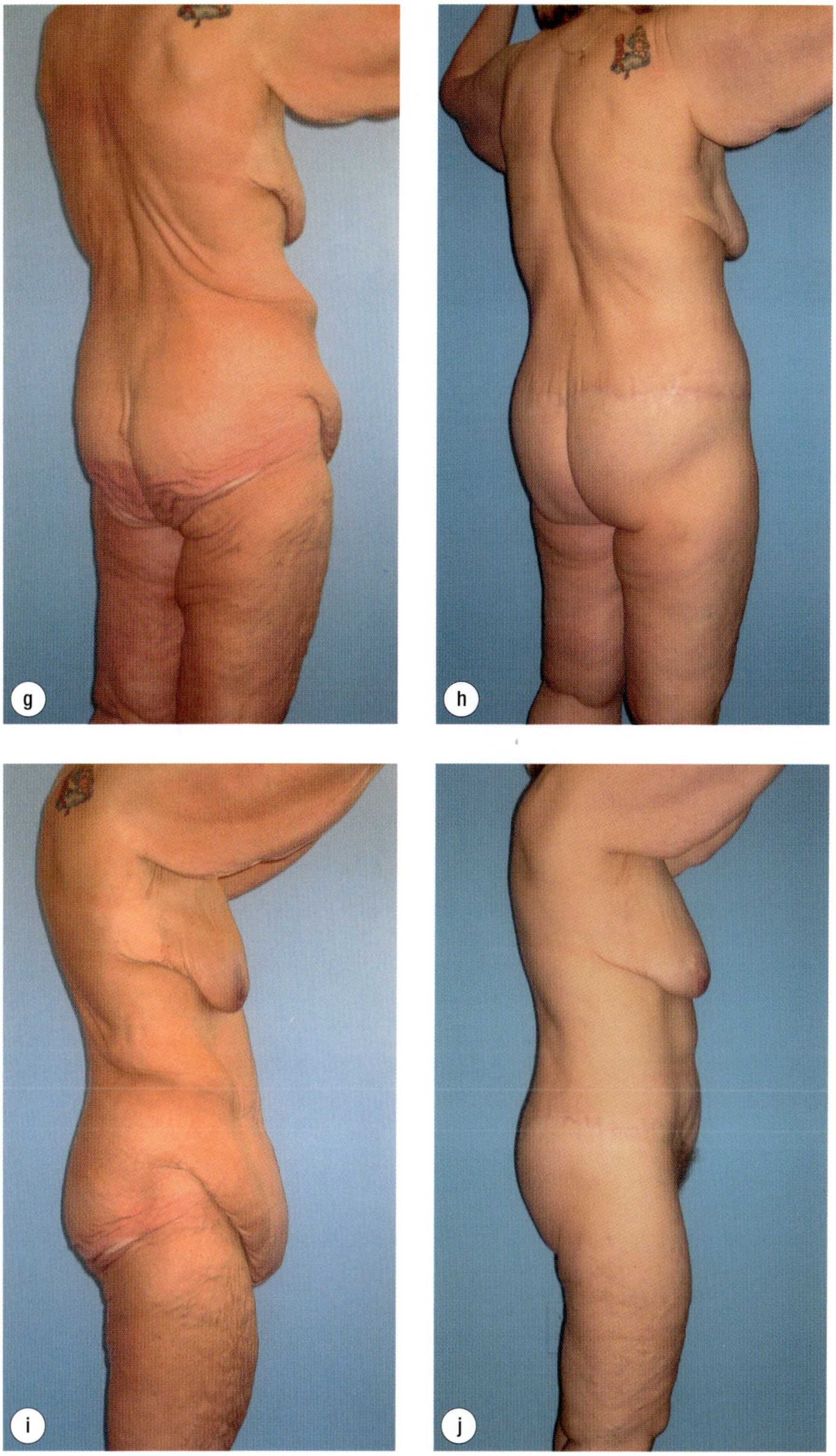

Figure 8.1 (*cont'd*)

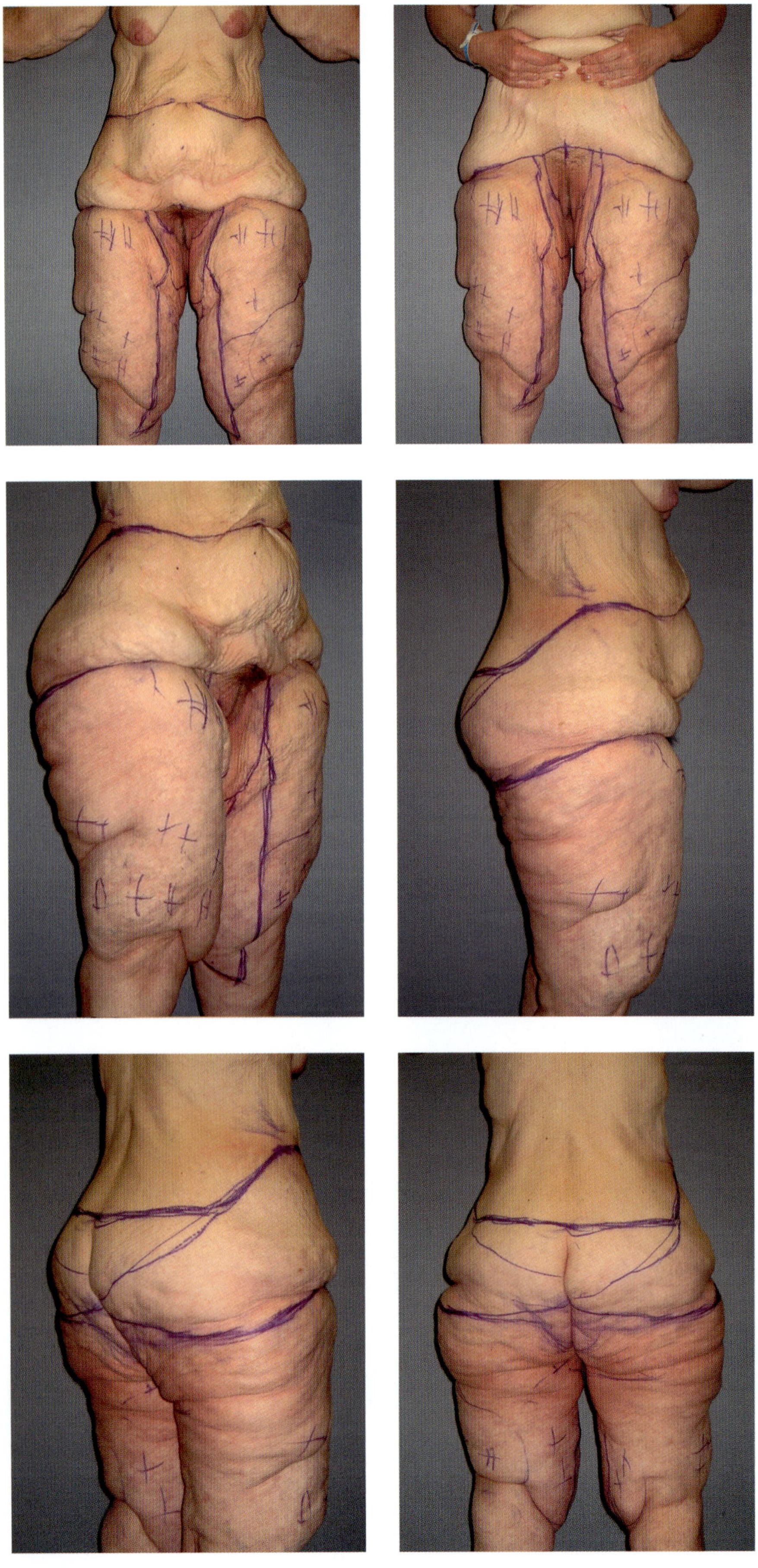

Figure 8.2 This 60-year-old, 5' 7" (1.70 m), 200-lb (91 kg) woman had persistent large and sagging thighs after gastric bypass and 150-lb (68 kg) weight loss. Her lower body lift, abdominoplasty, and L thighplasty were accompanied by ultrasound-assisted lipoplasty of over 1000 cc of fat on each side. Fat excess billows out everywhere but most prominently along the medial thighs, hips, and saddlebags. The markings for her operation have just been completed. The plus signs indicate anticipated relative amounts for liposuction.

can be simulated by having the patient pull up on her lower abdomen, buttocks, and saddlebags. The lateral thigh should be tight and the residual thigh redundancy mainly anterior and medial.

With the patient standing, observe overall thigh skin drape, excess, bulges, and tension. If the patient varies from the usual deformity, adjustments from routine planning should be considered. If a concomitant abdominoplasty is to be performed, the examination continues with the patient suspending the abdominal apron. This aids visualization and simulates anticipated tension on the upper thigh. Note the distance between the medial thighs. Observe the pattern of sagging. Loose skin of the inner thigh tends to be greatest proximal, like a scarf draped around the neck. Note the relationship of skin to underlying adipose. There is a continuum of skin excess from wrinkled layers to bulging from underlying fat. Thin tissues need no discontinuous undermining. Bulging fat suggests the need for concomitant liposuction, preliminary lipoplasty or further weight loss.

After simulating the anticipated crescent excision by firmly pulling up the sagging skin of the upper thigh skin to the labia majora, one examines the remaining inner thigh. If the patient still objects to her distal thigh laxity, explain that an upper lift will be inadequate. If the distal thigh is acceptable, then the vertical band extension is unnecessary. Grab the patient's distal excess and shake it to be sure that she understands what will be left behind if a vertical lift is not done. Skin laxity and bulges about the knee should be pointed out and will not be adequately treated in the primary operation. If the medial thigh skin bulging still touches, adjuvant liposuction will be needed.

For the overweight thigh, excess fat is removed with as little bleeding as possible. Hemorrhage is indicative of vascular injury, which may compromise flap survival. I believe that carefully performed ultrasound-assisted lipoplasty is more selective for fat and sparing of vasculature. I have considerable experience with both the LySonics ultrasound lipoplasty (Mentor Corporation, Santa Barbara, California) and Vaser LipoSelection (Sound Surgical Technologies, Boulder, Colorado) systems for concomitant defatting of large skin flaps. When used with care, both these systems are more gentle than traditional liposuction, but my preference is for Vaser. The postoperative recovery appears quicker and less painful. I believe that Vaser is the better technology. With the assistance of the VentX aspiration system, thermal injury and the destruction of supportive subcutaneous tissue appears less. On the other hand, Vaser is slower in its effect. I declare a potential conflict of interest, as I was an original scientific adviser for Sound Surgical Technologies and have unexercised stock options.

For excessively thin and loose skin thighs, multiple vertical band excision is necessary. For extreme cases, an additional lateral band excision is required (Fig. 8.3).

Preoperative markings

For these complex operations to be aesthetic, inconspicuous and predictable scar location is essential. Scar position relates to the extent and location of skin excision, as well as the closure tension. The magnitude of skin removal is determined through tissue-gathering maneuvers, preferably of the most redundant areas. Gender-specific contour is enhanced by attention to appropriate retention of subcutaneous tissue. Regimented planning gives confidence to judge the position and width of each skin resection, assuring accurate scar location. Then the adjacent dependent region can be planned. For example, the drawing for the crescent medial thighplasty begins only after the design for abdominoplasty is complete. Likewise, the medial thigh vertical excision extension follows design of the upper crescent (Fig. 8.4).

Preoperative incision markings are customarily sighted while the patient is standing. However, the sheer magnitude of massive weight loss hanging pannus, buttocks, and thigh skin is awkward and confounding. Hence I developed a sequence of recumbent body and limb positioning for orderly, unrestricted, and painless tissue gathering and incision drawing. In the usual case, I combine the medial thighplasty with an abdominoplasty and lower body lift.[5,9–12]

Markings start with the abdominoplasty.

1. The patient is reclined and evenly pulls up on her pannus until the ptotic mons pubis is fully effaced.
2. A 14-cm long transverse line is centered over the mons about 7 cm superior to the commissure of the labia majora.
3. With the patient's pannus then pulled obliquely toward the opposite costal margin, the lateral inferior skin incision is drawn straight to the anterior iliac spine.
4. The patient then turns on her side and her leg is abducted.
5. With the loose skin messaged to her hip, the line is drawn over the upper buttocks straight to her intergluteal fold.
6. Along the midaxillary line, the widest lower torso resection is marked by tissue gathering and pinching.
7. From that point, a tapering line is drawn to the umbilicus and lower midback.

The upper crescent medial thighplasty markings are made the same whether or not a vertical band extension is performed (Figs 8.4 and 8.5).

1. With the loose inner thigh skin pushed toward the knee, the upper incision line is drawn between the labia majora and thigh. This line is a continuation of a perpendicular dropped from the transverse lower abdominoplasty incision.
2. Posterior to the labia, the upper line veers beyond the ischial tuberosity.
3. The point of maximal resection along the midmedial thigh is determined with the thigh flexed and adducted.
4. After pushing all loose skin beneath the pubic ramus, the inferior resection line is marked at the level of the labia majora.
5. With the leg again abducted, the crescent-shaped inferior incision line from this inferior resection mark is extended anterior to the outer mons pubis line and posterior to the buttock thigh junction line. This outer mons pubis line is a second perpendicular line made several centimeters lateral to the first lateral mons pubic line. The width of this

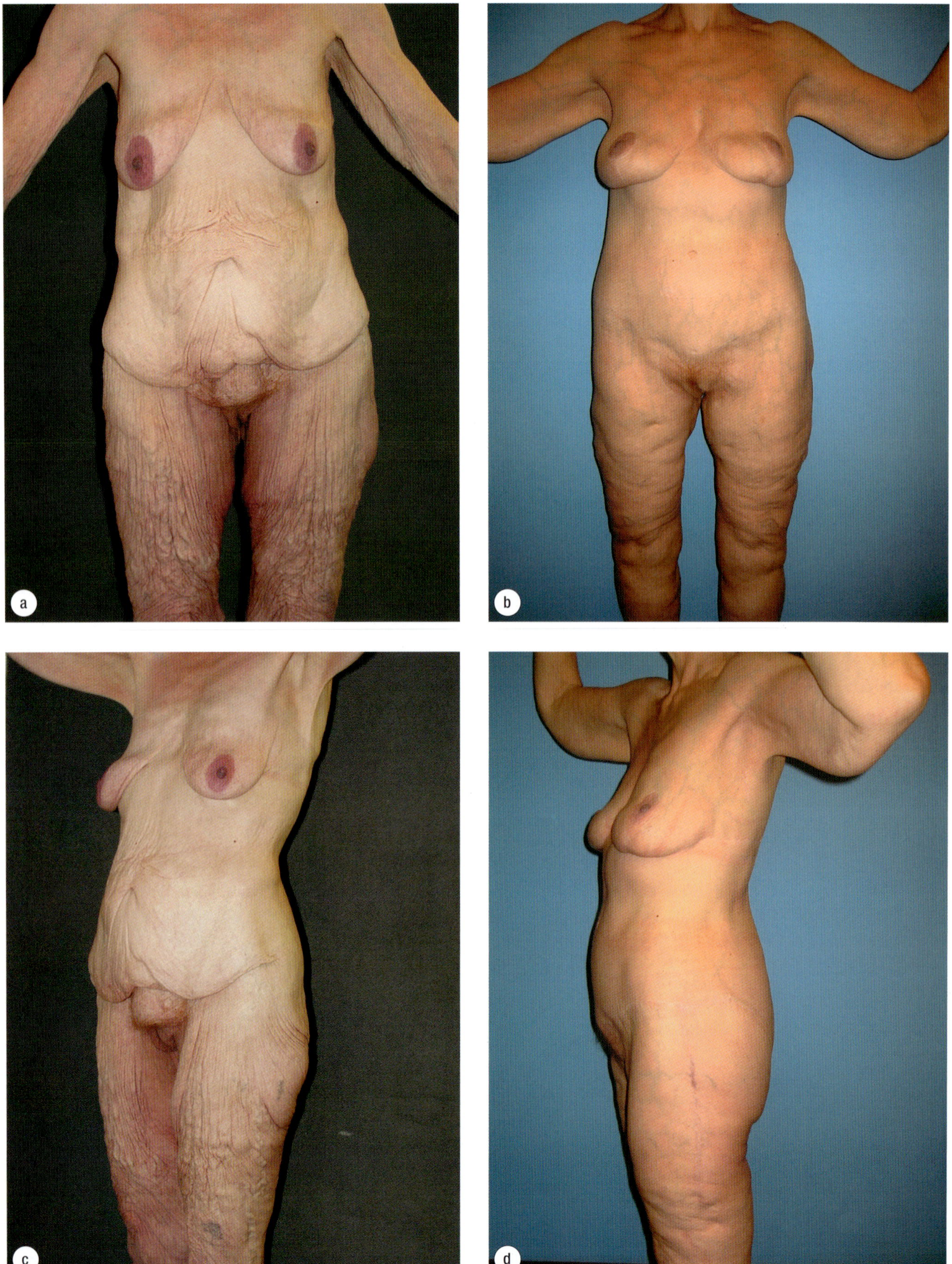

Figure 8.3 This 58-year-old, 5' 7" (1.70 m) woman weighed 130 lbs (59 kg) after losing 188 lbs (85 kg), and had dramatic loose skin circumferentially around her thighs. Extreme wrinkling of the anterior thighs, looking like melted wax, is seen on these standing views (**a** and **c**). A year after the L thighplasty, a vertical lateral thigh ellipse of skin was removed to complete the correction seen 6 months later (**b** and **d**).

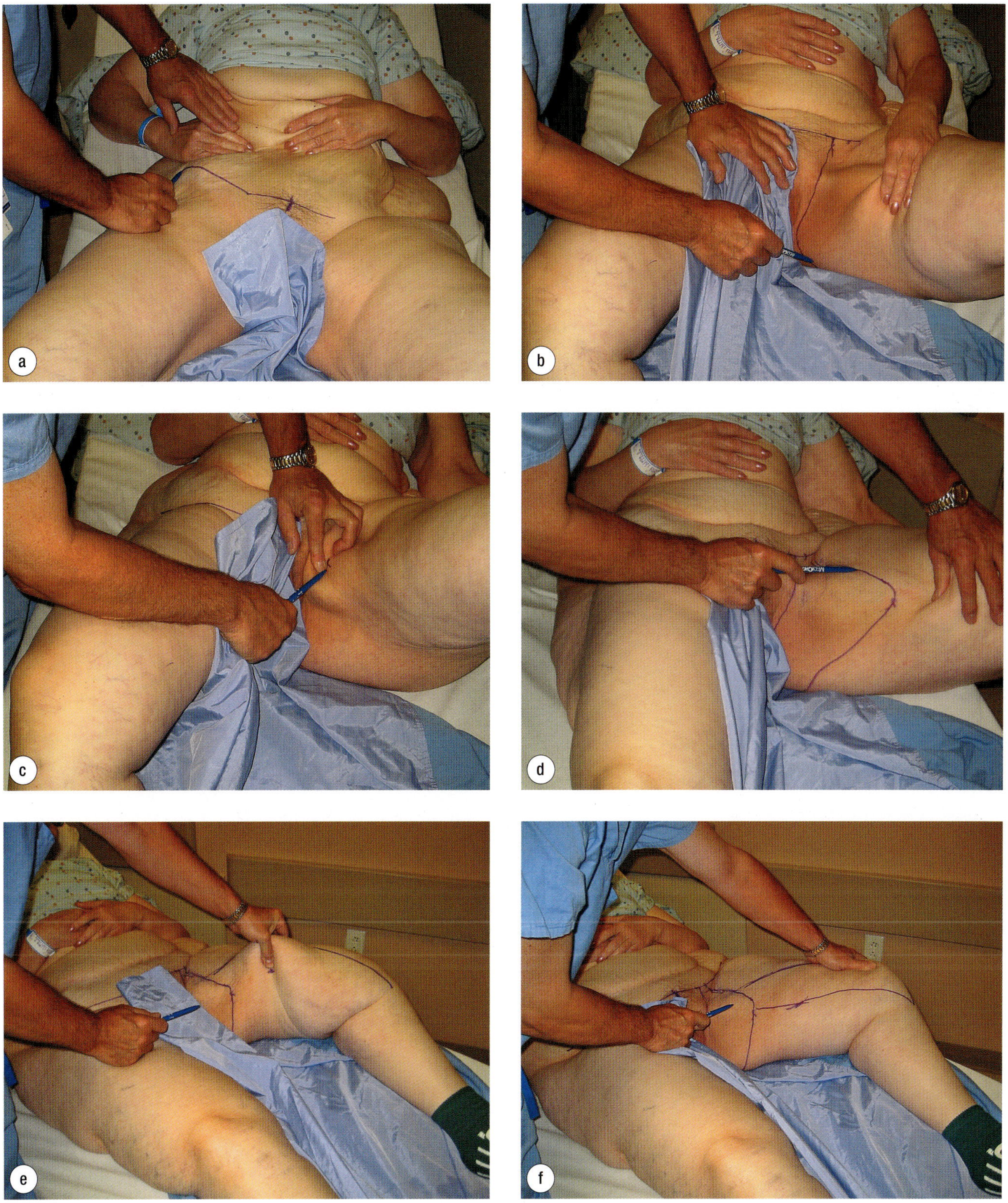

Figure 8.4 The essential steps in marking the L thighplasty. (**a**) By appropriate cephalad traction on the abdominal pannus, the lower incision line of the abdominoplasty is drawn. (**b**) The leg is moderately abducted as the loose inner thigh skin is pushed toward the knee to mark the upper incision line between the labia majora and thigh. (**c**) The point of maximal resection along the midmedial thigh is determined with the thigh flexed and adducted. After pushing loose skin beneath the pubic ramus, the midmedial thigh inferior resection line is marked. (**d**) With the leg again abducted, the crescent-shaped inferior incision line from this inferior resection mark is extended anterior to the outer mons pubis line and posterior to the buttock thigh junction line. Later, while the patient is standing and with the lifted buttock position simulated, the 'dog ear' triangular inferior gluteal thigh resection is made. (**e**) The patient remains supine during planning of the long limb of the vertical band extension to the knee. With medial drag on the anterior thigh skin, the anterior excision line is drawn along the midmedial line. Then gather the width of maximal resection at the midthigh as shown and mark this point. (**f**) From this midthigh mark, a widening posterior incision line is drawn from below knee to the ischial tuberosity. Finally, the angle between this vertical limb and the upper crescent excision is narrowed by edging the superior portion of the anterior line further posterior. The patient then stands to adjust the markings.

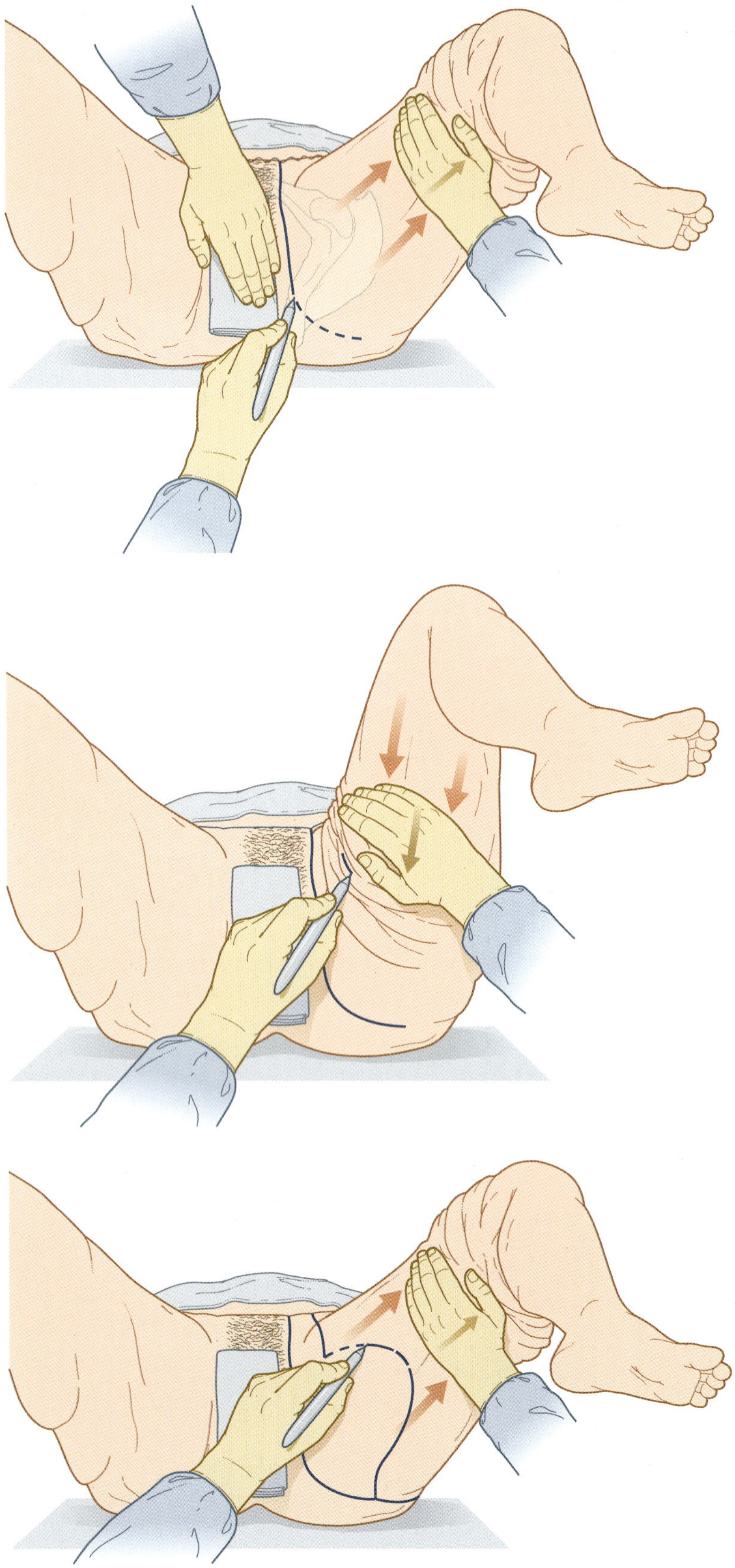

Figure 8.5 The upper medial thighplasty. (**a**) In this perineal view, the patient flexes her left hip and abducts the thigh. As an assistant pushes the loose thigh skin toward the knee, I draw the superior incision line between the labia majora and thigh. (**b**) The point of maximal resection along the midmedial thigh is determined with the thigh flexed and adducted. (**c**) As the thigh is again abducted, the crescent-shaped inferior incision line is extended from this inferior resection mark anterior to the outer mons pubis line and posterior to the buttock thigh junction line. See text for details.

resection of paramedian pubic skin is just enough to efface the mons pubis.

6. While the patient is standing and the lifted buttock position simulated, the 'dog ear' triangular gluteal thigh resection is marked.

The vertical excision extended medial thighplasty is called an L thighplasty because the resections and subsequent scar form the letter 'L' from pubis to knees.

1. The short limb of the L plasty (crescent upper thigh excision) is planned first, with the patient supine and the thigh flexed and abducted as just described.
2. The long limb of the L (vertical band extension to the knee) is also planned supine (Figs 8.4 and 8.6). With the leg on the bed, and superior and medial drag on the anterior thigh skin, the anterior excision line is drawn from medial knee up the thigh to the apex of the crescent excision line.
3. Then gather the width of maximal resection at the midthigh and mark this point.
4. From this midthigh mark, a widening posterior incision line is drawn from below knee to the ischial tuberosity.
5. Finally, the angle between this vertical limb and the upper crescent excision is narrowed by edging the superior portion of the anterior line further posterior. This change in position moves the scar slightly posterior, which creates an L shape.
6. For symmetry, the lines are emphasized and then the thighs are rubbed together to imprint one on to the other.
7. The accuracy is confirmed by tissue gathering.
8. The patient then stands to adjust the markings as needed (Fig. 8.7).

SURGICAL TECHNIQUE

The thighplasty begins with the lower body lift. The surgeon stands to the right side of the prone patient, facing the buttocks. Along the suture lines and the anticipated planes of dissection, she or he liberally infuses dilute vasoconstrictor and anesthetic (1 mg of adrenaline [epinephrine] and 20 cc of 1% lidocaine [Xylocaine] per liter of saline). In three or four swipes, the inferior posterior incision is made down to muscular fascia with a scalpel from anterior superior iliac spine (ASIS) across the buttocks, the lumbar spine, and the opposite buttocks to the opposite ASIS. Electrocautery cutting is avoided because thermal injury may reduce the suture holding of the subsequent tightly closed subcutaneous fascia. The buttock incision stops at the gluteus maximus muscle and continues laterally to the fascia lata. Scattered fascial adherences from the fascia lata to the lateral thigh deep dermis are released to beyond the palpable lateral trochanter.

Ultrasound-assisted lipoplasty of the lateral thighs debulks overly full subcutaneous tissue. Discontinuous undermining is provided as needed by forceful thrusts of Lockwood dissectors (Padgett Instruments, Kansas City, Missouri) over the fascia lata to nearly the knee. After mobilizing the lateral thigh skin, the superior incision line is confirmed. There needs to be enough mobilization of the lateral thigh so that the skin, not the underlying fascial extensions, is limiting cephalad advancement. The previously marked superior incision along the lower back is now incised to lumbodorsal fascia and external oblique muscles.

The skin and adipose between the superior and inferior incisions is resected at the desired depth. Usually, most of the large globular lumbar fat is preserved. If fat flap buttock augmentation is planned, then only a beltlike band of skin is removed (Fig. 8.8). The buttock skin is elevated off the upper two-thirds of the gluteus maximus muscle for a space for the adipose flap. The retained lower back mobile pad of adipose can be advanced and sutured inferiorly to augment the buttocks (Fig. 8.9). The lower buttock skin flap is then sutured to the lower back superior incision.

The lower torso midlateral wide resection with tight closure effaces the saddlebag deformity. In order to close the gap under the least tension, the leg is abducted on a wide arm board rotated out about 45°. Large, deeply placed absorbable sutures secure the lateral thigh deep dermis to the fascia lata of the thigh. The beltlike excision is closed with very large, absorbable braided sutures in the subcutaneous fascia, followed by an intradermal closure with long-lasting monofilament absorbable sutures.

While assistants close the lower body lift, the surgeon removes the anticipated infragluteal dog ears of the medial thighplasties under the buttock folds. In the unusual situation, when the posterior thigh is very loose, this excision can be as wide as 8 cm. The infragluteal excision cannot be made until the buttock lift is completed. The width of the triangular excision is adjusted inferiorly as needed. One should rely on the premarked superior incision line, which appears to curve superiorly. The depth of resection of this posterior dog ear is superficial to the facial lata, lateral to the ischial tuberosity, to avoid injury to buttock sensory inferior cluneal nerves and nutrient vasculature. If there is a vertical band excision and it is wide, then the posterior limbs are now incised through deep subcutaneous fascia. The terminal incision is more superficial to avoid injury to major lymphatics and may fishtail anterior and inferior to the knee or posterior toward the popliteal fossa. Medial to the ischial tuberosity, the posterior thigh skin and fascia lata is anchored to the bony prominence periosteum with two to three braided sutures. Then the triangular infragluteal wound wedge is closed in two layers of absorbable sutures. Prior to turning the patient supine, the posterior vertical thigh incision is temporarily approximated with staples.

The patient is wrapped into a surgeon's gown and turned supine. Larger patients are rolled over on to a gurney. Then the gown and patient are dragged back on to the operating room table. To relieve tension on lower abdominal skin, the patient is frog-legged. After a second antiseptic preparation, dilute anesthetic and vasoconstricting fluid is again injected into anticipated incisions and areas for liposuction and undermining. The abdominoplasty is resumed with the inferior incision from ASIS across the groins through the mons pubis, and completed

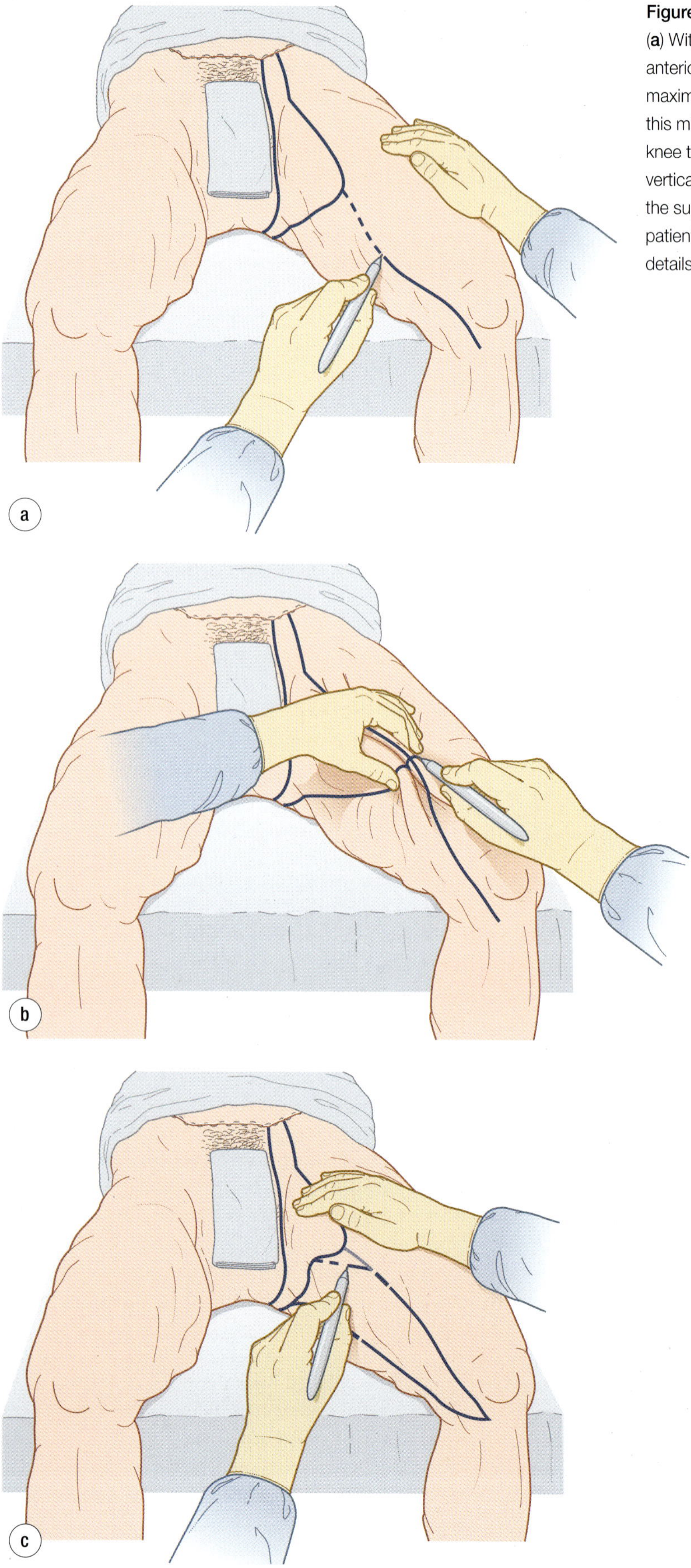

Figure 8.6 The vertical excision band extension to the knee. (**a**) With the leg on the bed, and superior and medial drag on the anterior thigh skin, the anterior excision line is drawn. (**b**) The width of maximal resection at the midthigh is gathered and marked. (**c**) From this midthigh mark, a widening posterior incision line from below knee to the ischial tuberosity is drawn. The angle between this vertical limb and the upper crescent excision is widened by edging the superior portion of the anterior line posterior. After marking, the patient then stands. Adjustments are made as needed. (See text for details.)

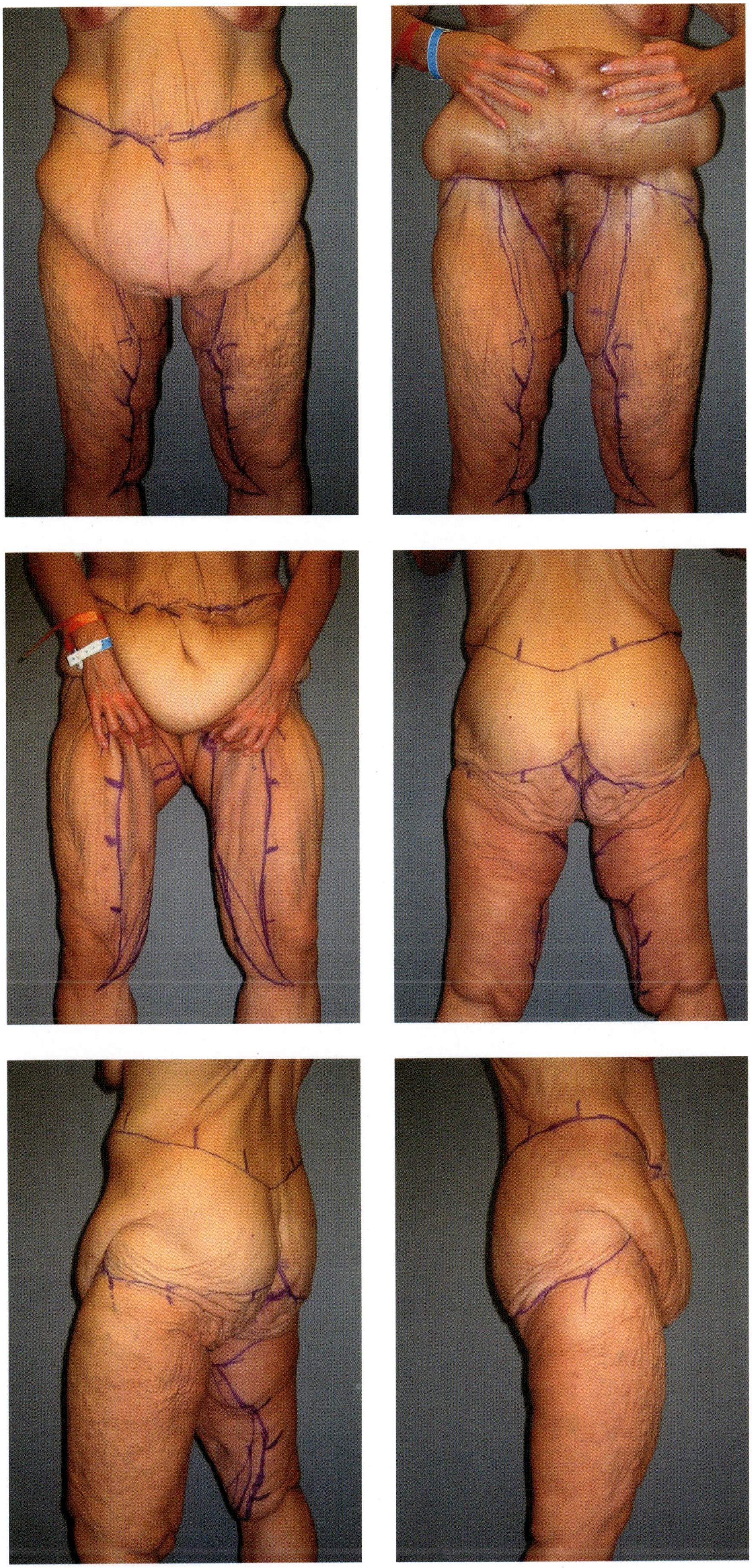

Figure 8.7 Preoperative markings for the patient in Figure 8.1. Her severely redundant thigh skin is worse medial, and least upper anterior and lower lateral thigh. The patient holds up her pannus to simulate the anticipated abdominoplasty, mildly effacing the upper anterior and medial thigh. Simulating the upper crescent excision, she suspends her vertical excision. The buttocks are flat, and lower gluteal skin folds extensive. A very broad lower back and upper gluteal excision with an intergluteal V excision is drawn. The effect of the posterior cephalad pull can be imagined after the lax lower gluteal skin is raised by the lower body lift. Remove most of the remaining upper posterior thigh wrinkling through a triangular infragluteal posterior extension of the crescent upper medial thigh lift.

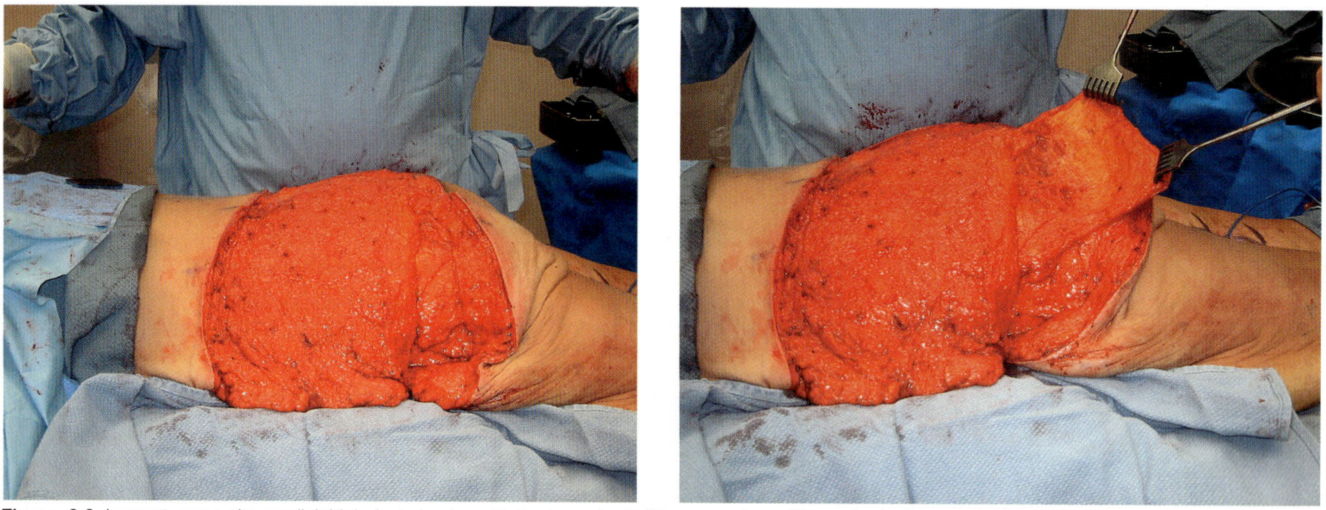

Figure 8.8 In most cases, the medial thighplasty begins with the lower body lift, as seen here. The patient of Figure 8.1 is prone on the operating room table, with the inferior and superior incisions made and removal of the intervening skin as described in the text. An inferiorly based buttock skin flap is elevated over the gluteus maximus muscle. (From Hurwitz 2005,[5] with permission of the *Aesthetic Surgery Journal*.)

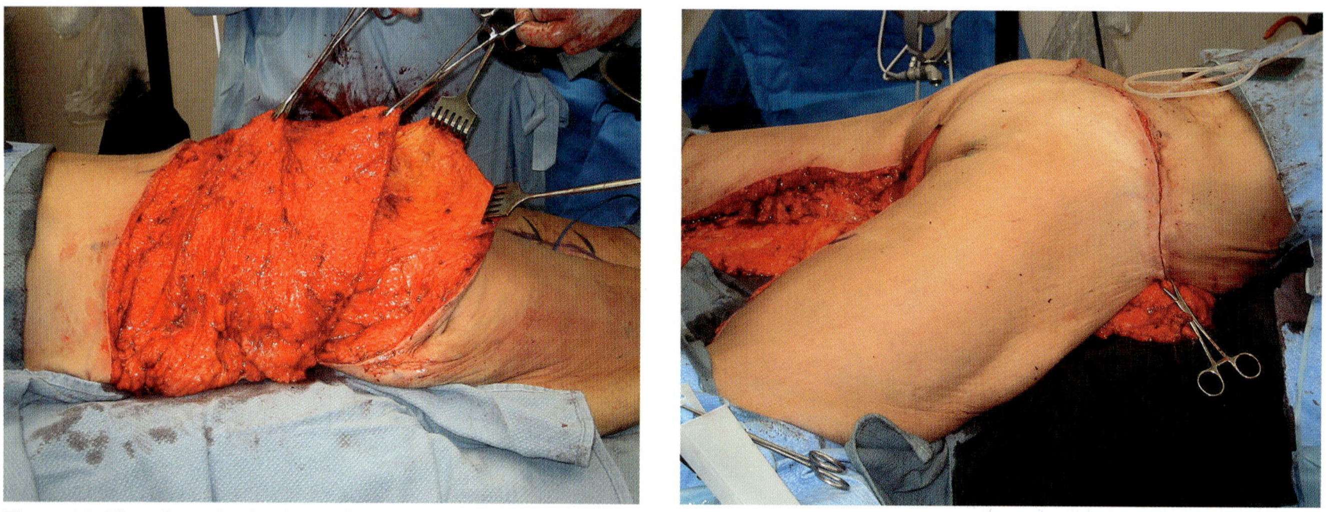

Figure 8.9 The adipose flap is advanced over the gluteus muscle and imbricated for buttock augmentation. Then the inferior buttock skin flap is advanced over the adipose flap, revealing the pleasing new buttock convexity. Because the vertical band extends far posterior, the posterior incision is made while still in the prone position. The 'dog ear' extension of the medial thighplasty along the inferior gluteal crease is resected and closed. (From Hurwitz 2005,[5] with permission of the *Aesthetic Surgery Journal*.)

across the other side. Groin adipose with rich lymphatic system is preserved. Broad suprafascial dissection continues to the umbilicus. The umbilicus is cut out as an inverted triangle. The dissection continues as a narrow midline band to the xyphoid. After removing excess from the superior abdominoplasty flap, the operating room table is flexed. Towel clips approximate the abdominal flap along the groins and mons pubis.

As assistants suture close the abdominoplasty, the surgeon resumes the medial thighplasty. The frog leg position suspends the thighs, which has two favorable consequences.

1. On closure of the abdominoplasty, loose upper thigh skin is unrestrained, as it is pulled into the abdomen.
2. There is freedom to circumferentially again estimate the extent of vertical band excision and closure.

For narrow-band extensions, the posterior incision is now made. If the band is wide, the posterior incision would have been better made when the patient was prone.

Next, the vertical band anterior line is incised through skin and subcutaneous fascia. Several centimeters of undermining present a subcutaneous edge for suture closure. Skin and underlying adipose is raised from knee to labia superficial to the fascia lata. Over the medial knee, most of the adipose is retained because of the rich plexus of lymphatics (Fig. 8.10). The medial thigh lymphatic vessels may be best preserved by preliminary thorough liposuction of the planned vertical excision followed by skin removal only. The saphenous vein is often transected distally but preserved under the anterior thigh flap. The vertical extension is approximated with towel

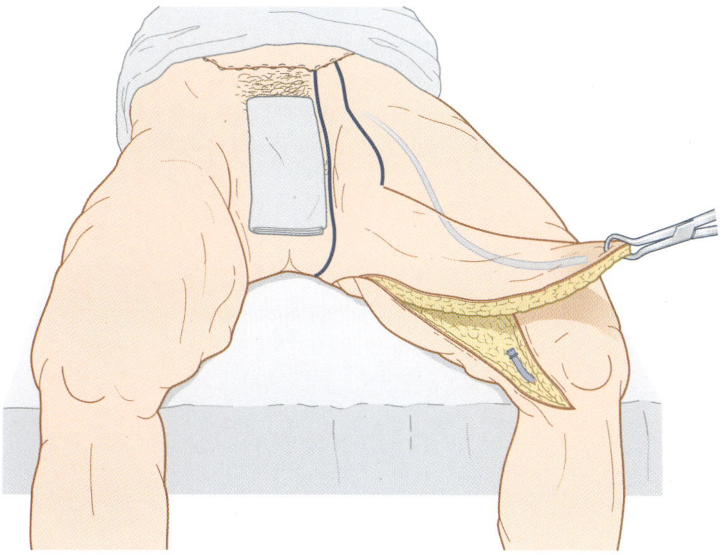

Figure 8.10 Excision of the vertical excision extension after the patient is turned supine. The posterior incision was made while the patient was still prone. After checking the accuracy of the width in the frog leg position, the anterior incision is made and then the band is resected over the fascia lata. At the level of the medial knee, the flap is cut thin to preserve underlying lymphatics. Midthigh transection of the saphenous vein is likely, but it can be preserved if so desired.

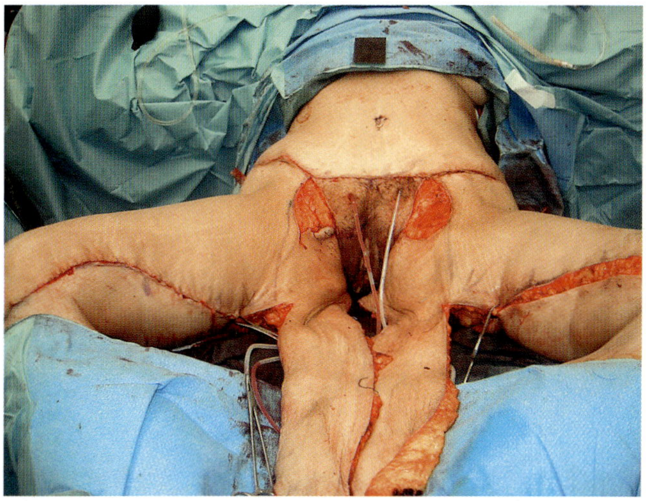

Figure 8.11 The patient has been turned supine and the abdominoplasty completed. The planned vertical band excision was rechecked, excised to subcutaneous fascia, and closed in two layers of continuous absorbable suture. The horizontal crescent can now be excised after reevaluation.

clamps and closed from knee to upper inner thigh in two long-lasting absorbable monofilament sutures (Fig. 8.11).

The final step of the L vertical medial thighplasty is resection of the transverse proximal crescent. The width of that resection is now adjusted as appropriate. Adduction of the thigh helps gauge this resection. The resection tapers alongside the mons pubis to reach the abdominoplasty closure. The para mons vertical resections start 6–7 cm from the midline, and each are about 3 cm in width. The paramedian mons pubis skin resections are only skin deep to avoid injury to bridging groin lymphatics.

A large, multiprong rake retractor elevates the lateral edge of the incised labia, and blunt-tipped scissors expose Colles fascia along the lateral pubic bone. The round ligament or spermatic cord may need to be pushed out of the way. Avoid cutting any structures, as the genitofemoral nerve also travels this path. With your helping hand finger palpating the pubis as a guide, three heavy braided permanent sutures are placed into Colles fascia (even pubic tuberosity periosteum) deep to the labia majora (Fig. 8.12). I prefer 0 Brailon with a taper pop-off needle (US Surgical, Danbury, Connecticut). Then each stitch generously bites the anterior thigh subcutaneous fascia.

The thigh is adducted to tie the three deep braided sutures under mild tension (Fig. 8.12). Then the mons plasty is sutured closed in two more layers superiorly, and the medial thigh to labial junction to the ischial tuberosity inferiorly (Fig. 8.13). The completed thigh suture line resembles an 'L' with the long limb down the thigh and the short limb along the labia and mons pubis (Fig. 8.14). The tail lies along the buttock thigh fold. The skin should be tight throughout, but with no tension on the labia majora (Fig. 8.15). Two anterior abdominal suction drains are placed through pubic stab wound incisions and extended laterally over the flanks. A supportive below-knee elastic garment is worn without gauze dressings. The result 7 months later needs a little further resection about the medal knees (Fig. 8.1).

The traditional upper inner thigh crescent thighplasty is similar to the L thighplasty without the vertical extension. As just described, the posterior dog ear is resected with the patient prone. As the abdominoplasty is being completed, the crescent resection is confirmed. Returning to the frog leg position, the labial thigh junction incision is made through skin only. The looping inferior incision is made through skin and subcutaneous fascia of the thigh. Both incisions end at the prior dog ear repair. When I want maximum traction on the medial thigh uplift, I gently push the Lockwood dissector under the fascia lata of the medial thigh. This is more likely to result in damage to perforating vessels than when done laterally, so great care must be taken. By design, the inferior incision line is much longer than the superior (labial–thigh).

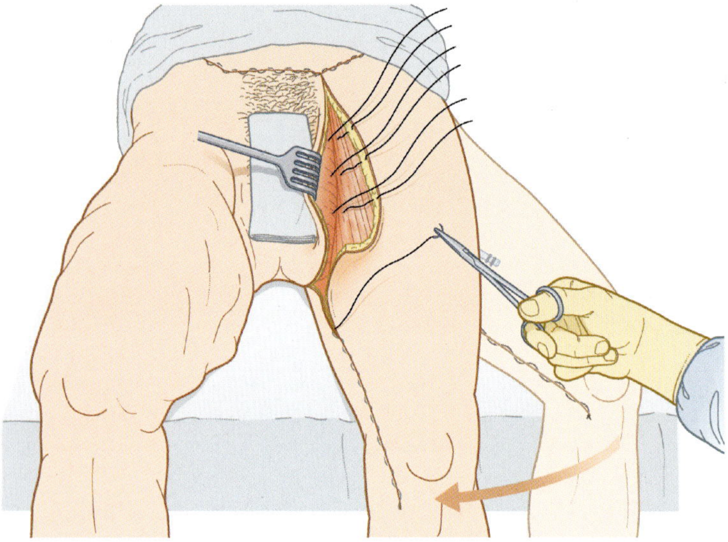

Figure 8.12 Closing the L thighplasty. The leg is adducted from the frog leg position to accurately determine the extent of upper crescent excision. After the excess skin is excised, large braided sutures approximate the subcutaneous fascia to Colles fascia, even pubic periosteum. The skin is sutured in two more layers.

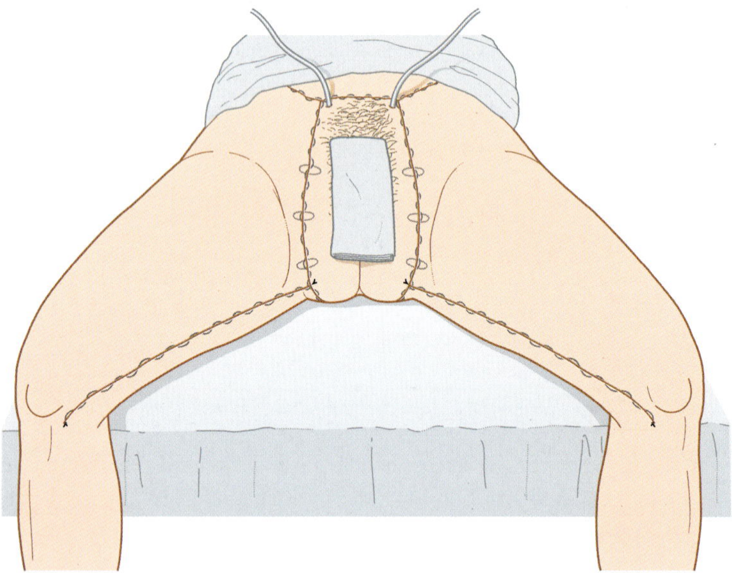

Figure 8.13 The completed L thighplasty closure, which resembles an 'L' that curves from the midthigh to the ischial tuberosity, and then ascends between the thigh and labia to the groin. The drains are abdominal.

Closure requires gathering of skin of the inferior line, which puckers it. If the discrepancy is considerable, then rippling persists (Fig. 8.14).

OPTIMIZING OUTCOMES

The operative technique just described is based on surgical principles. Technique will vary somewhat depending on the anatomy and surgeon preference, but the principles should not change. Accordingly, Table 8.1 lists the 10 principles or guidelines.

POSTOPERATIVE CARE

Throughout the procedure and during the 2- to 4-day hospitalization, automatic alternating pressure stockings function. Lower torso drains are removed when daily output is less than 50 mL each, which occurs around 10 days.

The patient will gain 5–10 lbs (2–5 kg) of weight due to large-volume fluid administration and postsurgical total body fluid retention. As this physiologic response makes patients look and feel poorly, they should understand its inevitability and be reassured that it will resolve shortly. Oral diuretics are started if diuresis is delayed beyond 3 days. To expedite edema resolution and improve skin quality, we prefer to start Endermologie (LPG, Miami, Florida) within 2 weeks. A month of home use of an automatic pressure device such as a Lympha Press (Mego Afek, Kibhutz Afek, Israel) can be helpful after the L thighplasty.

The suture lines are covered with Steristrips or dermal glue, obviating topical care. When gauze dressings are used, they need to be changed several times a day. All suture lines are inspected daily for skin vitality and separation. Large-gauge

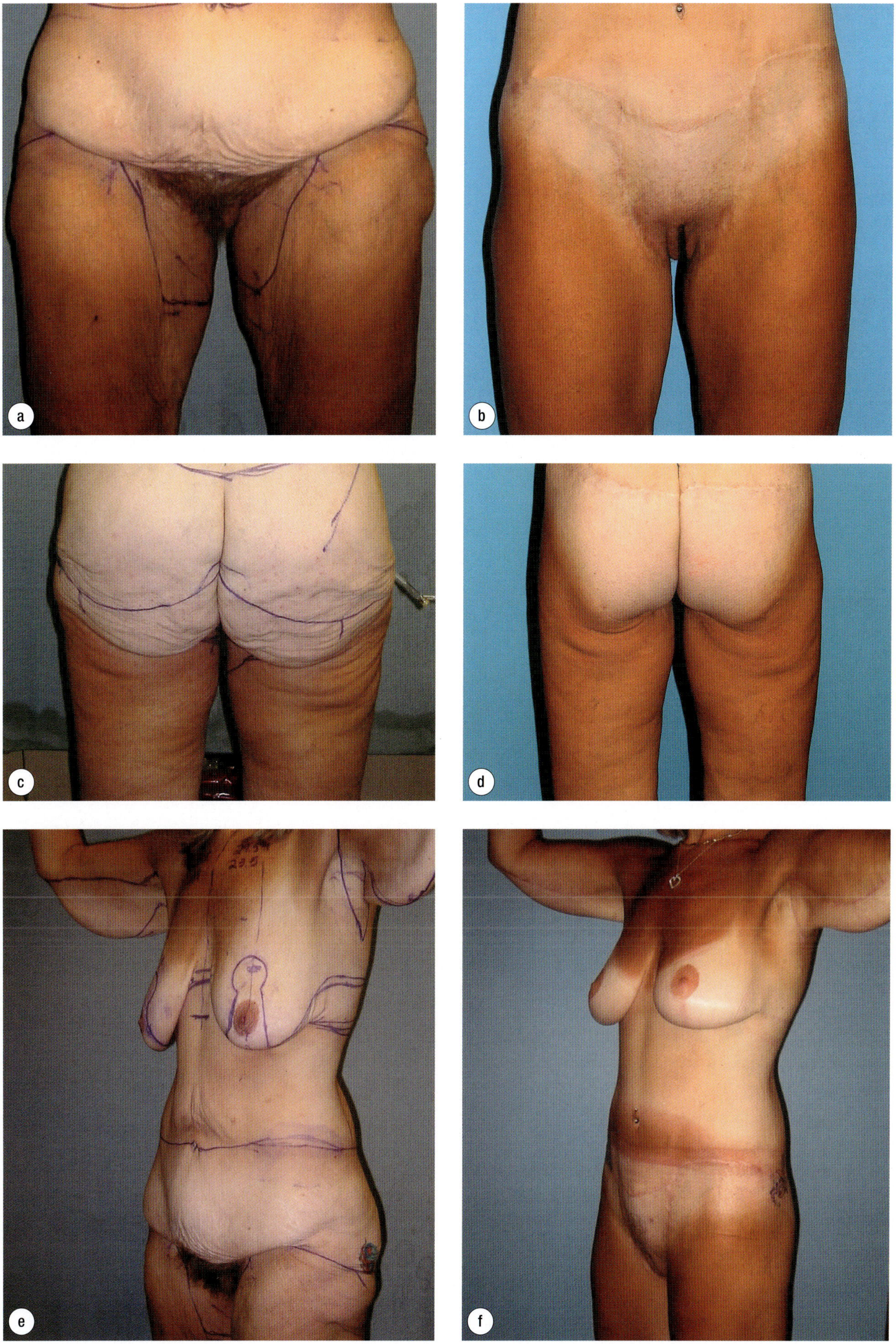

Figure 8.14 Close-up thigh and total body views (**a**, **c**, and **e**) before and (**b**, **d**, and **f**) 10 months after single-stage total body lift surgery with L brachioplasty. The patient is 37 years old, 5' 5" (1.65 m) tall, and weighs 137 lbs (62 kg) after losing 115 lbs (52 kg) from gastric bypass. She had moderate and mostly proximal medial thigh skin laxity. Her crescent-shaped medial thighplasty was designed as in Figure 8.6. The oblique full body views reveal the full impact of the 8-h operation without a transfusion. Spiral flaps shaped and augmented her breasts. (See Chapter 10.)

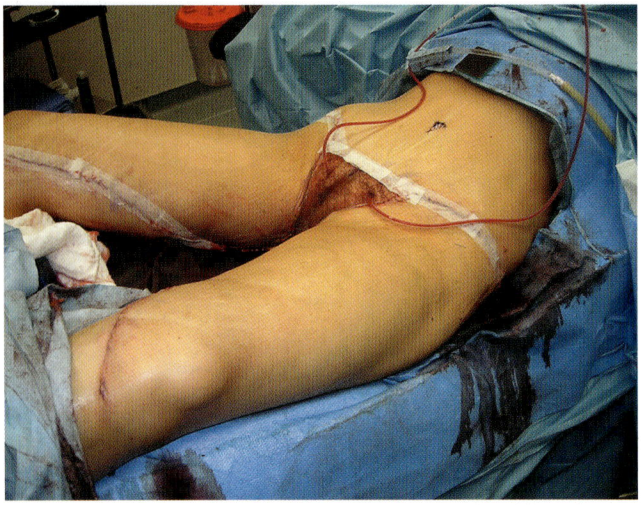

Figure 8.15 Intraoperative closure shows an intraoperative oblique view at the completion of the operation. There is no palpable laxity from umbilicus to knees. See Figure 8.1 for the before and 5 months after views.

monofilament sutures and a suture kit are readily available for the rare bedside repair of superficial dehiscence, which is most likely along the midlateral torso and ischial closures. I anesthetize the area with lidocaine (Xylocaine) injections and close with a continuous, baseball-type stitch. Routinely, the inner thigh to labial closure is moist, and despite best efforts for a secure closure small gaps are common. Meticulous wound care with bland soap cleansing and dry dressings reduces irritation and malodor. Antifungal creams may be helpful.

I favor postoperative compression garments, and currently use the black, lace-bordered long leg wraps by Inamed (Santa Barbara, California). The perineum opening exacerbates uppermost medial thigh and pubic swelling, which may become severe, requiring adjustments to or discarding the garment.

COMPLICATIONS AND THEIR MANAGEMENT

Suction drains drain serum and blood. Premature removal of these drains leads to seromas. Large-bore needle aspirations

Table 8.1 Ten surgical principles

No.	Principle	Notes
1	Properly analyze the patient and the deformity	Medical and psychologic issues must be minimized. For example, be wary of upper abdominal fullness due to excessive intraabdominal girth. It cannot be treated with abdominoplasty until there is further weight loss. Consider preliminary loss of excessive subcutaneous fat by diet or extensive liposuction.
2	Efficiency	A planned and deliberate approach avoids repetition in execution and unnecessary blood loss. Inefficiency lengthens an already long operation, thereby increasing hemorrhage, tissue trauma, surgeon fatigue, and costs, which promote prolonged convalescence with increased risk of medical and wound-healing complications. Develop a *consistent procedure* so that your assistants can anticipate your needs.
3	Excise skin transversely	Skin redundancy is predominantly vertical and lateral, so remove broad, horizontal bands of skin. Patients are made aware of anticipated residual transverse laxity, and few accept vertical torso excisions.
4	Plan incisions properly	Mark patients while they are recumbent and with leg positioning that takes advantage of gravity. Symmetric, transverse scars can be placed within underwear and are less likely to hypertrophy.
5	Focus on the tensions and contour left behind	The surgeon should not be preoccupied by the magnitude of the skin excision, but rather should plan on the resulting tissue tensions. In anticipation of contour depression along excessively tense long suture lines, leave extra deep adipose tissue during the resection of skin.
6	Gentle preservation of the incision line dermis and subcutaneous fascia	Limit the use of tissue-burning electrocautery and incise perpendicularly through the tissues with a scalpel. The subsequent tight closure will be more secure because of the reduced inflammation and necrotic tissue. Stitch abscesses and wound separation are less likely.

Table 8.1 (*cont'd*)

No.	Principle	Notes
7	Limit liposuction of flaps, and keep it as gentle as possible	This means prior generous saline infiltration of lidocaine (Xylocaine) and adrenaline (epinephrine), and a limited course with ultrasound probe before vented liposuction. Stop suction on the onset of bleeding.
8	High-tension, two-layer skin flap closure	High-tension, two-layer skin flap closure due to the poor skin elasticity, expedited by relieving the tension during closure by preliminary approximation of skin edges with towel clips and most favorable repositioning of limbs or body.
9	Close wounds as expeditiously as possible over long-dwelling suction catheters; respect larger lymphatics and use strategic quilting sutures	This is to reduce swelling, infection rate, phlebitis, and seroma. Preliminary liposuction of the medial vertical band excisions with skin only removal pressures lymphatics. A secure two-layer closure is optimal. Elasticized garments with minimal pressure over the lower abdomen are comfortable and reassuring.
10	Continuously analyze aesthetic results	Systematically compare standard before and after photos and solicit standardized patient comments. At the University of Pittsburgh, we have developed a standardized deformity and outcome grading scale.

are both diagnostic and therapeutic. Local compression with a sponge and elastic wrap is tried for about a week. If serum reaccumulates, then aspiration is repeated or preferably a percutaneous drainage catheter is inserted, sutured in place, and connected to a suction bulb. It is removed 7–10 days later. These catheters can initiate serious infections, so meticulous care is essential. On rare occasions, a drain is reinserted several times. Once a scarred seroma cavity is formed, compete resolution may require injection of sclerosing agents or surgical excision with quilting suture closure.

Several weeks after surgery, a firm, deep, slightly tender mass may be palpable above the medial knee. On aspiration, this invariably yields straw-colored, watery fluid, which refills to firmness within a day, suggestive of a lymphocele. Prolonged closed suction drainage usually resolves the problem. A small residual mass is left alone, as it tends to resolve by fibrosis.

Delayed distal medial thigh abscess has required incision and debridement in four limbs over the past 5 years. All healed secondarily. A recent patient had sepsis from a *Streptococcus viridans* abscess of the proximal thigh 1 week after her total body lift with L thighplasty and extensive Vaser® LipoSelection®. With the onset of high fever and obtundation, immediate operative drainage and intravenous antibiotics restored her health.

Inadequate care and excessive activity can lead to troublesome thigh swelling. Skin edge necrosis will be followed by suture line dehiscence. Because of the tightness of the closure and persistent swelling, a conservative wound care approach is taken. There may be a long line of necrotic and inflammatory tissue. Thorough debridement is performed. Topical papain-urea agents such as Accuzyme followed by Panafil are applied. Be vigilant for undrained areas that may lead to abscesses. Increasing redness and fever require investigation. Once a granulating bed is cultivated, the wounds tend to contract and epithelialize within weeks. Attention to meticulous hygiene, clipping of irritating hairs, and offending sutures are essential.

Descent of the labial thigh scars and distortion of the labia are recognized long-term complications. With the introduction of the Colles fascia stitch, I believe that this problem has become uncommon.[4] Nevertheless, overresection of medial thigh skin cannot be overcome by those sutures. Skin grafts are the most expedient means to correct the labial deformity, but they may be rejected as unsightly by the patient. Theoretically, tissue expansion, although awkward in this location, should yield more skin. If there is residual transverse laxity of thigh skin, then a limited vertical band excision can raise the scar and take distorting tension off the labia majora.

There is no operative solution to excessively heavy, thick thighs, as they are prone to abscess infections and pulling through of sutures. Further weight loss or preliminary lipoplasty is indicated. Some thighs appear too heavy but are actually primarily sheets of sagging skin. Pull the skin superiorly and palpate the thickness. If it is not too thick, proceed with thighplasty but plan for an exceptionally broad resection of skin (Fig. 8.3).

Weight loss patients with the following are not candidates for this surgery:

- unstable chronic illnesses,
- cardiovascular disease,
- postphlebtic syndrome, and
- lymphedema.

Also, patients with unresolved depression or unrealistic expectations should be avoided.

CONCLUSION

The crescent medial thighplasty reduces upper thigh laxity. A vertical midmedial excision extension reduces the remaining distal two-thirds of oversized thighs. The L thighplasty runs the long limb the length of the medial thigh, and the short limb lies between the labia majora and inner thigh and the mons pubis and groin. This thorough resection of excess tissue on heavy thighs minimizes descent of the upper medial thigh scar and recurrence of saddlebags.

For the crescent medial thighplasty, a properly positioned labia–thigh scar is an acceptable trade-off for objectionable loose upper inner skin. In the L thighplasty, the vertical scar is better accepted when it lies posterior to the median line of the thigh. Most scars mature nicely.

Concomitant abdominoplasty and lower body lift with the L thighplasty improve severe lower torso and thigh laxity with reasonable scars and minor complications. Accurate presurgical marking is essential. The prone and supine positions expedite symmetry and efficiency. The lower body lift raises the lateral thighs and buttocks through a circumferential, wide beltlike excision of skin and discontinuous undermining of the lateral thighs. The high lateral tension abdominoplasty suspends proximal anterior and medial thigh. The lateral portion of the lower body lift is closed under high tension. This tension is temporarily relieved during closure by full abduction of the thighs. On completion of the lateral closure, the thighs are adducted, which transmits tautness along the entire lateral thigh.

Closure of the crescent portion of the medial thighplasty is completed with the leg adducted, forcing the vector of body lift pull cephalad. This is the optimal time for the medial thighplasty, because of maximal cephalad pull of the lower body lift and abdominoplasty. Figure 8.16 diagrams the vectors of combined surgery.

The combined lower body lift, abdominoplasty, and L thighplasty is complex elective correction of a difficult clinical problem. Consistently good results can be obtained, with complications minor and patient satisfaction high.

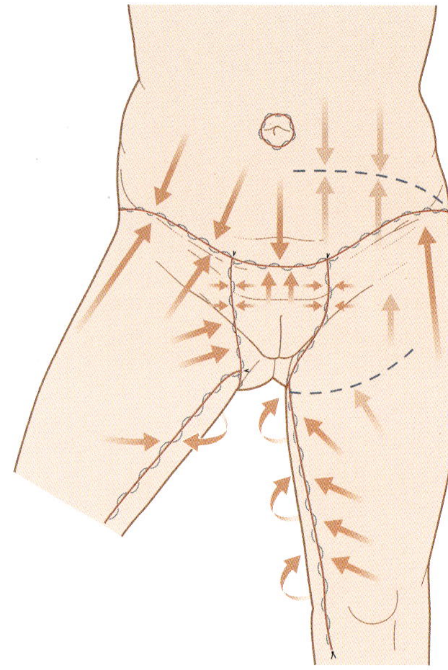

Figure 8.16 The tension vectors following combined circumferential abdominoplasty, lower body lift, monsplasty, and the L medial thighplasty are shown. The strongest lift is along the lateral torso and thighs, followed by the medial thigh to Colles fascia. The monsplasty is aided by superior and lateral distracting forces. The vertical excision extension reduces drag on the lateral lift. The median thighplasty is synergistic to the superior lift from the abdominoplasty and lower body lift.

REFERENCES

1. Lewis JR. The thigh lift. J Int Coll Surg 1957; 27(3):330–334.
2. Schultz RC, Feinberg LA. Medial thigh lift. Ann Plast Surg 1979; 2:404–410.
3. Regnault P, Daniel RK. Lower extremity. Massive weight loss. In: Regnault P, Daniel RK. Aesthetic plastic surgery: principles and techniques. Boston: Little Brown; 1984:655–678,705–720.
4. Lockwood T. Fascial anchoring technique in medial thigh lifts. Plast Reconstr Surg 1988; 82:299–304.
5. Hurwitz D. Medial thighplasty for operative strategies. Aesthetic Surg J 2005; 25:180–191.
6. Lockwood T. Lower-body lift. Aesthetic Surg J 2001:355–370.
7. Lockwood T. Maximizing aesthetics in lateral-tension abdominoplasty and body lifts. Clin Plast Surg 2004; 31:523–537.
8. Aly AS, Cram AE, Chao M, et al. Belt lipectomy for circumferential truncal excess: the University of Iowa experience. Plast Reconstr Surg 2003; 111:398–413.
9. Hurwitz DJ, Zewert T. Body contouring surgery in the bariatric surgical patient. Oper Tech Plast Surg Reconstr Surg 2002; 8:87–95.
10. Hurwitz DJ. Single stage total body lift after massive weight loss. Ann Plast Surg 2004; 52:435–441.
11. Hurwitz DJ, Rubin JP, Risen M, et al. Correcting the saddlebag deformity in the massive weight loss patient. Plast Reconstr Surg 2004; 114:1313–1325.
12. Hurwitz D, Rubin P. Body contouring after bariatric surgery part 2—surgical principles and techniques. Plastic Surgery 2003, instructional DVD 0383-03. Available: http://www.plasticsurgery.org.

APPROACH TO THE ARM AFTER WEIGHT LOSS

9

Berish Strauch and David Greenspun

Key Points

- A careful analysis of skin laxity and adiposity in all four aesthetic zones of the upper extremity is paramount.
- A posteriorly placed scar is less visible to the patient.
- Sinusoidal incisions contribute to good scar quality and help avoid the pitfall of proximal and distal underresection.
- A Z plasty in the dome of the axilla prevents bowstringing of the scar.

The well-documented rise in the popularity of *bariatric* (from the Greek *barys*, meaning heavy, and new Latin *iatria*, meaning related to medical treatment) surgical procedures for the morbidly obese has been associated with a sharp rise in the number of patients seeking consultation for post–weight loss body-contouring procedures.[1–3] The group of patients who have lost massive amounts of weight, defined as loss in excess of 100 lbs (45 kg), presents a number of unique challenges to the plastic surgeon. Some of these challenges are related to the patient's psyche, some to the underlying health status of these patients, and some to body habitus itself. This chapter outlines our approach to the correction of upper extremity and axillary contour deformities that result after massive weight loss.

Various techniques for surgical management of upper extremity contour deformities have been suggested since aesthetic brachioplasty was first described in the 1950s.[4] Early techniques for the rejuvenation of the upper extremity appear to have been developed to address the aesthetic changes that are commonly associated with aging or 'normal' weight loss. Such techniques were typically based on elliptic resections centered over the proximal brachium.[5,6] Later, techniques that placed a second elliptic resection over the axilla oriented at 90° to the long axis of the arm were described.[7] Satisfactory results of reasonable normal body habitus can be achieved using these approaches in appropriately selected patients. However, we do not believe that optimal results can be achieved in the massive weight loss patient using these techniques. They fail to address the unique anatomical deformities found after massive weight loss.

APPROACH BASED ON ZONES

To better understand and address the deformities found after massive weight loss, it is helpful to conceptualize the upper extremity based on four zones (Fig. 9.1).[8]

- Zone 1 extends from the wrist to the medial epicondyle.

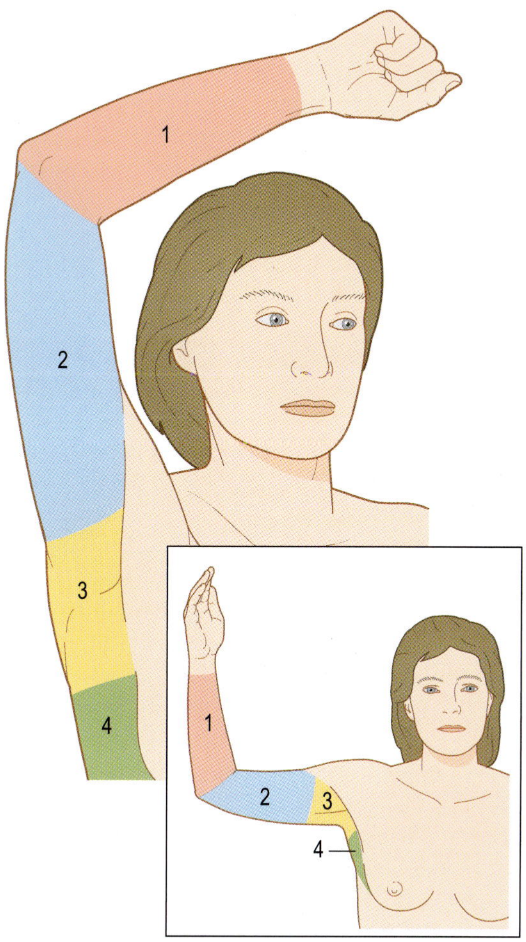

Figure 9.1 Zones of treatment. (After Strauch et al. 2004,[8] with permission.)

- Zone 2 extends from the medial epicondyle to the proximal axilla.
- The anatomical borders of the axilla proper define zone 3.
- The subaxillary upper lateral chest wall is termed zone 4.

Systematic evaluation of each of these zones allows the surgeon to develop a rational treatment plan.

Zone 1 deformities

It has been our experience that massive weight loss patients do not typically present with severe deformities of zone 1. When deformity is present, it is most often characterized by a mild excess of subcutaneous fat without skin redundancy. This type of deformity can be well managed with suction-assisted lipectomy alone. We have not found it necessary to perform direct excision for zone 1 deformities.

Zone 2 deformities

Isolated zone 2 deformities can be divided into two types. Some patients will present with a zone 2 deformity characterized by excessive fat only, while others will have both excessive fat and skin. It is important to recognize the degree to which the fat, and the degree to which the skin, contribute to the overall deformity. This is because the relative contribution of excess ptotic skin dictates the type of procedure that will achieve optimal contour.

Although it is the exception rather than the rule, some massive weight loss patients will present with a proportionately greater excess of zone 2 fat compared with skin. If such patients have good skin tone, they may be candidates for treatment with suction-assisted lipectomy and not require direct excision. More commonly, however, patients with zone 2 deformities have redundant ptotic skin far in excess of the extent of excess fat. These patients may be treated with direct excision, if restoration of upper extremity contour is to be achieved.

Deformities of zones 2 and 3

The majority of massive weight loss patients present with a deformity that spans both zones 2 and 3. The characteristics of the tissues associated with this type of deformity are such that a wing or web is formed that spans the upper brachium and axilla. In these cases, excess skin is present in abundance, while relatively little fat is present. Careful evaluation will reveal that the excess ptotic skin hangs from the posterior axillary fold of the axilla and from the posteriomedial aspect of the arm, posterior to the bicipital groove. This can readily be demonstrated when the patient is examined with the arms abducted 90° from the trunk and the elbows flexed at 90°. Within zone 3, the excess does not hang from the central portion of the axillary dome, but rather from the posterior axillary fold. This anatomical finding has important implications in the design of the surgical procedure.

Patients with deformities of both zones 2 and 3 invariably require direct excision to restore a natural contour to both the arm and the axilla. Our surgical strategy combines a sinusoidal pattern of resection along the brachium with a Z plasty in the region of the axilla. The incisions are planned so that the resultant scar lies more posterior than the traditionally described location along the medial bicipital groove. This location proves to be far less noticeable to the patient. A generous Z plasty in the axillary portion helps restore a natural concavity to the axilla. The details of our surgical approach to brachioplasty are described later in this chapter.

Deformities of zones 2–4

For those patients with deformities of combined zones 2, 3, and 4, direct excision is required to help restore contour to the arm, axilla, and upper lateral chest wall. Although severe deformities of zone 4 may sometimes require a separate surgical thoracoplasty, we have found that more moderate deformities can be addressed with an extension of the brachioplasty. Specifically, the sinusoidal pattern of excision used in zones 2 and 3 is carried more proximally into zone 4. The Z plasty is then placed in the axilla, as described above.

THEORETIC BASES OF THE PROCEDURE

Previous techniques of brachioplasty have been associated with postoperative residual contour deformities, hypertrophic scars, widened scars, and patient dissatisfaction with scar location.[9,10] We have sought to overcome the limitations of previous techniques by applying several basic plastic surgery principles to the problem of upper extremity contour deformity.

First, we have recognized that not all scars heal equally. A scar placed on the upper eyelid will almost always heal better than a scar placed on the brachium. This is a fact of nature that we do not, as yet, have the ability to change. In recognition of this fact, and in order to make the resultant scar acceptable to the patient, we rely on placing the scar in a location where it is relatively difficult to see. By placing the scar posterior to the medial bicipital groove, it is not readily seen by patients when they look in the mirror or by others interacting with the patient during the course of most routine activities.

It is also important to consider the effect of tension on a healing surgical scar. We believe that a longer undulating scar will heal more kindly than a shorter scar under tension. To this end, we have adopted the use of sinusoidal type incisions that converge at their proximal and distal ends. Moreover, the use of the sinusoidal incisions helps us to avoid the pitfall of proximal and distal underresection that can be associated with the use of elliptic pattern brachioplasty techniques.

A straight line scar placed across a concave body part is prone to forming a bowstring. The axilla has a domelike concave form, and procedures designed to restore its natural form must respect this architecture. The generous Z plasty that we employ recruits excess lax tissue from either side of the long axis incisions, and allows the tissues to fall into the natural concavity of the axilla. This is analogous to the use of a Z plasty to recontour the cervicomental junction after a burn injury or the medial canthal region. An alternative approach to the Z plasty is to use a T or L pattern in which the axillary and arm scars converge at an angle in the dome of the axilla.

THE PROCEDURE

The patient is marked first in the standing position, and the markings are refined and finalized when the patient is under general anesthesia. A reference line is visualized along the axis of the arm from a point midway between the olecranon and the medial epicondyle, respectively, points A and B, and the end of the excess tissue on the arm itself, in the axilla, or on the chest wall. In other words, the line is visualized along the inferior margin of the ptotic skin as it hangs from the arm and posterior axillary border when the arms are held abducted.

Sinusoidal incisions are planned on either side of the visualized reference line. The two incisions converge at both their proximal and distal ends. The incisions are planned so that the central oscillations will interdigitate after the intervening excess is resected. This is analogous to the separation of syndactylous digits. The margins of resection are determined by eyesight and a pinch test. With this design, the final scar will take the shape of an undulating scar that lies posteriomedial on the arm. The markings are made on both upper extremities (Figs 9.2a and 9.3).

The skin and superficial subcutaneous tissue are sharply incised along the planned markings down to the level of the underlying muscular fascia of the arm, leaving a thin layer of fat on the fascia. The soft tissue between the sinusoidal incisions is subsequently elevated off the muscular fascia using face-lift scissors in a pushing–cutting manner. The ulnar nerve and medial antebrachial cutaneous nerve must be protected during this stage of surgery. The laxity of the remaining skin and soft tissue allows closure without the need for undermining beyond the surgical margins. If the closure is too loose, residual deformity may persist postoperatively. If the closure is too tight, tissue necrosis and loss may ensue. A snug but not tight closure should be the surgeon's goal.

For those patients with deformities that also involve zone 3 or zones 3 and 4, a Z plasty is used to restore the contour of the axillary dome. The long axis incision is temporarily tacked closed to simplify the design of the axillary Z plasty. The upper and lower limbs of the Z are marked at approximately 60° angles to the central limb on either side of the long axis incisions. The central limb of the Z will ultimately lie in the transverse axis of the axillary concavity, with the other limbs running parallel to the direction of the anterior and posterior axillary folds. For those patients with zone 4 deformities, the sinusoidal incisions extend on to the upper chest wall medial to the Z plasty.

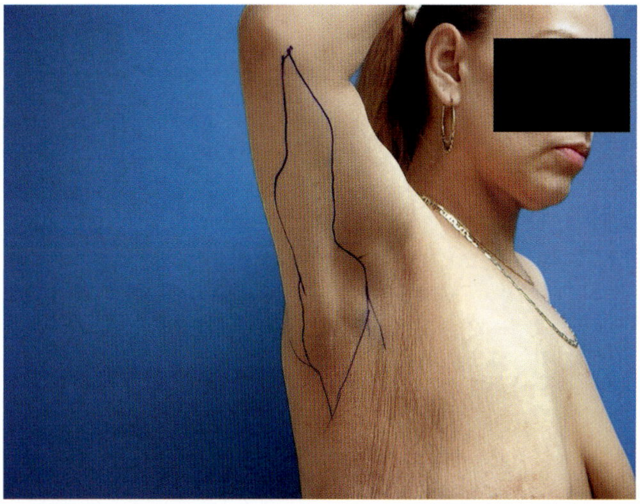

Figure 9.3 Brachial excess extending down from the posterior axillary line. A double-interdigitating pair of lines drawn from the region of the olecranon to the region of the excess. This is similar to division of syndactylized digits.

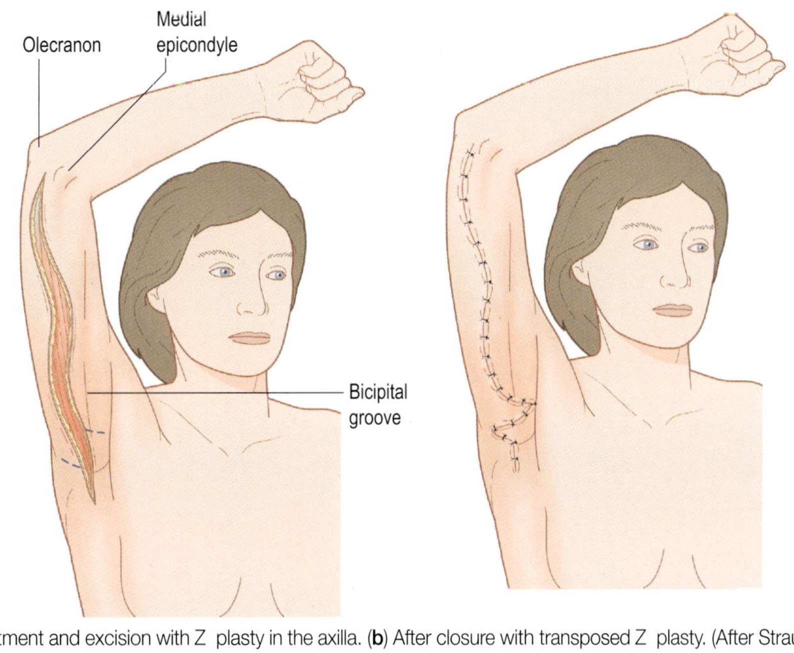

Figure 9.2 (a) Planned treatment and excision with Z plasty in the axilla. (b) After closure with transposed Z plasty. (After Strauch et al. 2004,[8] with permission.)

The limbs of the Z plasty are incised and transposed. The Z plasty permits the tissue to conform to the dome of the axilla and, at the same time, allows an anteroposterior tightening of the skin closure along the long axis of the arm (Fig. 9.2b).

All incisions are closed over Jackson–Pratt drains. The closure of the sinusoidal incisions is begun at both ends and proceeds toward the central portion of the surgical wound. Anchoring sutures placed in the depth of the deep tissues of the axilla are *not* used or advisable, as vital structures may be injured. Wounds are dressed with Xeroform (Sherwood Medical, St. Louis, Missouri) and gauze. Each extremity is then wrapped from the wrist to the axilla with Kling (Johnson & Johnson Medical, Arlington, Texas) and an Ace bandage (DE Healthcare Products, Denver, Philadelphia). A Spandage (Medi-Tech International, Brooklyn, New York) dressing is then placed over the Ace wrap from one wrist to the other; this holds the entire compressive dressing in place until the first follow-up visit. Drains are removed when drainage is less than 30 cc/24 h on each side. No liposuction is used or needed for this technique.

DISCUSSION

We believe that this technique of brachioplasty is ideal for previously morbidly obese patients who have achieved massive weight loss and present with deformities of zones 2, 3, and/or 4. It allows the surgeon and patient to avoid many of the recognized pitfalls of previously described techniques of arm rejuvenation.

By creating a final scar that is sinusoidal in shape, the likelihood of developing a linear scar contracture is reduced. Likewise, the added length achieved with undulating incisions (compared with a straight line incision) helps reduce the tension that is oriented perpendicular to the long axis of the arm at any given point along the final scar. This reduction in tension may help contribute to the relatively low rate of hypertrophic scars that have been reported in previous series.

By utilizing portions of the central long axis incisions in the Z plasty, a naturally shaped axilla is formed and the aesthetically important anterior and posterior axillary folds are recreated. Finally, by carrying the resection on to the upper lateral chest wall in patients with zone 4 deformities, it is sometimes possible to correct contour deformities in this anatomical region without performing a separate thoracoplasty.

The position of the final scar, slightly posterior to the medial bicipital groove, is acceptable to patients. When a patient stands with arms at the side, the scar is impossible to see. We believe that placing the scar in a location where it is not readily seen is critical. Ultimately, patient satisfaction is the most important goal, and we have found an extremely high satisfaction rate among our patients using this approach to brachioplasty (Figs 9.4–9.7). Some surgeons advocate placing scars in the bicipital groove. While a posterior placement is less visible to the patient, it may be noticed by other people and draw unwanted comments. This is an area of ongoing debate.

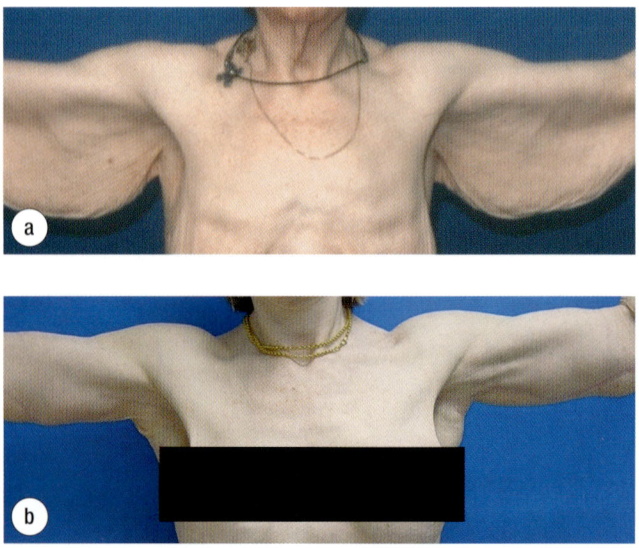

Figure 9.4 (**a**) A 300-lb (136 kg) weight loss. (**b**) One year postbrachioplasty.

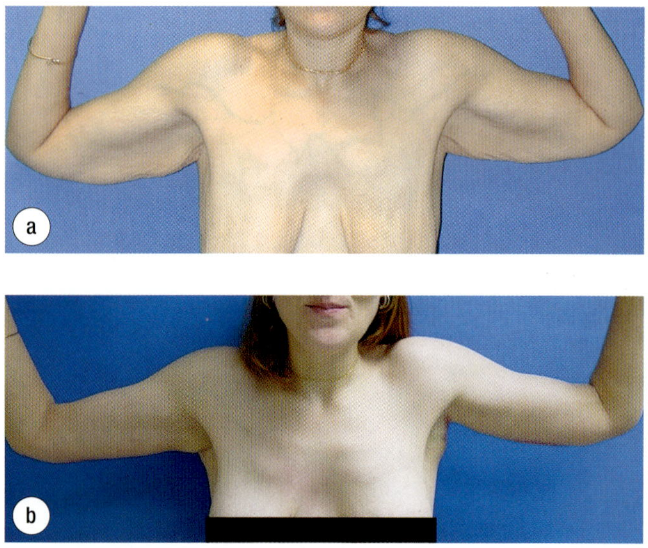

Figure 9.5 (**a**) A 120-lb (54 kg) weight loss. (**b**) One year postbrachioplasty

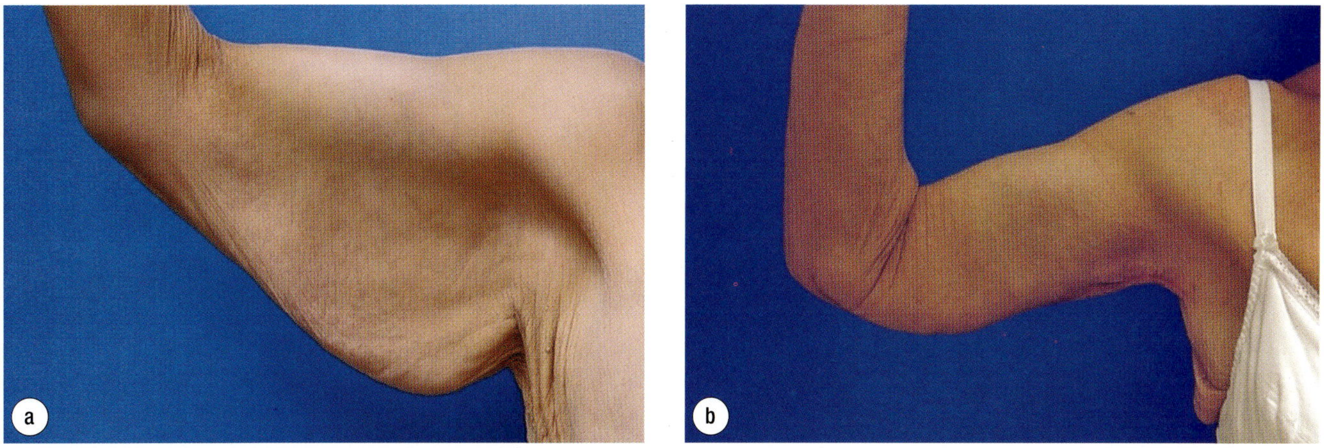

Figure 9.6 (**a**) A 175-lb (79 kg) weight loss. (**b**) Two years postbrachioplasty.

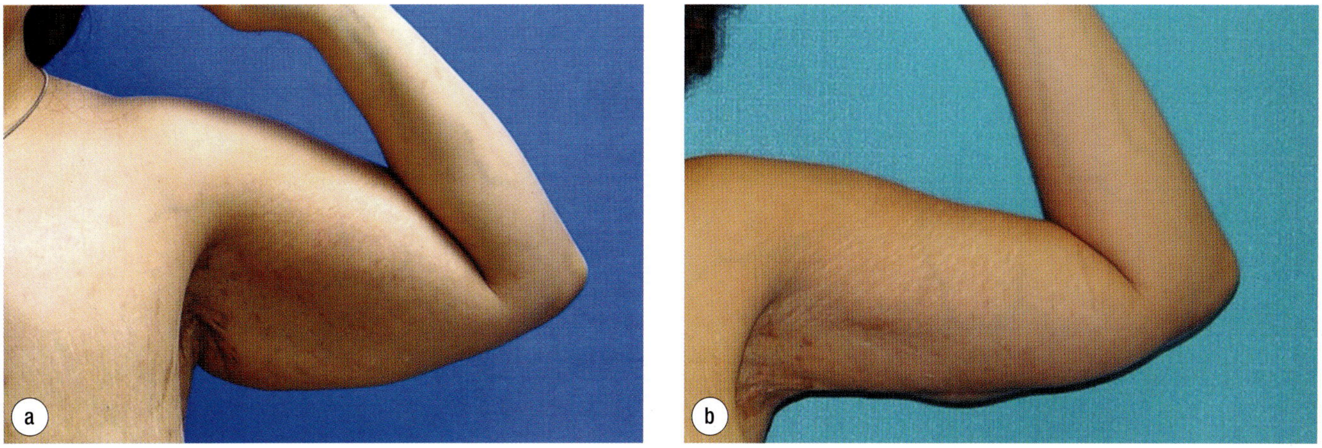

Figure 9.7 (**a**) A 250-lb (113 kg) weight loss. (**b**) One year postbrachioplasty.

REFERENCES

1. Livingston EH. Procedure incidence and in-hospital complication rates of bariatric surgery in the United States. Am J Surg 2004; 188(2):105–110.
2. Cottam DR, Nguyen NT, Eid GM, et al. The impact of laparoscopy on bariatric surgery. Surg Endosc 2005; 19(5):621–627.
3. American Society of Plastic Surgeons. 2004 quick facts. Cosmetic and reconstructive plastic surgery trends. Online. Available: http://www.plasticsurgery.org
4. Correa-Inturraspe M, Fernandez JC. Demolipectomia braquial. Prensa Med Argent 1954; 34:24.
5. Guerro-Santos J. Brachioplasty. Aesthetic Plast Surg 1979; 2:1.
6. Lockwood T. Brachioplasty with superficial fascial system suspension. Plast Reconstr Surg 1995; 96(4):912–920.
7. Lockwood T. Contouring of the arms, trunk and thighs. In: Achauer BM, Eriksson E, Gyuron B, et al, eds. Plastic surgery—indications, operations, and outcomes, vol 5. Aesthetic surgery. St. Louis: Mosby Year-Book; 2000.
8. Strauch B, Greenspun D, Levine J, et al. A technique of brachioplasty. Plast Reconstr Surg 2004; 113(3):1044–1048.
9. Goddio A-S. A new technique for brachioplasty. Plast Reconstr Surg 1990; 35:202.
10. Gilliland MD, Lyos AT. CAST liposuction: an alternative to brachioplasty. Aesthetic Plast Surg 1997; 21(6):398–402.

APPROACH TO TOTAL BODY LIFT SURGERY

10

Dennis J. Hurwitz

Key Points

- Massive weight loss patients complaining of skin redundancy should have a comprehensive evaluation of all skin deformities and a treatment plan.
- Healthy, athletically fit, and highly motivated patients are candidates for a single-stage total body lift, which is the combination of lower trunk and extremity contouring with a circumferential contouring of the upper trunk and possible brachioplasty.
- Reliable preoperative markings are made in multiple positions, including supine, lateral decubitus, sitting, and standing.
- An aesthetic result follows the consistent placement of level, symmetric, and hidden scars with the retention of adequate adipose tissue for creation of gender-specific contours.

While the combination of circumferential abdominoplasty, a modified lower body lift, and medial thighplasty adequately treats skin laxity of the lower torso and thighs (see Ch. 8), the glaring persistent deformity of the upper torso and breasts leaves incomplete patient transformation. Hence staged total body lift (TBL) surgery was designed. The second stage, called the upper body lift, removes epigastric and midback rolls of skin, adjusts the inframammary fold (IMF), and reshapes the breast, leaving behind a near-circumferential transverse scar hidden by a brassiere. For the correction of gynecomastia, the least intrusive scar remains.

When dramatic improvement could be reliably achieved by separate operations of the upper and lower body, it was inevitable that single-stage TBL surgery be considered.[1] TBL surgery treats sagging tissues of the torso and thighs.[2] TBL surgery sculpts the body by excision of excess and reconstruction of what remains into pleasing, gender-specific contours in as few stages as safely possible. More than a linked series of operations, TBL surgery is a paradigm shift from minimalist to comprehensive.

Women achieve a narrower waist than otherwise possible. The optimum female patient is young (<45 years old), not obese (BMI < 30 kg/m²), physically fit, and mentally balanced. Energetic, accomplished individuals who disdain the double-recovery periods entailed in two major stages are excellent candidates. Single-stage TBL has unique biomechanical advantages for the correction of gynecomastia after massive weight loss as well.[1] Over the past 3 years, except for a greater number of blood transfusions, no increased morbidity has been found in the single over the multistage TBL.[1]

Over 25 years of personally performing craniofacial surgery confirms that prolonged and complex operations are more efficiently and safely performed by an experienced and organized surgeon with well-prepared assistants, working together as a team.

In 1975, Elvin Zook proposed that once all indicated surgical procedures were identified in a weight loss patient, a surgical plan was coordinated 'so that as many (procedures) as possible can be done simultaneously'.[3] With two or three teams working simultaneously, the arms and breasts were contoured at the same time as the circumferential abdominoplasty was done.[3,4] He considered loosely hanging breasts 'an extremely difficult problem'. He cited his experience that normally discarded flaps should be deepithelialized and placed behind the breasts.[3] He favored the Pitanguy mastopexy with deepithelialization of the keyhole and the entire inferior breast, which was then turned upward to give the breast bulk and projection. An inferior incision was carried around the trunk to correct undesirable rolls and bulk.[3]

About the same tine, Palmer et al. advocated limiting procedures to only one area at a time.[5] To this day, the debate continues as to the advisability of multiple combined procedures. In his approach to the breast, Palmer recognized the availability of undesirable skin folds below and lateral to the breasts, and rebuilt the breast 'using the loose tissue surrounding it'.[5] He favored the Wise pattern[6] and popular McKissock[7] vertical deepithelialized bipedicle mammoplasty to gather the remaining glandular tissue under the nipple. In three patients, his group combined this 'with a wide excision of the submammary fold'.[5] In 1979, Shons simply preferred the McKissock technique with removal of excess skin through the Wise pattern for weight loss patients.[8]

In 1984, Paule Regnault described 'total body contouring', which included a batwing torsoplasty of midlateral wide excisions of skin from the upper arms to the hips.[9] Fred Grazer described secondary correction of upper abdominal skin laxity by reverse abdominoplasty along the IMFs.[10] Zienowicz has championed using nearby excess tissue for cosmetic breast enlargement by augmentation by reverse abdominoplasty.[11] The reverse abdominoplasty crosses the sternum and is suspended by deepithelialized dermal tabs sutured to chest fascia.[12]

THE TOTAL BODY LIFT

Fundamental to my TBL is Lockwood's elucidation of the superficial fascial system and securing this subcutaneous multilayer fascia for high-tension skin closure.[13] For tightening the loose IMF and improved breast projection, he fixes the IMF at 'the appropriate elevated position by non-absorbable sutures from the superficial fascial system of the inferior skin wound edge to the underlying muscular fascia'.[13]

Most massive weight loss patients have bizarre midtorso rolls of excess skin, flat drooping breasts, and oversized axillae that lead into batwinged arms.[14] There are four intertwined components to an upper body lift:

1. reverse abdominoplasty,
2. positioning of a secure IMF,
3. removal of midtorso excess skin, and
4. reshaping and augmenting the breasts.

The upper body lift is optimally combined with the L brachioplasty to reduce lateral chest and oversized axilla, and raise the ptotic posterior axillary fold (described below).[15]

In the following sections, the aim of each component of an upper body lift is elaborated.

Reverse abdominoplasty

Number 1, and fundamental, is the reverse abdominoplasty, which removes residual excess skin of the upper abdomen. When associated with a well-defined midtorso transverse roll, standard abdominoplasty fails to efface loose epigastric skin.

Positioning of a secure IMF

Component no. 2 is upward repositioning and securing the descended IMFs. The new IMF repositioning and the reverse abdominoplasty are integral. A properly located and secure IMF is essential to success. The reverse abdominoplasty remains tight, and the breast is better situated and supported. In the male patient, the goal is opposite. The IMF is obliterated. The tightened upper abdomen is suspended by the upper chest boomerang pattern excision and pulled down by the abdominoplasty.[1,2]

Removal of midtorso excess skin

Component no. 3 is removal of the midtorso back skin rolls, which is essentially a posterior continuation of the reverse abdominoplasty. A lower body lift does not correct prominent midback rolls unless the excision level is raised unacceptably cephalad.

Reshaping and augmenting the breasts

Component no. 4 is reshaping the breasts. If the breasts have adequate or excess volume, they are reshaped or reduced using a Wise pattern and pedicle of choice. If the breasts are small and misshapen, they may be reconstructed with implants and mastopexy. Unfortunately, the reshaped breasts rarely conform well to the implants. Over time, the larger implants sag and ripple. These atrophied breasts are better rebuilt with a Wise pattern mastopexy and a deepithelialized spiral flap.

In essence, excess skin and fat of the epigastrium and midtorso back rolls is deepithelialized in continuity with the central breast mount. The epigastric flap is flipped on to the inferior breast, and the lateral extension is twisted around the breast mound over the pectoralis major muscle. Created from torso discard, the spiral flaps are mobile enough to permit artistic creativity in shaping and augmentation. The breasts are not only enlarged and well shaped, but are also soft and shift naturally with change in body position. The constricted inferior breast is filled and supported with redundant deepithelialized epigastric tissue. Tapering of the lateral breast along the anterior axillary line into the axilla is possible for the first time.

In men, the excess midtorso tissue is excised transversely except at the nipple areolar complex (NAC). Here, two oblique ellipses rise to meet over the descended NAC. A continuous horizontal scar is avoided with accurate repositioning of the NAC, removal of gynecomastia, smoothing out lower chest and upper abdomen, and obliterating the IMF by ultrasound-assisted lipoplasty (UAL).

PREOPERATIVE PREPARATION

Body contouring can start approximately 1 year after bariatric surgery if weight loss has stabilized for 4 months. Rapid weight loss of about 70% of excess weight is completed by 1 year after a Roux-en-Y bypass. This is regularly followed by a 20% weight gain over the next 3 years. Skin quality will not improve by waiting longer, although patients should be warned that body contouring followed by further weight loss may result in undesirable skin sagging.

A compulsive review of recognized comorbidities of obesity and their change after bariatric surgery may reveal unacceptable, inadequately or overly treated chronic medical conditions.

- Smoking and narcotic drug dependence are contraindications.
- Depression is ubiquitous in the obese and will be reduced in 50% of the weight loss patients. Candidates with persistent, disabling depression or personality disorders should be rejected.
- Albumin levels should be checked in all candidates. Protein deficiency should be suspected with selected dietary limitations, a wide range of food allergies, and recurrent vomiting. Hypoproteinemia leads to delayed healing and chronic edema.
- Inadequate vitamin K absorption may follow intestinal bypass, and supplemental treatment may improve blood coagulation.

A comprehensive body evaluation is mandatory. The presentation varies according to genetics, prior fat stores, and rate of weight loss. Skin elasticity is poor, probably due to poor amino acid absorption and catabolism of elastin and supportive collagen in the subcutaneous tissue. Functional skin issues should be isolated from aesthetic ones. The location of transverse rolls of fat-laden skin demarcated by skin to fascia adherences is noted. On the torso, the rolls are larger laterally than medially, and on the thigh the deformity is reversed.

Prior scars on the abdomen must be considered, particularly subcostal scars, or major distal flap necrosis is likely.[14] Undermining beyond the scar is limited and/or incision design is altered. A well-executed lower body lift and thighplasty are integral to a successful TBL, which was described in Chapter 8 and elsewhere.[16–18] When staged, the upper body lift is usually performed at the second stage. For single-stage planning, the upper body lift is marked after the lower.[1,2,18] Candidates for single stage must accept increased risk of infection, thrombophlebitis, and more blood transfusions. Further major procedures and some revision may still be necessary.

Surgical markings for TBL are accurately made 30 min prior to surgery, after the patient has had a thorough antibacterial scrub. Once the decision is made to start prone and finish supine, one has to be confident that the lateral extent of the resection will be appropriate after the patient is turned to the supine position.

The markings for the circumferential abdominoplasty, modified lower body lift, and medial thighplasty are drawn first with the patient reclined and standing as noted in Chapter 8. Drawing for the upper body lift begins with the patient standing, which allows the torso skin to descend by its own weight (Figs 10.1 and 10.2). Follow the numbering on Figure 10.2. The sagging end of the breast is elevated off the chest wall to sight and mark the current IMF. The level is registered on the lower sternum. Commonly the breasts lie low, at or below the seventh rib. A higher IMF level is selected about the sixth rib. The revised level is sighted and marked (1) over the sternum. There should not be more that several centimeters difference from the old IMF.

Factoring in this new IMF location, the new nipple position along the mammary nipple line is marked (2). A narrow-angled Wise breast 'key whole' pattern with medial and lateral extensions is drawn (3). The pattern removes loose skin, raises the nipple, and cones the breast. With the anticipated tissue fill, the descending vertical limbs are drawn narrow and long. The usual IMF incision line of the Wise pattern (4) is now

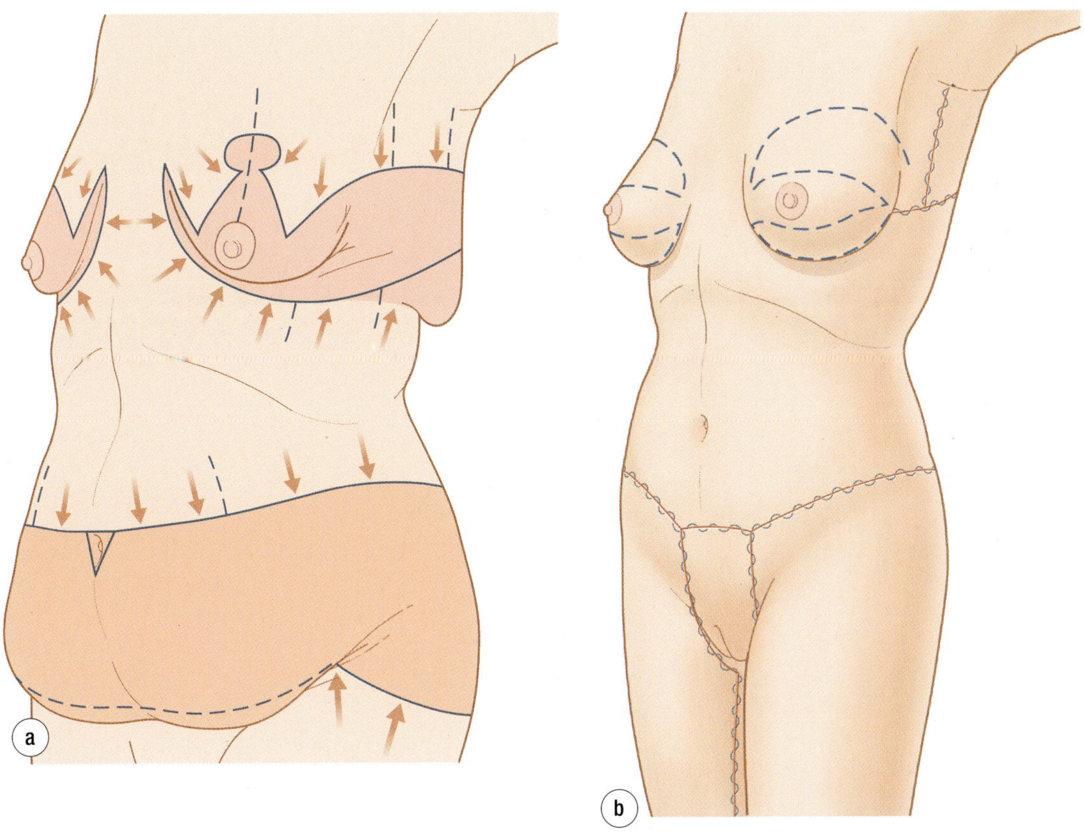

Figure 10.1 The incisions and closing scars for the total body lift. (**a**) The upper body lift incisions are drawn after the lower lift and abdominoplasty. The new inframammary fold is established as the boarder between the reverse abdominoplasty and the mastopexy. Using the gathering technique, the midtorsal back roll is removed along the bra line. There is a beltlike excision of the lower body lift and abdominoplasty. The upper body lift is deepithelialized for mastopexy and spiral flap elevation. The arrows represent vectors of tension. (**b**) Except for the arms and down the thighs, the final scars are seen to lie under underclothes and along the medial inner thigh. The spiral flaps positioning is shown.

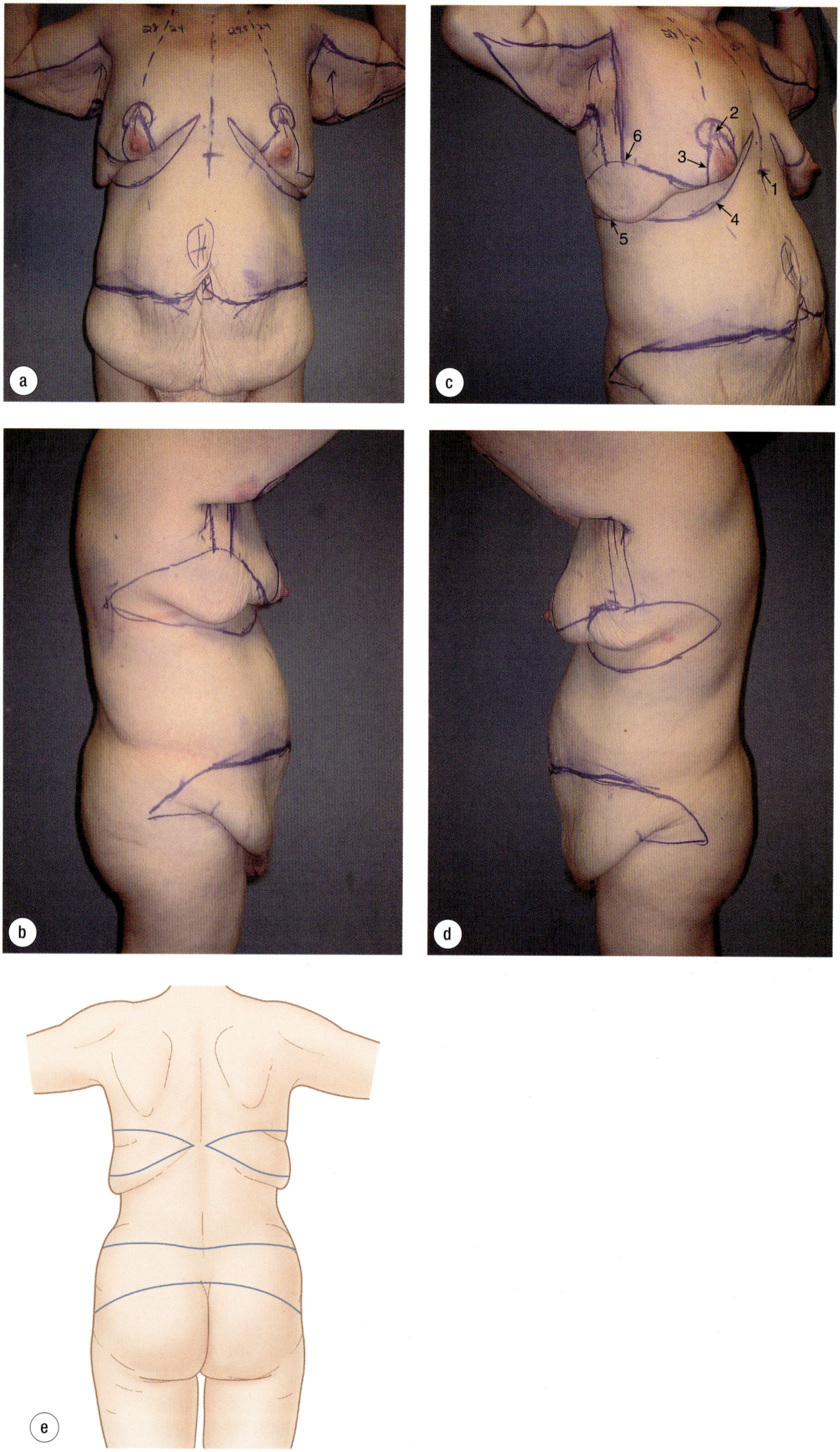

Figure 10.2 (**a–d**) The frontal and right lateral oblique photographs after completing markings for a total body lift in a 38-year-old massive weight loss patient. Follow in the text the description of the markings by the numbering in (c). The lower body portion is an extended abdominoplasty, monsplasty, and limited vertical thighplasty. Marking for the upper lift begins with sighting the inframammary fold and registering a new one over the sternum. The loose skin of the upper abdomen is pushed up and obliquely posterior over the costal margin. The epigastric excess is pushed into the lower poll of the breast. (**e**) Locations of scars after surgery.

dropped inferiorly on to the lower chest to include anticipated excess skin flap to be removed during the reverse abdominoplasty. To determine this area of skin, have the patient lift her breast mound to the new level. Then push epigastric skin upward and lateral until the umbilicus moves superior. Then ink dot the raised lower chest skin on the convergence of the nipple line and an imaginary horizontal extension of the new IMF marked on the sternum (1). From the ink dot, a tapered line (4) sweeps medially to meet the medial line of the Wise pattern near the sternum, and laterally and horizontal to about the midaxillary line. This advanced reverse abdominoplasty flap establishes the new IMF.

Next, the breath and length of the transverse lateral chest and back skin roll removal is determined. If needed for breast autoaugmentation, this roll will be deepithelialized and used as a laterally based fasciocutaneous flap. The width of the tissue removed is determined by pinch and gathering of local redundancy, while eyeing upward movement of the lower body lift incisions. The alignment of the excision (between lines 5 and 6) aims to leave the closure along the brassiere line. If there was a prior lower body lift, watch when the transverse scar pulls superior. While holding the raised skin in place, the roughly parallel superior incision line (6) is estimated by skin gathering and marked. The transverse lower line (5) meets the upper line (6). These two lines continue into the previously marked reverse abdominoplasty lines and lateral limb of the breast reduction pattern. The lines (5 and 6) are tapered in the back to close the ellipse near the tip of the scapula. It is alarming how narrow the skin band is that remains along the midtorso between the upper and lower body lift.

Unless there is synmastia and the breast reduction pattern takes us there, these reverse abdominoplasty incisions do not cross anterior midline, even though some midline laxity remains. Avoid transsternal scars, which are easily seen and frequently hypertrophy. An identical marking procedure is done on the opposite side. Differences in level of markings are reconciled due to asymmetry or drawing error. For the most redundant skin problem, an oblique elliptic excision, similar to the latissimus dorsi myocutaneous donor site for breast reconstruction, is drawn to gather excess skin in both the transverse and vertical dimensions. I have only resorted to oblique and vertical excisions in two severely deformed patients. The usual excision runs transversely toward the middle of the back, necessitating removal while the patient is prone.

UPPER BODY LIFT: THE INVERTED L BRACHIOPLASTY

For most, the upper body lift is completed with an L brachioplasty.[15] The L brachioplasty treats the four component deformities of the upper arm, axilla, and lateral chest.

1. The upper arm has massive hanging skin, which is worse centrally.
2. There is ptosis of the posterior axillary fold.
3. There is axillary enlargement.
4. There is lax lateral chest skin.

The L brachioplasty not only reduces upper arm excess tissue, but also raises the posterior axillary fold junction with the axilla, reduces the oversized axilla, and completes the lateral chest shaping. Other techniques ignored the hanging folds and chest excess, and leave unnatural T- or Z-shaped flaps in the axilla that are susceptible to skin necrosis, thickened scars, or geometric shape.

I excise excess skin and fat in the form of an inverted L with the long ellipse situated along the medial aspect of the upper arm and the short ellipse along the anterior half of the axilla and midlateral chest (Fig. 10.2). The upside-down closed angle bridging these short and long ellipses crosses the dome of the axilla. With healing, the final scar courses along the inferior medial arm, rises to the axillary dome, and then drops vertically to the chest, forming an inverted L. The two excision limbs are nearly perpendicular ellipses.

The brachioplasty markings are made with the patient sitting.[15] The arm and forearm are abducted 90° with the palm forward as if the patient were taking an oath. The superior incision line of the arm ellipse rises from the medial elbow along the bicipital groove to the deltopectoral groove. By gathering and pinching the center of the arm, the maximum width of resection can be determined. The inferior incision line of the arm ellipse runs from the medial elbow along the posterior margin of the arm to rise toward the midaxilla. When there is fatty excess, one has to compensate for the volume reduction subsequent to liposuction. Approaching the axilla at the posterior axillary fold, the inferior incision line rises toward the deltopectoral groove. The second ellipse drops vertically from the deltopectoral groove to include approximately the lateral half of the axilla and excess lateral chest wall skin. The chest portion of this ellipse is coordinated with the transverse removal of a back roll performed during an upper body lift. The width between lines is adjusted later, depending on the amount of expansion of the breast from autoaugmentation.

An inferiorly based triangular flap is formed as the inferior arm incision meets the lateral incision of the vertically oriented axillary ellipse. The ability to advance this triangular flap to the deltopectoral groove is checked by pinch approximation. This maneuver elevates the ptotic posterior axillary fold and tapers the arm toward the axilla. The markings are reevaluated with the arm and forearm fully extended above the head. The incision lines are then crosshatched for proper alignment.

SURGICAL TECHNIQUE

In one or several stages, TBL combines lower and upper body lifts. UAL removes excess fat. Medial thighplasty and L brachioplasties can be concomitant. When staged, the upper lift follows a prior circumferential abdominoplasty lower body lift and medial thighplasty. If immediate, upper lift planning considers the patient positioning, operative sequencing, tissue tensions, and blood supply inherent in the first part of the operation. The overriding principle is to leave as few scars as possible; however, the further the skin is from the line of closure, the less effective is the correction of laxity and contour deformity, especially if there are intervening lines of adherence between the dermis and muscular fascia.

For small, ptotic breasts, reshaping and fill is provided by spiral flaps. Figures 10.3–10.6 show the sequence. Anesthesia is provided by tertiary care university hospital anesthesiologists and their nurse anesthetists, who are experienced with my TBL surgery. They evaluate the patients the day of surgery or weeks sooner if we identified relevant medical issues. Unexpected adverse events during the procedure would curtail the scope of the operation, but that has not yet happened. Patients are started on broad-spectrum prophylactic antibiotics prior to the induction of anesthesia.

Special considerations for the anesthesiologist are head holding while prone, turning the patient supine, and fluid and body temperature management. The patient is induced under endotracheal anesthesia on the stretcher while alternating pressure stockings are functioning. Unless there are special indications, my patients do not receive anticoagulation for thrombophlebitis prophylaxis. The endotracheal tube is secured, and the eyelids padded and taped closed.

After the Foley catheter is inserted, the patient is turned prone on to an operating room table covered with a sterile drape. Soft chest rolls and a lower abdominal pillow lay under the drape to aid in respiration and alleviate pressure points. I check their position prior to the antiseptic preparation. The head is nestled into a foam rubber cutout and slightly turned toward the exiting endotracheal tube. Often, a warming pad is on the operating

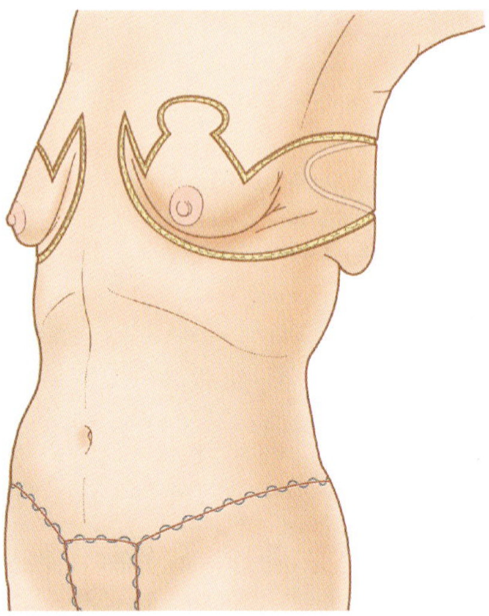

Figure 10.3 The Wise pattern is incised on the left breast with its epigastric and lateral chest extensions.

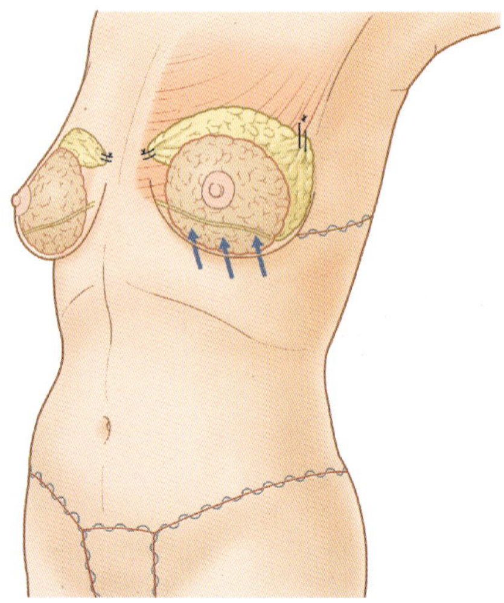

Figure 10.5 The lateral extension has been spiraled around the breast and over the pectoralis major muscle. The distal portion is sutured to the fifth costocartilage. The epigastric extension is folded 180° to fill the inferior pole of the breast.

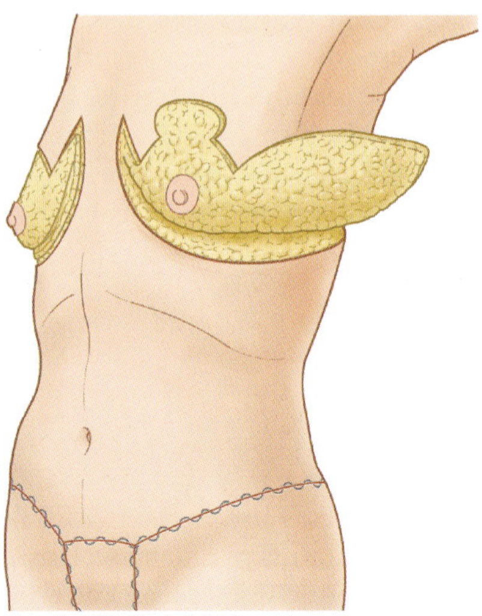

Figure 10.4 Except for the nipple areolar complex, the entire pattern is deepithelialized.

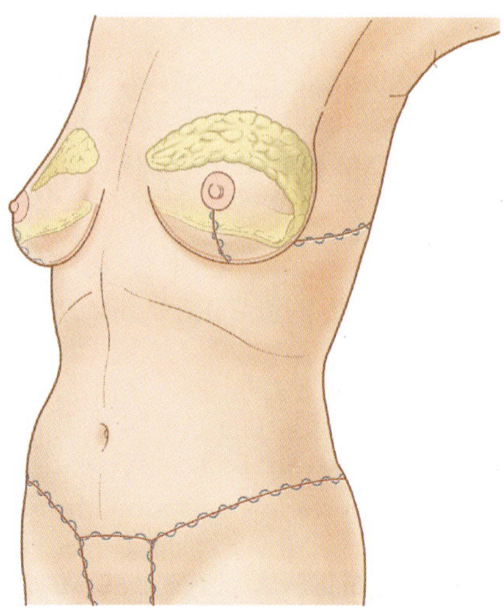

Figure 10.6 The closure of the Wise pattern helps cone and shape the breast.

room table and usually a forced hot air blanket covers the shoulders, arms, and head. Intravenous irrigation and infiltration fluids may be warm through microwave heating. Only areas immediately being operated on are exposed, and once closed they are covered with sterile drapes. If the patient's temperature falls, the operating room temperature is elevated.

The usual method of safely turning the patient back to the supine position returns the stretcher next to the operating room table. Except for the arms, the patient is wrapped with a sterile gown and then rolled over into my waiting arms, over the underside arm. That arm is then carefully pulled cephalad as the patient is nestled on to the stretcher. Finally, the now supine patient is slid back to the operating room table by pulling the now underside surgical gown like a hammock.

Prior to incision, saline with 1 mg of adrenaline (epinephrine) and 20 cc of 1% lidocaine (Xylocaine) is infiltrated with narrow, multiholed cannulas liberally along the markings, intended levels of dissection and liposuction. Thus bleeding from scalpel-created full-thickness incisions is minimized and early postoperative pain reduced. Crystalloid fluid is run at a rate to maintain appropriate pulse rate, blood pressure, and urine output, with constant monitoring of blood loss and frequent checks of blood hemoglobin. Typically, over an 8-h operation 6000–7000 cc of crystalloid and 500–1000 cc of hetastarch (Hespan) are given. Packed cell blood transfusions may start with over 800 cc of blood loss, hemoglobin under 8 g/dL, and difficulty in maintaining preoperative blood pressure and pulse. If possible, we delay transfusions until the end of the case so that the most dilute blood is lost during incisions.

During a single-stage procedure, the upper body lift begins in the prone position with removal of midback excess skin after competing closure of the bikini line excision of the lower lift. If the back and lateral chest soft tissue is to be used to augment the breast, it is deepithelialized and elevated as a lateral thoracic, medially based fasciocutaneous flap from over the latissimus dorsi muscle first (Fig. 10.7). Deepithelialization is expedited with an electric dermatome. The flap must extend to the tip of the scapular to be able to reach the ipsilateral parasternal region when later tunneled over the pectoralis major muscle. If the lateral back excess tissue is too wide, the flap can be narrowed, but I cannot imagine that it could be safely thinned. With minimal undermining, the subcutaneous fascia is closed with large braided absorbable sutures, and monofilament absorbable sutures in the dermis, usually over a drain.

On completion in the prone position portion of the operation, the patient is turned supine. The deepithelialized lateral chest flaps are left attached to the central breast pedicle. The first step is the abdominoplasty portion of the circumferential incision across the lower abdomen. Redundant skin between the umbilicus and pubis is resected. The midline attenuated fascia is imbricated. After minimal lateral undermining, the upper abdominal flap is advanced to the pubis and groin. Preservation of some of the epigastric transrectus muscle perforators to the skin is important.

After the abdominoplasty, the estimated upper abdominal skin resection is rechecked by gathering and pinching tissues. With adjustments of the markings, the upper body lift, breast reshaping. and L brachioplasty can resume (see Figs 10.3–10.6).

After marking a 45-mm diameter NAC cutout, the extended Wise pattern mastopexy is deepithelialized, as much as possible, with an electric dermatome to the lateral dorsal extension and over the epigastric excess (Fig. 10.8). A Wise pattern breast reduction includes a vertical bipedical deepithelialized NAC. The deep side of the NAC continues to receive blood supply from the breast mound. Because there is considerable tissue laxity, only minimal undermining of the Wise pattern breast flaps is necessary.

The incision for the reverse abdominoplasty is made along the lower border of the deepithelialized extended Wise pattern flap from parasternum along the lower anterior chest to the medial base of the lateral thoracic flap. The deepithelialized central breast with its inferior flap extension is released cephalad to about the sixth rib. The inferiorly based chest wall flap is discontinuously undermined to below the costal margins with dissector dilators in order to preserve perforating neurovasculature.

The deepithelialized fasciocutaneous flap immediately lateral to the breast is prepared for advancement into a tunnel under the superior breast (Fig. 10.8). The lateral to medial supramuscular dissection of the flap is resumed over the serratus muscle with dissection halted to preserve larger neurovascular intercostal perforators. Dissection over the serratus proceeds superiorly to expose the lateral border of the pectoralis major muscle. In the heavier person, this muscle can be difficult to locate, and it is just as easy to fall into the subpectoral plane. For easier anatomical orientation, I turn to the parasternal pectoralis muscle. That muscle is exposed through a 4- to 6-cm long skin incision through the most medial aspect of the Wise pattern. The medial breast is undermined over the pectoralis muscle under the superior pole of the breast rather easily. At the end of the dissection, one breaks through the lateral border of the pectoralis muscle to enter the space over the serratus muscle. Taking care to leave an adequate base to the breast, the space is enlarged to receive the lateral thoracic flap extension.

After the distal tip of the flap is cut back until there is bright red bleeding (Fig. 10.8), a suture is placed through the dermal end. With a long clamp inserted through the parasternal exposure, that suture is grasped and the flap pulled and pushed through the dissected submammary space. If need be, further lateral release is done. The large pulling suture at the end of the lateral thoracic portion of the flap is then sutured to the sixth costochondral junction, which secures the flap behind the breast. While in situ, the flap is adjusted to best augment and reshape the breast. Generally it lies flat, but it may be rolled on itself. The spiral flap may be secured to the lateral border of the pectoralis muscle with large absorbable sutures. After suturing the apex of the NAC to its higher chest position, the deepithelialized medial portion of the breast is advanced and secured to the costochondral junction. Finally, the deepithelialized epigastric extension of the lower breast is flipped upward and sutured to the lower pole of the breast. Larger flaps are trimmed as necessary.

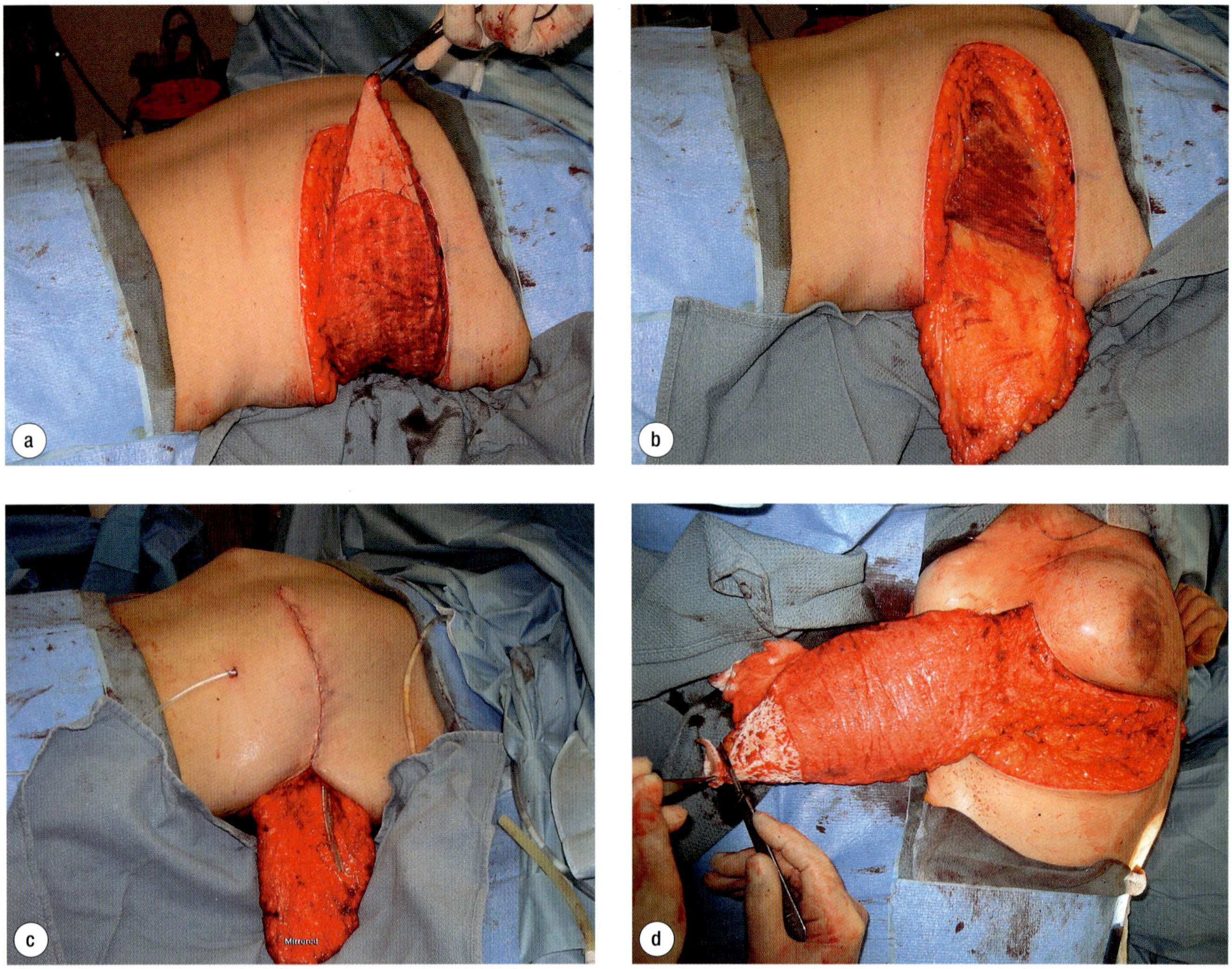

Figure 10.7 (a–d) These are the key steps of the back roll flap harvest in the prone position. Except for the most posterior triangle, the posterior ellipse is deepithelialized. A mechanical dermatome speeds the process. After the superior and inferior incisions are made, the flap is elevated from medial to lateral over the latissimus dorsi muscle. Dissection in this position stops just beyond the medial border of the muscle over the serratus fascia. The donor is closed with large absorbable sutures. A suction drain is placed to avoid a seroma. (d) shows the patient turned supine, and the lateral extension flap harvested from the back has the distal tip deepithelialized to reveal vigorous punctuate bleeding. The flap is ready for twisting around the breast.

After final positioning of the spiral flap, the reverse abdominoplasty is completed with a higher new IMF. The cephalad location for the new IMF has been registered over the sternum that guided the prior superior positioning of the central breast mound with its inferior pedicle. With the central breast pedicle out of the way, the inferior-based abdominal flap is advanced to this new IMF, about the fifth and sixth ribs. Approximately one dozen interrupted 0 braided polyester sutures are placed in the flap subcutaneous fascia and then into sixth rib cartilage and periosteum. The sutures are kept loose and held with hemostats until all have been placed. As all sutures are pulled superiorly simultaneously, the abdominal flap is pushed firmly upward to the new position and the sutures are sequentially tied. There may be some temporary dimpling of the skin. Obesity and/or excessive flare of the costal margins make this advancement difficult. The closure of the reverse abdominoplasty forms the new IMF. Most of the long scars are hidden under the breasts.

Once there is a secure IMF, positioning of the spiral flap is adjusted (Fig. 10.8). The spiral flap should form a crescent of volume in the medial, superior, and lateral breast. The epigastric portion of the flap then rolls on itself to fill and support the lower pole of the breast.

After securing the NAC into its new superior position, the medial and lateral Wise pattern flaps are approximated. The somewhat thin medial and lateral breast flaps are advanced over the breast mound to be sutured along the IMF to complete the reformation of the breast. The added flap volume can make this closure tight.

The most medial donor site of the lateral thoracic flap along the midaxillary line is closed tightly in layers, leaving high tension from the axilla to the IMF appropriately flattening this

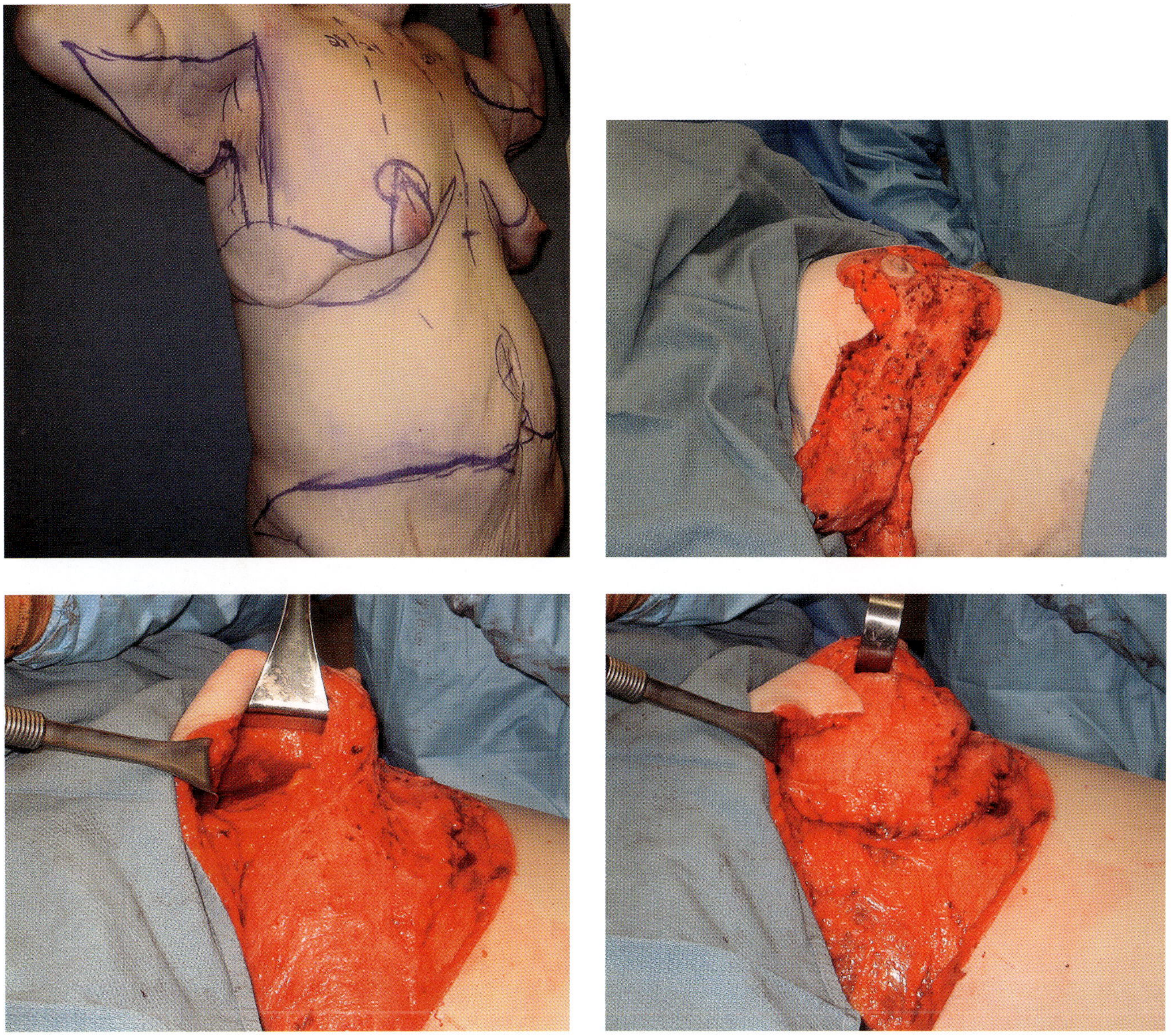

Figure 10.8 Returning to the patient shown in Figure 10.2, the steps in shaping and augmentation of the breast are shown. The deepithelialized and raised spiral flap is seen in situ. There is a retractor in the submammary space over the pectoralis muscle made for the lateral flap extension. Finally, the flap is rotated into the submammary space and folded against the inferior pole of the breast.

area, emphasizing the newly created lateral breast fullness and supporting breast projection. This lateral chest donor site closure is continuous with the advanced and stabilized new IMF. The firm fold also improves breast projection and eliminates bottoming out. Final contouring of the lateral chest awaits excision of the short limb of the L brachioplasty. A matching procedure is performed to the other side (Fig. 10.9).

If this soft tissue fill is too small, I have successfully placed small saline-filled silicone implants at this time, although I believe that, in general, implant augmentation is best left for another time. The time-consuming and complex tissue resections and rearrangements of the upper body lift, the tight skin envelope, and the additional devascularization intrinsic to creating a space for the implant make simultaneous implant and autoaugmentation procedures precarious. Moving the nipple upward requires excision of intervening skin, sometimes making the skin closure with precarious flaps over an additional volume of implant too tight.

The upper body lift is complete. The IMF is higher and secure. The reverse abdominoplasty has removed excess upper abdominal skin and left a scar hidden under the breasts. The scar continues laterally along the bra line instead of a mid-torso roll. The breasts are larger, with improved shape.

For the L brachioplasty, the upper arms have been prepared with antiseptic on operating room table arm boards. The unprepared forearm with a forearm blood pressure cuff is wrapped in sterile drapes. The width of resection is checked one more time. If there is any doubt, then a slightly narrower

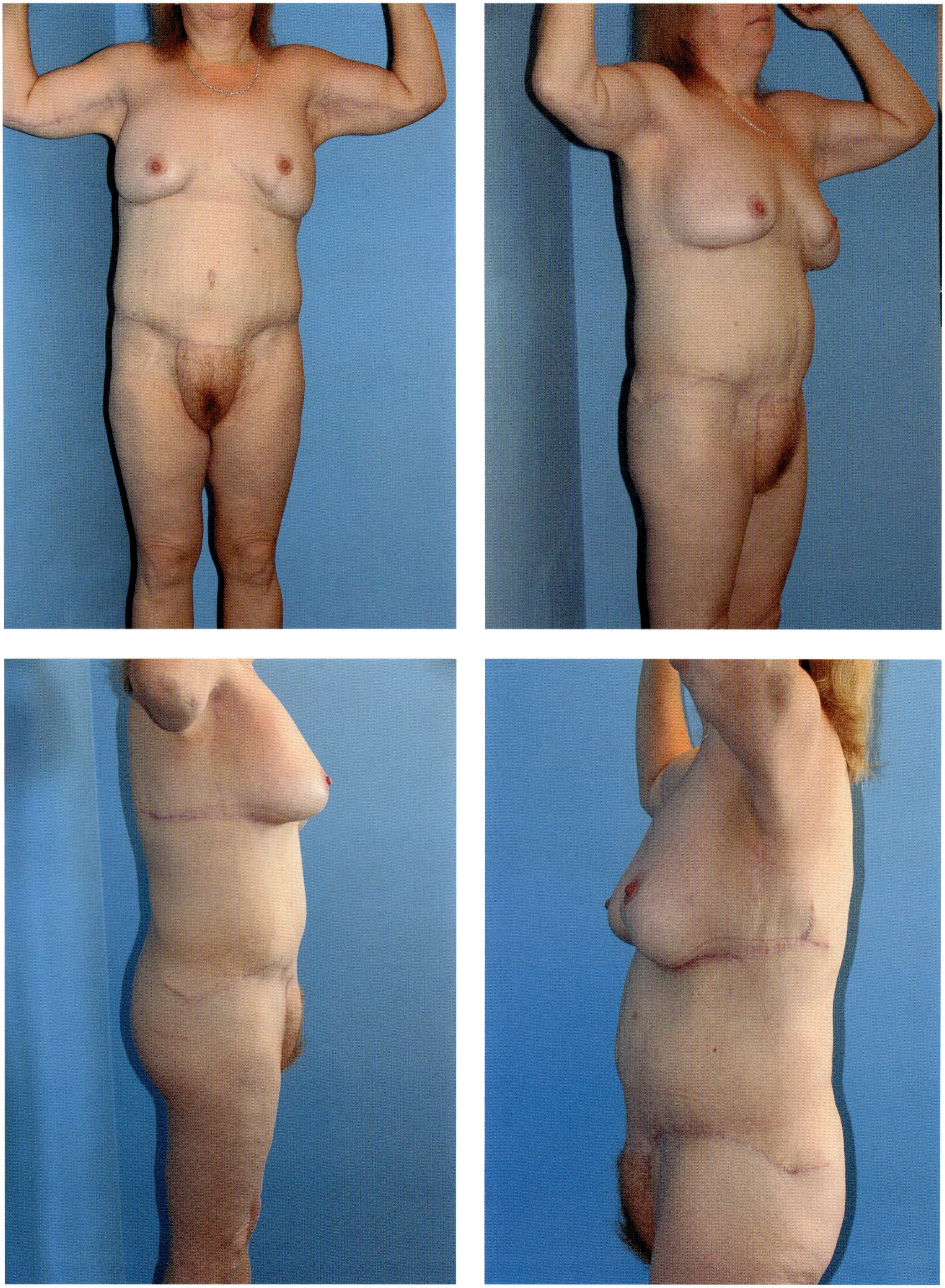

Figure 10.9 The 1-year postoperative result is seen after a single-stage total body lift performed entirely in the supine position. The preoperative markings are seen in Figure 10.2, and selected intraoperative views of the breast reshaping are seen in Figure 10.8. A lower body lift was not done—only an extended abdominoplasty and modified vertical thighplasty. There is improved breast shape and volume. The L brachioplasty complements the upper body lift. The exceptionally low left lateral IMF will need secondary elevation to improve breast symmetry.

ellipse is removed. In the manner previously described, I infuse several hundred cubic centimeters of saline with dilute adrenaline (epinephrine) and lidocaine (Xylocaine). After allowing 10 min for vasoconstriction, UAL is performed as needed.

With the medial skin rolled superiorly, the inferior incision is made to the level of the crural fascia enveloping the muscles. About 1 cm of undermining is done. Then the arching superior incision is made from the elbow to deltopectoral groove and also minimally undermined. Hemostasis is again obtained. I similarly incise the outline of the axillary chest ellipse, taking care to go just deep to the dermis in the axilla. The triangle of skin and fat at the elbow are grasped with the multitooth clamp or rake. The instrument firmly distracts the ellipse toward the chest so as remove the tissue, leaving a fine deep layer of subcutaneous fascia and fat over the subcutaneous nerves. Dissection stops to give electrocoagulation to patients with greater bleeding. The excision courses subdermal through the axilla, and then completes deeply over muscular fascia of the lateral chest. The clavipectoral fascia of the axilla is seen but not entered. Major veins and sensory nerves are not seen. The final decision on the width of lateral chest excision is made so as to remove all excess skin without lateralizing the breast.

Using the previously marked guidelines, the incisions are aligned with towel clamps. A continuous running 2-0 long-lasting but absorbable suture approximates the subcutaneous fascia. When approaching a towel clamp, a second clamp leapfrogs ahead before the first clamp is released. A second, smaller caliber continuous intradermal closure follows. Stern strips or dermal glue completes the operation. The arms are wrapped by an Ace wrap over a large ABD pad.

As the skin tensions equilibrate, the scar courses from the medial epicondyle to along the inferior medial arm, inferior to the bicipital groove. It gently rises to the axillary dome and then drops vertically to the chest, forming an inverted L. The inferior contour of the arm drops slightly at the midhumerus and then distinctly rises to a superiorly positioned posterior axillary fold. The suspended posterior axillary fold skin conforms well to the axillary hollow.

The breasts are placed in a surgical bra. No constricting binder is placed across the midabdomen, although for the lower body lift a long-leg lower body elastic garment is used. When only an upper body lift is done, patients are admitted for a single night's observation and care. The arm wrap is replaced with elastic sleeves several days later, taking care not to put direct pressure on the delicate triangular flap crossing the axilla. See Figures 10.10–10.12 for three cases of single-stage TBLs with L brachioplasty.

UPPER BODY LIFT IN MEN

In men, the objective of the upper body lift is to obliterate the IMF while correcting gynecomastia and redundant skin. Male upper body lift has definite synergistic effect when combined with the lower body lift and circumferential abdominoplasty. The upper lift in men also has four components.

1. A unique reverse abdominoplasty.
2. Obliteration of the IMF.
3. Removal of the midtorso roll.
4. Correction of the gynecomastia.

Male massive weight loss patients have loose upper abdominal skin, but too often a protuberant upper abdomen due to persistent intraabdominal epigastric obesity, which has to be considered in any reconstruction. A distinct IMF accentuates their disdainfully enlarged breasts. The midtorso rolls are lateral extensions of moderately ptotic gynecomastia. The gynecomastia is not only severe but also has inelastic skin that will not accommodate to a reduced volume.

The complete correction of weight loss grade 4 gynecomastia:

- properly positions NACs on pedicles;
- removes offending glands and skin, both vertically and horizontally; and
- leaves inconspicuous, long, anteriolateral chest scars (Fig. 10.13).

This is best accomplished with two elliptic excisions of skin wrapped around the areola, which I call a boomerang pattern excision correction of gynecomastia.

A common technique for loose skin gynecomastia is to remove the ptotic nipple. The gynecomastia is cut out along a long horizontal ellipse. Then the excised nipple is grafted on to the chest in the proper location. The take is not assured, and irregularity follows partial necrosis. But even with a 100% take, the nipple graft often looks like a skin graft, unnaturally flat and discolored. The long, straight scar is conspicuous, with a distinctly postsurgical appearance.

I have recently described the boomerang excision correction of gynecomastia. This procedure is an improvement over prior techniques because:

- the resection includes both vertical and horizontal excess;
- the NAC remains on a skin/glandular pedicle;
- the NAC is integrated into the upper body lift and TBL, and the long scar changes direction as it wraps around the repositioned areola.[1]

This gynecomastia correction considers biomechanical and aesthetic issues. There is a full-thickness triangular flap to support the nipple. That triangular base flap has excess fat and breast. I emulsify the fat and obliterate the IMF with UAL, followed by judicious liposuction. The resulting scar has a short limb that starts near the lower sternum, rises to arch the areola, and then descends toward the lower outer chest. Because the areola acts to break up the scar, it appears as if there were two smaller scars. The scar that wraps around the areola is less conspicuous than a straight line scar. The excision pattern resembles a boomerang, hence the appellation. In some cases, further reduction of the base was necessary at a later procedure. The ideal patient has a hirsute chest, which tends to be most dense around the areola and that obscures the scar.

Preoperative marking of the boomerang correction starts with sighting the new nipple position and registering it on the sternum. The ptotic breast and NAC are raised until the NAC falls in the correct position as agreed by the surgeon and

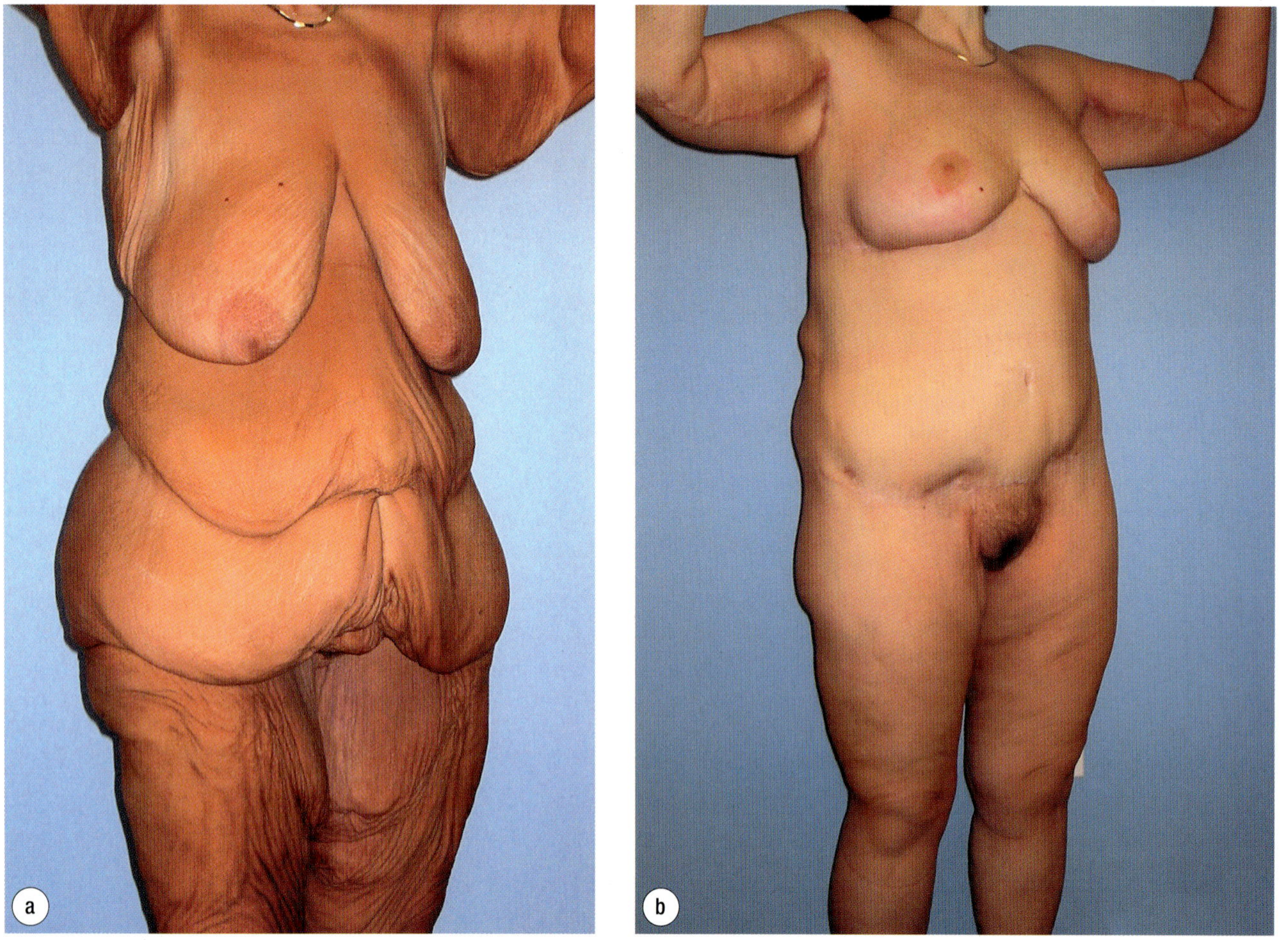

Figure 10.10 This right anterior oblique view is (a) before and (b) 1 year after three-stage total body lift (TBL) surgery and brachioplasties in a 5' 3" (1.60 m), 170-lb (77 kg) 47-year-old. She weighed over 400 lbs (181 kg) prior to her minimally invasive gastric bypass surgery. Her first-stage TBL was an abdominoplasty, lower body lift, and vertical inner thighplasty. Three months later, her second stage was an upper body lift with breast reshaping using mastopexy. Four months later, she had bilateral L brachioplasties and minor revisions of past procedures. While still a full-sized woman, she is thrilled with the loss of her hanging skin and the creation of voluptuous contours.

patient, remembering that the male nipple lies along the lateral pectoral border near the fourth interspace. The distraction effect of the abdominoplasty is taken into consideration, because there is a continuum of pull across the entire anteriolateral thorax. Visualization and the pinch-gathering technique of the excess tissue guides the planning of the width of the elliptic excisions that arch over the NAC at about an 80° angle. Bulky gynecomastia makes this judgment difficult. I prefer to slightly underresect and then take out more tissue superiorly if closure tensions dictate. The excision continues transversely around the posterior thorax to near the inferior tip of the scapula in order to capture the midtorso rolls.

During the course of a TBL, the upper body lift/gynecomastia correction begins after closure of the lower posterior incision in the prone position. The markings for the midtorso roll skin excision are reevaluated by gathering and pinching the marked roll, tugging on the just closed lower lift. The transverse triangle is excised and the wound closed in two layers of absorbable sutures. The patient is then turned supine and the abdominoplasty is completed. The appropriateness of the planned boomerang excision is checked. After UAL reduces excess fat and gland between the clavicle and boomerang excision, the two ellipses are excised. The NAC sits atop a triangular inferior pedicle. UAL of this pedicle removes the excess adipose and gland, discontinually undermines the flap into the abdominoplasty, and obliterates the IMF. NAC cephalad advancement is to a level indicated by the registered marks over the sternum. The NAC is carefully aligned during the layered closure of this superior reverse abdominoplasty (see Fig. 10.14).

OPTIMIZING SINGLE-STAGE TBL OUTCOMES

Contouring the entire trunk, thighs, and breasts with possible brachioplasty

- Total body lift surgery is for the surgeon experienced and confident in the component body-contouring operations.

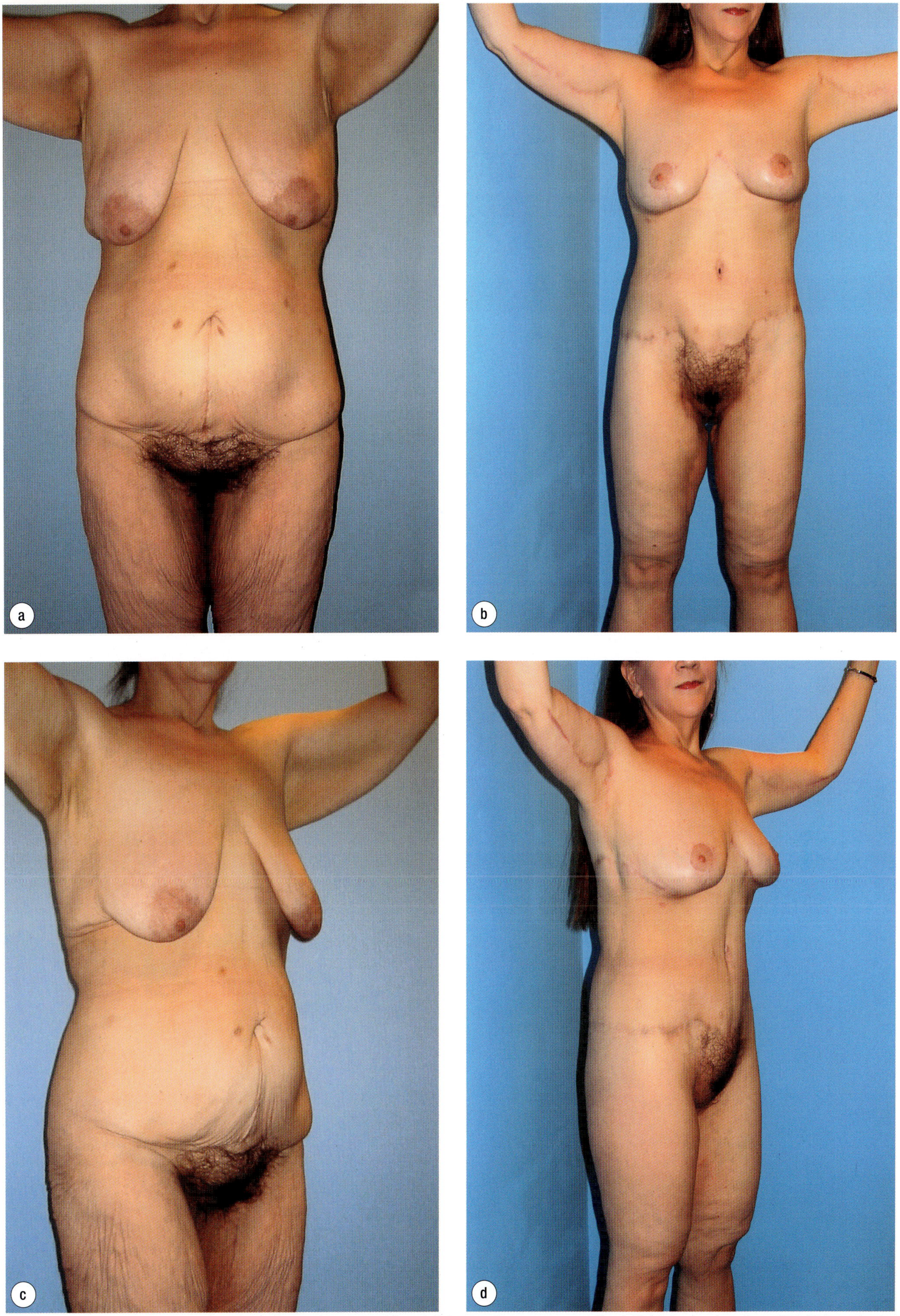

Figure 10.11 This right anterior oblique view is (**a** and **c**) before and (**b** and **d**) 1 year after one-stage total body lift (abdominoplasty, inner thigh lift, lower body lift, upper body lift, and breast reshaping with local flaps) in a 49-year-old woman. She is 5' 6" (1.68 m) and weighs160 lbs (73 kg), having lost 150 lbs (68 kg) after minimally invasive gastric bypass surgery. She hated her loose thighs and sagging breasts, and loved the improvement. She then focused on her severely sagging arms, face, and neck. Five months later, her second set of operations were face-lift, endoscopic assisted brow lift, and bilateral L brachioplasty.

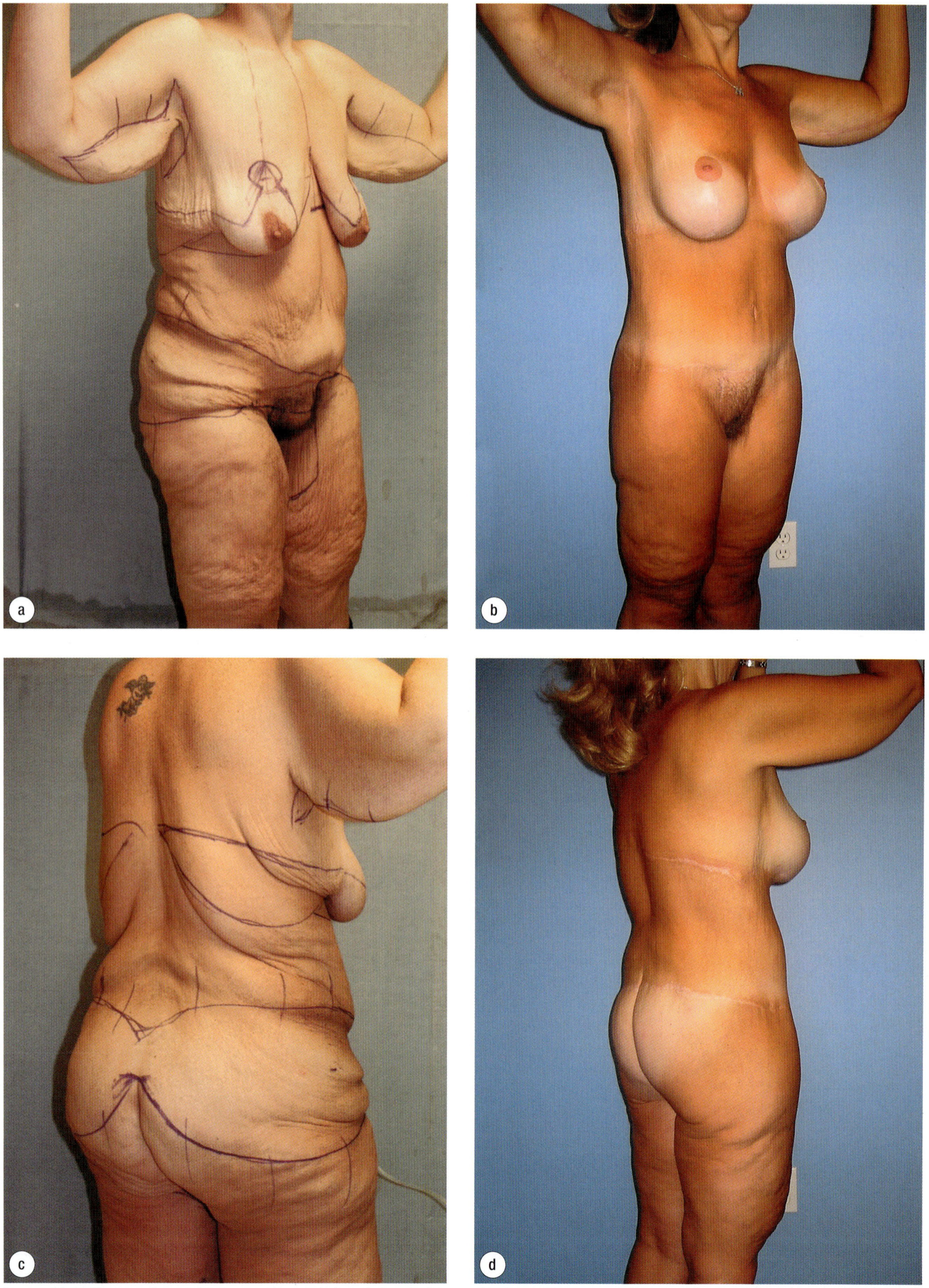

Figure 10.12 These are (**a** and **c**) before and (**b** and **d**) after photos of a 34-year-old who had laparoscopic Roux-en-Y bypass followed 3 years later by my total body lift with L brachioplasty. Her initial weight was 335 lbs (152 kg), and she now weighs 145 lbs (66 kg) (BMI 50–28 kg/m^2). One year after her lift, which removed 18 lbs (8 kg), her breasts were augmented with 300 cc of saline-filled implant, and L medial thighplasties were performed.

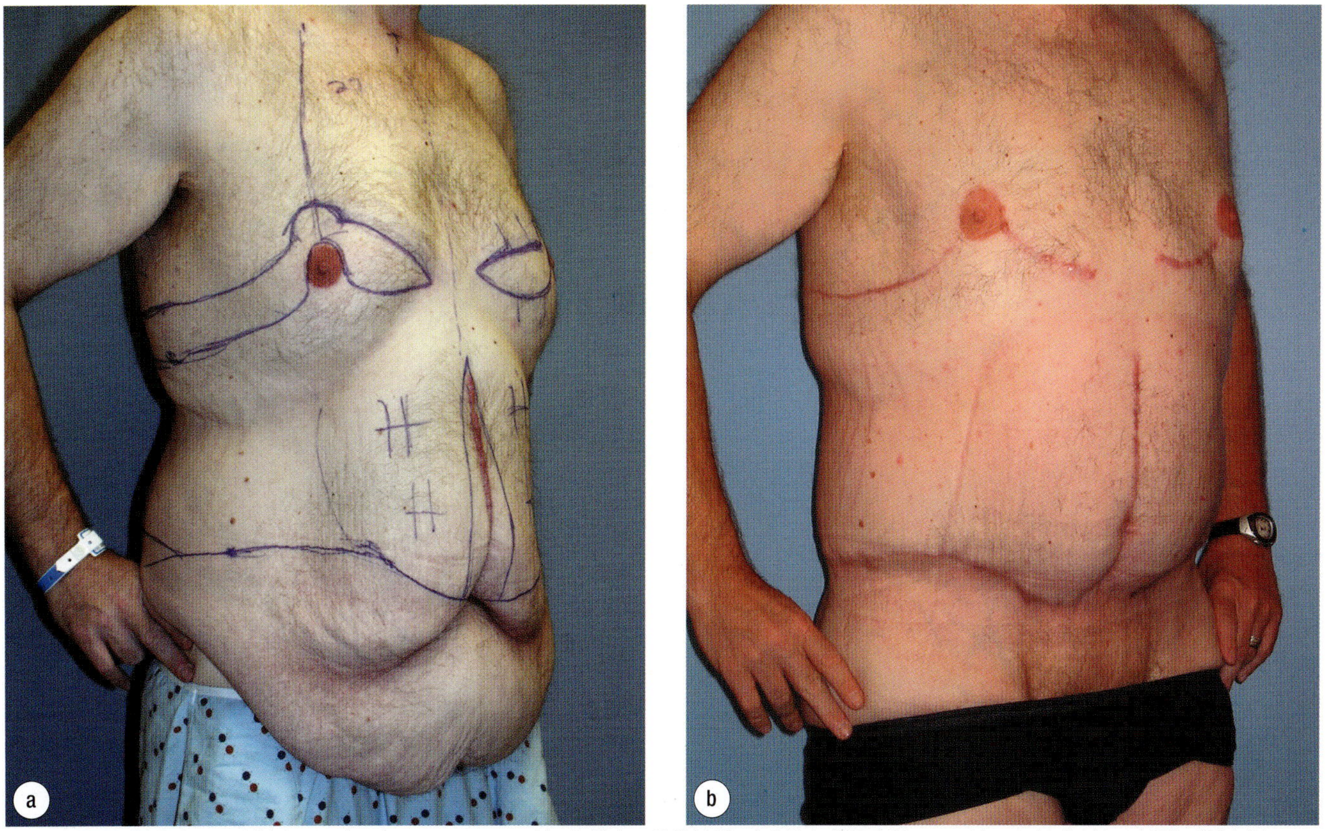

Figure 10.13 (a) Before and (b) 8 months after one-stage total body lift in a 6' 4" (1.93 m), 212-lb (96 kg) 26-year-old man. He had lost 150 lbs (68 kg) from gastric bypass surgery. The boomerang excision pattern is best seen in this frontal view.

- An experienced surgical team with multiple operators should be organized in a proper hospital setting.
- Candidates for single-stage TBL should be in good health and physically fit, not obese (BMI under 30 kg/m^2), and highly motivated.
- Markings for excision of skin are made with the patient recumbent for the lower body lift and thighplasty, sitting for breast reshaping and brachioplasty, and standing for the upper body lift, according to gravity and ease of marking. All markings are reassessed and adjusted while the patient is standing.
- With experience, markings can be reliably followed, but they should be checked as needed. Most scars should be transverse, level, and hidden beneath underwear.
- The prone then supine positions are the most efficient means of circumferential body contouring with symmetry.
- There is a sequential order of proceeding that accounts for the effect of one area on another. Starting prone, the lower body lift is closed with the thighs abducted, followed by closure of the lateral thoracic flap donor site. The thighs are then adducted for closure of the medial posterior thighplasty. After turning the patient supine, the abdominoplasty is closed while the table is flexed and frog-legged. Then the upper medial thighplasty is closed with the thighs adducted. With the table still flexed, the breast is reshaped and raised to allow for cephalad repositioning of the IMF at the end of the reverse abdominoplasty. The L brachioplasty ends with adjusting the width of the short vertical limb along the lateral chest.
- High-tension closure minimizes nearby skin redundancy. There is high tension when distracting wound edge forces need to be alleviated with relaxing limb or body positioning in order to achieve secure closure.
- High-tension closure flattens tissues so that the appropriate amount of underlying adipose is retained for optimum convexities.
- Assistants should be capable of closing wounds as the surgeon proceeds ahead.
- Changing limb position, preliminary application of towel clamps, and pushing tissues together relieve tension immediately prior to wound closure.
- Most weight loss patients prefer to avoid breast implants.
- Patients are very appreciative of a natural-appearing mons pubis, and object to descended inner thigh scars, as noted in Chapter 8.
- Patients are more accepting of residual laxity and undesirable scars when rounded buttocks and projecting curvaceous breasts are created.

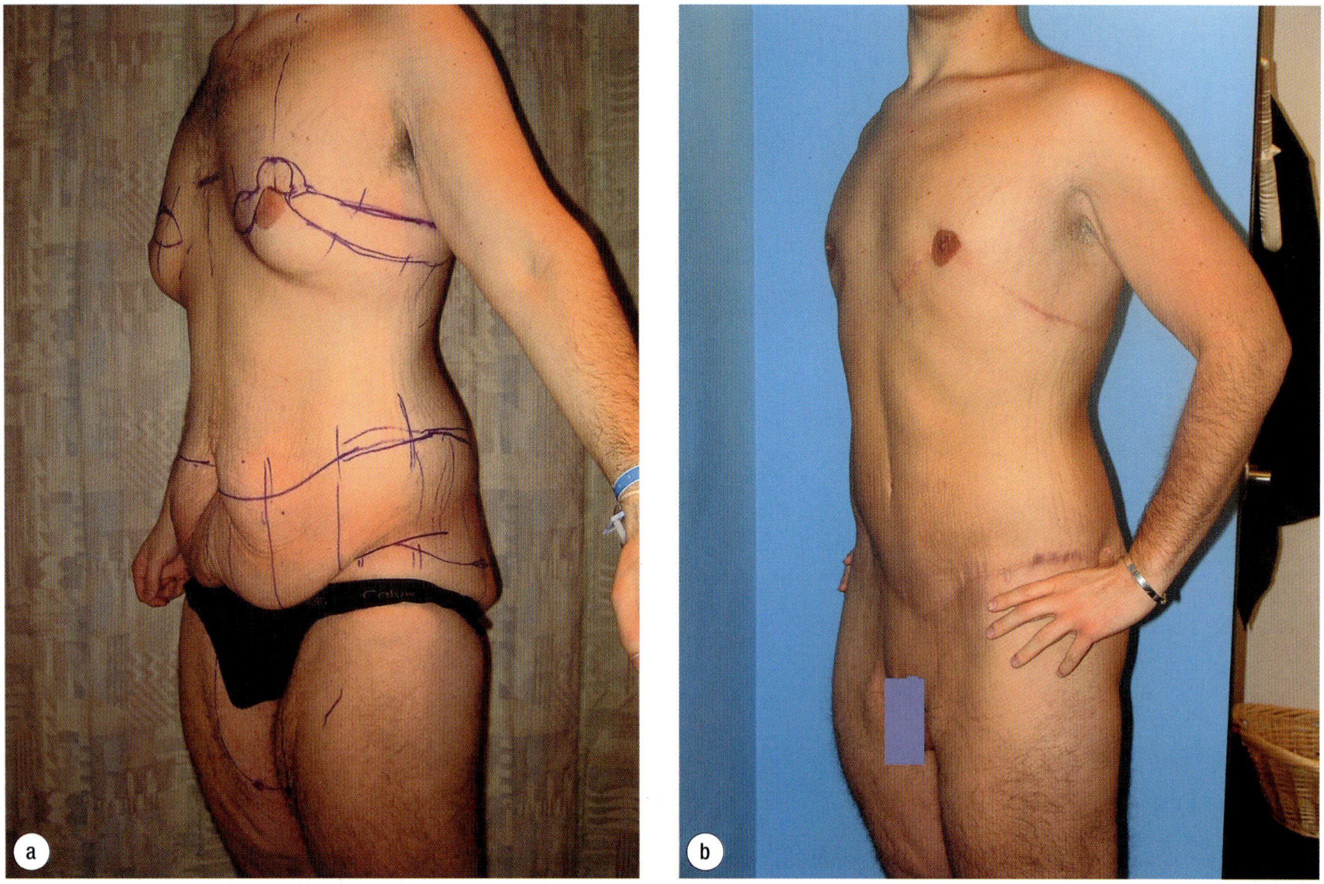

Figure 10.14 (a) Before and (b) 6 months after one-stage total body lift with correction of bilateral gynecomastia using boomerang excision correction. The patient is 5' 11" (1.80 m) and 190 lbs (86 kg), having lost over 100 lbs (45 kg) from open gastric bypass surgery. While troubled by his hanging abdominal apron, it was his sagging breasts that troubled him the most. He never exposed his chest in public. Following abdominoplasty, lower body lift, and upper inner thighplasty, I corrected his gynecomastia with removal of excess tissue and upward positioning of his nipples. He now goes shirtless on the beach.

- Gynecomastia correction is facilitated by the single-stage TBL.
- Severe gynecomastia after weight loss demands long broad areas of excision well treated with two obliquely oriented ellipses.
- The L brachioplasty completes the aesthetics of the upper body lift by sculpting the axillary folds into a reshaped lateral chest and breast.

POSTOPERATIVE CARE

Concurrent in the development of the upper body lift, measures were instituted to improve safety. By implementing a consistent and logical plan, we have been able to gain efficiency, reduce operative times, and improve outcomes. Attentive in-hospital 1 day of postoperative care for the isolated upper body lift allows for the early discovery and treatment of healing and medical problems. TBL patients require 3–4 days in hospital care. The designation of a dedicated nursing floor for bariatric patients at Magee-Women's Hospital of the University of Pittsburgh Medical Center has been instrumental in keeping our complications low. Accurate fluid management and conservative blood replacement, antiembolism prophylaxis with continuous use of pressure-alternating stockings, and patient warming by heating systems are essential.

It takes 4–6 weeks to recover from TBL surgery. Postoperative care begins with the activation of automatic intermittent calf pressure stockings prior to induction of anesthesia. Patient-controlled analgesia is available through push button control through the intravenous line. Prophylactic intravenous antibiotics are continued throughout the brief hospitalization.

Patients are transferred from the operating room table to their nursing floor bed similarly flexed. Vital signs including body temperature and the intake and output are compulsively monitored. Patients are warmed with heated blankets and, if need be, forced hot air. I usually show the emerging patients their improved body contour, which relieves some of the early stress and pain. The use of dilute lidocaine (Xylocaine) in the preparatory infusion reduces pain for up to 6 h.

After several hours in a tertiary care hospital recovery room, the patient is transferred to a furnished, well-staffed private hospital room in a designated postsurgical nursing unit. Immediate care is provided by experienced house staff and nurses. Sutures are available at the bedside to repair minor dehiscence. Patients start using the incentive spirometer but do not ambulate until the next morning. I insist on full return of sensorium before moving.

If a patient's condition deteriorates, transfer to an intensive care unit is immediate for continuous monitoring and care. Strict monitoring of fluid intake and output through an indwelling bladder catheter and suction drains is essential throughout the stay. Hemoglobin and serum chemistries are monitored daily, with appropriate treatment until stable. Fluid retention due to traumatic swelling and stress hormone release is expected over several weeks. Edema, particularly of the legs, is common and is usually treated with diuretics, leg elevation, and compression wrappings. Recently, we have initiated extremity suction/massage therapy prior to discharge with the use of the Well Box (LPG, Miami, Florida) with success.

When the patients' condition is stable and they are ambulating, the Foley catheter is removed. Prior to discharge, the patient is showered and discharged in properly sized elastic garments. After discharge, we encourage our patients to increase progressively non-taxing light activity. Within 4 weeks, most patients can resume daily functions such as driving and desk work. Elastic garments are worn for 6 weeks to encourage proper healing and provide support for the incisions. The first office visit is 10 days after surgery. The dramatic improvement in body contour becomes evident. Stitches around the umbilicus are removed. I will remove suction drains with output less than 50 cc per day. Many patients can resume vigorous exercise after 6 weeks. Minor wound-healing problems, especially along the medial thighs, are common and will require the patient to regularly change dressings.

COMPLICATIONS AND THEIR MANAGEMENT

Complex and lengthy surgery over a large portion of the body understandably entails medical and surgical risks. TBL surgery may be performed in several stages or in a single stage depending on the patient presentation and desire. Optimal candidates for single-stage TBL are physically and mentally stable. Highly motivated patients are willing to accept theoretic greater chance of morbidity and mortality for the efficiency and satisfaction of a single-stage operation. They accept that revision surgery is possible. Refined metabolic and inflammatory tissue markers are being considered to identify ideal candidates. Individuals having multiple stages did not fulfill these criteria or were under treatment before the single stage was regularly offered. Since regularly offering a single-stage operation in 2002 to optimal candidates, 53% (38 of 72) of the patients having TBL had a one-stage procedure.

Regarding complications, points to note are as follow.

- High-risk patients have nutritional disorders, obesity, undertreated or unstable chronic medical conditions, coagulation issues, mental disorders, and unrealistic expectations.
- Patients over 55 years of age are probably at higher risk of medical complications.
- Patients with insulin-dependent (type 1) diabetes, poorly controlled hypertension, unstable cardiac condition, and arrhythmias, or who are chronic smokers, should be avoided or have limited procedures.

Disregarding these admonitions may result in extensive wound-healing problems, postoperative intensive care unit admissions, prolonged or rehospitalization, and death.

After the first 72 patients with a single- and two-stage body lift, there have been no cases of thrombophlebitis. There has been one single-stage TBL patient with sepsis requiring readmission a week after her surgery. I emergently drained an upper medial thigh abscess that grew *Streptococcus viridans* and *Haemophilus influenzae.* A week of intravenous antibiotics and wound care cleared up the infection, and she was discharged to home 1 week later; within 4 weeks, the thigh incision wounds healed. She had 3000 cc of fat removed from her thighs using UAL lipoplasty during her TBL. I suspect that contamination must have been introduced at that time. Six months later, she is troubled by recurrent stitch abscesses. In two other patients, I have drained two midthigh abscesses 1 month and 3 months after their TBL.

The most common dilemma is the persistently overweight patient, having a BMI from 31 to 35 kg/m^2. The operations are more bloody and lengthy. High-tension closure of heavier tissues may dehisce or stretch out and depress, with loss of carefully created contours. Fat necrosis, wound infections, and suture abscesses are common. For these and general medical issues, oversized patients are encouraged to lose weight. An in-office nutritionist with an accepted rapid weight loss program is helpful. Through the cooperation of Drs El Hassane Tazi of Casablanca, Morocco, and Trudy Vogt of Zurich, Switzerland, we have used the A.W. Simeon severe caloric restriction diet with low-dose, off-label, daily human chorionic gonadotropin hormone (hCG) injections.[19] Dozens of our patients have lost from 15 to 30 lbs (7–14 kg) without suffering hunger in 6 weeks, making them better candidates for body-contouring surgery. While this rigorous low-caloric/hCG injection program has had high success without morbidity in Switzerland and Morocco, it has not yet been submitted to recent clinical trials in the USA. As such, the Simeon method is considered investigational. Confident of its advantage in preparing borderline patients for body contouring, I feel obligated to implement it with the aid of my physician assistant.

For the still oversized, optimal body contouring includes extensive liposuction, which is traumatic to the patient and flaps. I believe UAL to be the least injurious. The greater the amount of liposuction, the lesser should be the extent of excision surgery. Vacuum suction drainage is mandatory when liposuction and flap elevation are extensive (Fig. 10.15). Because of her excessive weight and an occult lateral thigh seroma cavity, outpatient readvancement of the lateral hips were needed in the patient in Figure 10.15. When there is excessive fat deposition and limited skin laxity, then a preliminary staged liposuction may be indicated.

On the flip side is the dramatically thin patient with circumferential layers of hanging skin. On the torso, transverse

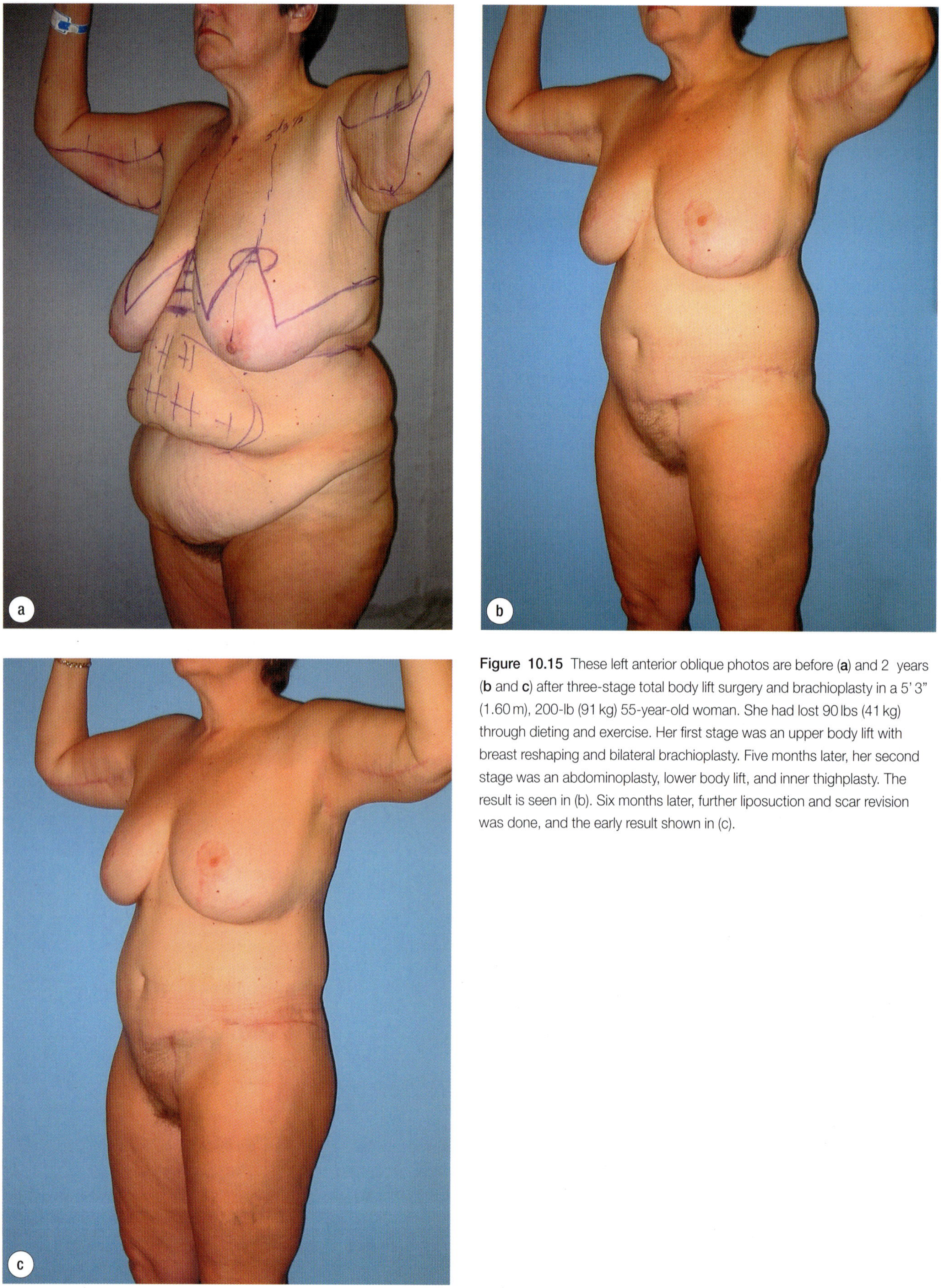

Figure 10.15 These left anterior oblique photos are before (**a**) and 2 years (**b** and **c**) after three-stage total body lift surgery and brachioplasty in a 5' 3" (1.60 m), 200-lb (91 kg) 55-year-old woman. She had lost 90 lbs (41 kg) through dieting and exercise. Her first stage was an upper body lift with breast reshaping and bilateral brachioplasty. Five months later, her second stage was an abdominoplasty, lower body lift, and inner thighplasty. The result is seen in (b). Six months later, further liposuction and scar revision was done, and the early result shown in (c).

excision only will leave too much loose skin vertically. On the thighs, the vertical extension excision needs to be precariously broad, and even then, secondary strips of excision need to be done.

All patients are informed of the inherent risks of TBL surgery. Our written informed consent document is instructive and covers the following major points:

- change in plans during the operation;
- bleeding;
- infection;
- thrombophlebitis and pulmonary embolism;
- change in nipple and skin sensation;
- long-term effects due to aging and weight change unrelated to the surgery;
- chronic pain;
- suture spit;
- anesthesia risks;
- allergic reactions to tape, suture material, or topical preparations;
- aesthetic shortcomings; and
- pregnancy and breast-feeding concerns.

SUMMARY AND CONCLUSION

Total body lift surgery is an original and boldly comprehensive correction of skin sagging, demanding insight, artistry, skill, stamina, and teamwork. TBL surgery was created to meet the unique challenge of body contouring after massive weight loss, and has been extended to treat the consequences of pregnancy and aging.

The single-stage TBL is an artistic tour de force, made possible by thoughtful surgical experience and innovation, modern anesthesia, and widespread patient education.[2] Effectiveness and safety are intertwined and directly related to the surgeon's outlook, temperament, and experience. There is a synergism at the midtorso level with improved narrowing of the waist and better effacement of gynecomastia. With proper organization, I believe that motivated plastic surgeons can reliably and safely offer TBL surgery to their patients.

Total body lift surgery is analogous to craniofacial surgery. Craniofacial surgery was introduced in the 1970s as a dramatic new discipline for the congenitally deformed. After 25 years of practicing craniofacial surgery, I consider that field complex and a dramatic, high-risk aesthetic facial reconstruction. Before craniofacial surgery, corrective operations for the congenitally deformed were limited in scope. Neurosurgeons reshaped congenially deformed craniums. Later, plastic surgeons advanced the jaws and bone grafted the midface and orbits. As a boundary between the cranium and face, the orbits were poorly treated. There was no comprehensive and coordinated planning and treatment. With the advent of craniofacial surgery, the entire deformity, including the orbits, could be approached in a coordinated single stage. Plastic surgeons, uniquely experienced in body contouring, can organize a team to treat the entire massive weight loss deformity.

As the craniofacial approach to the congenitally deformed became routine, enormous progress was made in elective aesthetic facial surgery. Similarly, once I developed a routine, coordinated total body approach for the weight loss patient, my aesthetic body contouring expanded and improved. As I became confident in the essential elements of skin excision, I could concentrate on the aesthetic details that make a difference. TBL surgery is as grand in scope as craniofacial surgery.

Total body lift surgery is a time-tested way to improve the abdomen, thighs, buttocks, midback, and breasts. Commonly, a first stage corrects the abdomen, thighs, and lower body. I position the patient prone and remove a large beltlike segment of skin above the buttocks, up to the lower back. On closure of this broad wound, the thighs and buttocks are lifted. Then I turn my patient supine to complete the anterior and medial thighs and the abdomen.

If it is not done immediately, I will correct the upper body deformity in stage 2 as early as 3 months after the first operation. By that time, all minor wound-healing issues, the threat of thrombophlebitis, and chronic edema are resolved. The patient should be on a healthy diet, restoring protein and correcting anemia. The upper body lift consists of a reverse abdominoplasty (from umbilicus to breasts), removal of midback rolls, and reshaping of flattened and hanging breasts. If the patient desires, the upper arms are included.

The upper body lift hides the upper scar under the breast and along the bra line. The breasts are beautifully shaped as the nipples are raised to the optimal position. A distinct new fold is secured under the breast to help maintain breast shape and a flat upper abdomen. Then I complement the upper body lift with an L brachioplasty. I remove excess skin and fat of the upper arm, axilla, and side of the chest roughly in the form of an L. The scar may take many months to mature, leaving a sweeping and as inconspicuous scar as possible because it lies between the bicipital groove and the posterior margin of the arm (see Fig. 10.16).

By coordinating several surgeons and skilled assistants, the TBL takes approximately 8 h, with additional time needed for larger patients. On average, three units of blood transfusion are needed. There has been no recognized thrombophlebitis or pulmonary embolism. Consistent with our initial report, there have been no increased complications as compared with the multistaged approach.[1]

The final contour relates to the deep fat, the extent of undermining, the tension of the closure, and the elasticity of the skin. In the massive weight loss patient, the skin is inelastic, so that only in areas that it is pulled taut is there no looseness in that direction. Transverse pull corrects vertical laxity only. Nevertheless, I had hoped that the combined superior and inferior tension at the bra and bikini line excisions would create a Chinese finger trap effect, thereby narrowing the waist; this is best seen in thinner patients.

By limiting the undermining and using gentle liposuction, removal of skin from both the upper and lower ends of the abdomen does not lead to flap edge ischemia. It is clear that patients with prior abdominoplasty and considerable upper

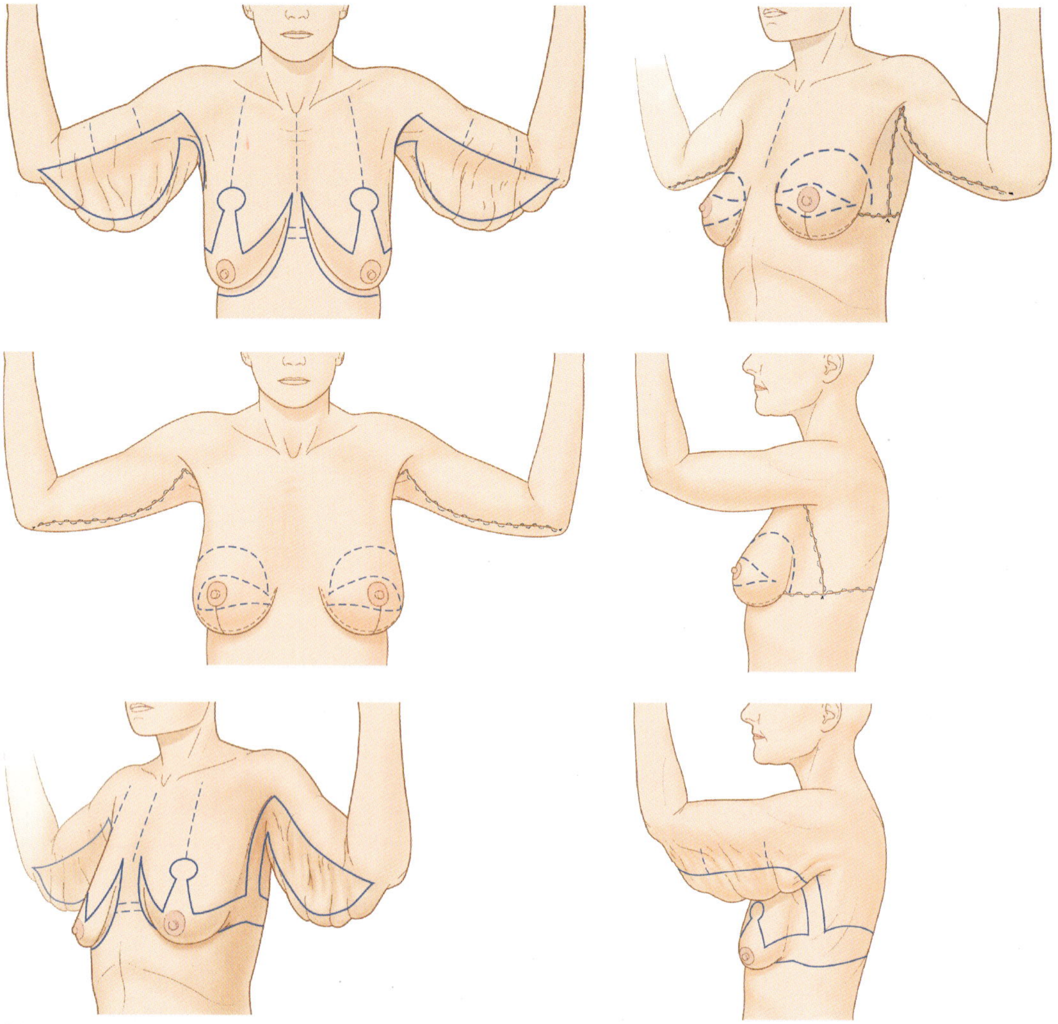

Figure 10.16 Multiple views of the combined upper body lift with spiral flap reshaping of the breasts and brachioplasty. Also demonstrated are the final scars and spiral flap positioning.

abdominal skin laxity are inadequately treated by traditional secondary abdominoplasty and are better served by a single-stage TBL. Otherwise, the advantage of a single stage in women primarily seems to be in limiting the number of operative sessions, which are onerous when considering face-lift, blepharoplasties, brachioplasties, leg reductions, etc. Some patients poorly tolerate the waiting period necessary before operating on the upper body deformity. During that time, patients find increasing fault with the results of the first stage and many never advance to the second.

The extensive scarring that follows these procedures has been more than offset by the dramatic improvement in the breasts, torso, and arms. While some patients have scars that become raised or irregular, most scars will fade over several years. An active scar treatment program with a variety of modalities is essential.

We have established that a single-stage TBL can be effective and safe. Accepting the theoretically increased risk, some patients prefer one major operative intervention instead of two or more.

REFERENCES

1. Hurwitz DJ. Single stage total body lift after massive weight loss. Ann Plast Surg 2004; 52(5):435–441.
2. Hurwitz DJ. Total body lift: reshaping the breast, chest, arms, thighs, hips, waist, abdomen and knees after weight loss, aging and pregnancies. New York: MDPublish; 2005.
3. Zook EG. The massive weight loss patient. Clin Plast Surg 1975; 2(4):57–466.
4. Zook EG. Discussion of 'Abdominoplasty following gastrointestinal bypass surgery' by RC Savage. Plast Reconstr Surg 1983; 74:508–509.
5. Palmer B, Hallberg D, Backman L. Skin reduction plasties following intestinal shunt operations for treatment of obesity. Scand J Plast Reconstr Surg 1975; 9:47–52.
6. Wise RJ. A preliminary report on a method of planning the mammaplasty. Plast Reconstr Surg 1956; 17:367–369.

7. McKissock PK. Reduction mammoplasty with a vertical dermal pedicle. Plast Reconstr Surg 1972; 49:245–252.
8. Shons AR. Plastic reconstruction after bypass surgery and massive weight loss. Surg Clin North Am 1979; 59:1139–1152.
9. Regnault P, Daniel RK. Massive weight loss. In: Regnault P, Daniel RK. Aesthetic plastic surgery: principles and techniques. Boston: Little Brown; 1984:705–720.
10. Grazer FM. Abdominoplasty. In: McCarthy et al, eds. Plastic surgery, vol. 6. The trunk and lower extremity. Philadelphia: Saunders; 1994:3929–3963.
11. Zienowicz RJ. Augmentation mammoplasty by reverse abdominoplasty. Presented at Emerging Technologies and Techniques in Plastic Surgery, New York University Medical Center, May 20–21, 2005.
12. Lockwood TE. Superficial fascial system (SFS) of the trunk and extremities: a new concept. Plast Reconstr Surg 1991; 87:1009–1015.
13. Lockwood TE. Reduction mammaplasty and mastopexy with superficial fascial system suspension. Plast Reconstr Surg 1999; 103:1411–1420.
14. Hurwitz DJ, Golla D. Breast reshaping after massive weight loss. Semin Plast Surg 2004; 18:179–187.
15. Hurwitz DJ, Holland SW. The L brachioplasty: an innovative approach to correct excess tissue of the upper arm, axilla and lateral chest. Plast Reconstr Surg 2006; 117(2):403–411.
16. Hurwitz DJ, Zewert T. Body contouring surgery in the bariatric surgical patient. Oper Tech Plast Surg 2002; 8:87–95.
17. Hurwitz DJ, Rubin JP, Risen M, et al. Correcting the saddlebag deformity in the massive weight loss patient. Plast Reconstr Surg 2004; 114(5):1313–1325.
18. Hurwitz D. Medial thighplasty for operative strategies. Aesthetic Soc J 2005; 25:180–191.
19. Vogt T, Belluscio D. Controversies in plastic surgery: suction-assisted lipectomy (SAL) and the hCG (human chorionic gonadotropin) protocol for obesity treatment. Aesthetic Plast Surg 1987; 11(3):131–156.

COMBINED PROCEDURES AND STAGING

11

Loren J. Borud

Key Points

- There is no current consensus on an optimum strategy for combining and staging body-contouring procedures in the massive weight loss patient.
- Advantages of combining procedures include patient satisfaction, financial savings, and reduction in total recovery time and time out of work.
- Disadvantages of combining procedures include lengthy operating time and higher risks of blood transfusions. Potentially, risk of deep venous thrombosis, pulmonary embolus, and other complications may be increased. When procedures are staged, there is generally less pain from each stage, and thus patients are more mobile in the postoperative period. Staged procedures allow built-in opportunities to revise unpredictable skin relaxation in previously operated areas. Finally, some procedures, such as upper body lift and lower body lift, have vectors of pull in opposite directions and may interfere with each other if performed simultaneously.
- An individualized approach for each patient is advocated, with assessment of patient priorities, general medical risk, and patient work and lifestyle considerations.
- Surgeons are encouraged to develop their own individualized approach based on experience, availability of personnel, and level of assistance, tracking recent operative times for component procedures, and estimated total operating time and transfusion risks for proposed combinations of procedures.

> *You are ambitious, which, within reasonable bounds, does good rather than harm.*
>
> Abraham Lincoln

Whether in philosophy, politics, business, love, war—or surgery, examples abound of the conflict between the strategy of the rapid, quick, decisive move versus the prudent, stepwise, conservative process. In plastic surgery, this yin and yang is nowhere more evident than in the massive weight loss (MWL) patient undergoing body-contouring surgery. How much is too much? Should one 'get it over with' in one or two long operations? Or is it safer to divide the job into multiple stages?

Advances in laparoscopic techniques, anesthetic management, and establishment of comprehensive bariatric centers have transformed bariatric surgery from an extreme, risky treatment of last resort reserved for only the most morbidly obese patients into a widespread, established series of techniques applicable to vast numbers of patients in the USA and across the world. In the past 10 years, the number of such procedures performed in the USA has increased an astonishing 644%.[1] As recently as a decade ago, it was extraordinary to encounter a patient who had lost 100 lbs (45 kg), usually through diet and exercise. Now, plastic surgeons are faced with these scenarios on a daily basis.

Such MWL is associated with multiple areas of substantial skin excess that are of medical and aesthetic concern to most patients. The MWL patient is frequently a candidate for multiple body-contouring procedures from head to toe, including:

- face/neck lift;
- mastopexy/breast augmentation or reduction;
- brachioplasty;
- panniculectomy/abdominoplasty;
- belt lipectomy/buttock lift;
- thigh lift; and
- various combinations and permutations of these, such as lower body lift, total body lift, and other procedures.

Individually, the various body-contouring procedures can be extensive, lengthy procedures. In no other realm of plastic surgery are the surgeon and patient confronted with such vexing questions of how such varied anatomical regions and procedures should be combined and/or staged. Intense media exposure in recent years has popularized the 'extreme makeover' mentality. While some patients are well-informed and extremely sophisticated in terms of understanding the risks of prolonged surgery, some other patients view body contouring as merely an extended cosmetic makeover.

At this time, there is no generally accepted consensus on the right or wrong ways of combining or staging body-contouring procedures in the MWL patient. Any dogmatic formula or policy for this complex problem is intrinsically flawed, because it could not be applied to all patients, nor could it be useful to a diverse group of surgeons with varied practice settings and levels of experience. This chapter seeks instead to outline the risks and benefits, the pros and the cons, of combining or staging various combinations of body-contouring procedures.

It is designed to assist plastic surgeons in formulating their own optimum strategy for treating individual patients.

PREOPERATIVE PREPARATION

Evaluating surgeon experience and practice setting: expected operating room time

Body-contouring operations in MWL patients can generally be described as lengthy, complicated, technically demanding, and time-intensive versions of the standard body-contouring procedures familiar to most plastic surgeons. They require specialized knowledge and expertise, as well as an appropriately trained surgical team of assistants, nurses, and anesthesiologists. Even prior to evaluating the patient, careful surgeons will evaluate:

- their own level of experience with these procedures,
- the availability of appropriate first or second assistants, and
- the availability of efficient and experienced nursing and anesthesia team members.

Surgeons should be able to estimate fairly accurately, based on their own practice situation and carefully maintained records from recent body-contouring cases, factors such as the expected duration and blood loss for the various proposed combinations of body-contouring procedures for a particular patient. As outlined below, there is evidence that the risk of the most substantial complications is related to the total time under general anesthesia. Therefore the expected operating room time should include the surgery time plus the typical anesthesia induction, preparation, and emergence time in the surgeon's practice setting.

Evaluation of the MWL patient

Evaluation of the MWL patient is discussed in greater detail elsewhere in this text. A detailed history, physical examination, and photographs form the foundation of this evaluation. A thorough discussion of the various body areas that could be treated follows. The surgeon's most important task at this time is to provide a detailed discussion of the various procedures and to ensure that the patient gains an understanding of realistic expectations of each procedure. The anticipated degree of skin resection, the location of incisions, and the expected appearance of the resulting scars and contour are discussed. The duration of hospitalization, potential for blood transfusion, and expected duration of recovery should be emphasized, as well as the possibilities of:

- deep venous thrombosis,
- pulmonary embolus,
- hematoma,
- seroma,
- need for return to the operating room,
- pneumonia,
- fat necrosis,
- cellulitis,
- lymphocele, and
- lymphatic injury leading to lymphedema.

The informed consent should potentially include a rough estimate of the duration of the procedure.

It is vital to focus on the chief complaint and, after detailed discussion of each possible component procedure, the patient and surgeon should make a written list of the patient's priorities. The most common areas treated and their associated procedures are summarized in Table 11.1. Of course, the amount of surgery involved in a given procedure can vary tremendously from patient to patient, because there is a broad spectrum of skin excess within the MWL patient population. Our practice is to classify patients into three broad categories, summarized in Table 11.2, based on their skin excess, which is the difference between the body surface area (BSA) at maximum weight minus their expected BSA at their current weight. The Mosteller formula shown below is the most commonly used formula for BSA,[2] and easy-to-use calculators are readily available on the Internet:

BSA (m^2) = (height [inches] × weight [lbs])/3131$^{1}/_{2}$

This classification is helpful in estimating the degree of the procedure and in determining the various staging options. Finally, the surgeon must take special note of any other additional procedures that must be done at the time of body contouring, such as repair of a large ventral hernia, and any medical conditions that present an increased anesthetic risk to the patient.

Table 11.1 Body-contouring procedures

Body area	Procedure
Face/neck	Rhytidectomy
Breast	Breast reduction
	Mastopexy
	Mastopexy and augmentation
Arm	Brachioplasty
Trunk/back	Panniculectomy
	Abdominoplasty
	Belt lipectomy
	Lower body lift
	Upper body lift
Buttock/thighs	Thigh lift
	Lower body lift
	Buttock lift
	Total body lift (all areas)

Table 11.2 Classification of skin excess in the massive weight loss patient

Class	Skin excess	Excess surface area (m^2)
1	Moderate	<0.4
2	Large	0.4–0.7
3	Extreme	>0.7

Overview of staging strategies

After the informed consent process is completed, if the patient is interested in combining a number of body-contouring procedures, our practice is to then develop two or more options for combining and staging the procedures. This process begins with the patient priority list and takes into account the classification of skin excess, other concomitant procedures (such as hernia repair), and the overall anesthetic risk of the individual patient. The advantages and disadvantages of combining versus staging are summarized in Table 11.3. In our experience, most MWL patients can be treated in either one or two major stages, as outlined below.

Two-stage body contour strategy

This strategy involves a multiprocedure first stage that combines procedures in one or more anatomical regions. The abdomen/lower body lift or belt lipectomy is generally the patient's first priority. This can be done alone as a substantial first stage, or combined with a smaller procedure, such as brachioplasty, medial thigh lift, or mastopexy with or without augmentation. Some surgeons choose to set a time limit for a single anesthetic, such as 6–8 h, and minimize the risk of blood transfusion, deep vein thrombosis, pulmonary embolus, and other complications. There is no current evidence to support a specific time limit, but surgeons should be guided by their level of experience, stamina, and degree of technical assistance. The second stage would typically involve a thigh lift with brachioplasty or mastopexy, or upper body lift if not done at first stage. Face-lift, if indicated, would usually be done at the second stage or at a separate stage altogether.

One-stage body contour strategy

Three or more major body areas are treated at one sitting:

- abdomen/lower body lift,
- mastopexy/augmentasion with or without brachioplasty, plus or minus thigh lift.

The strategy here is to combine all the patient priorities into one operation, accepting lengthy operative time and possible need for blood transfusion. A face-lift, if indicated, would generally be done as a separate procedure, because the one-stage body lift is an aggressive, all-day-long procedure in and of itself, even for the most experienced surgical team.

Operating time and maior risks

While the two-stage approach is more conservative and is the prevalent strategy in most centers, the one-stage approach is becoming increasingly popular in some centers. The one-stage approach, in our view, should be offered only by an experienced surgeon with the availability of an experienced operative team and substantial anesthesia or critical care resource, and is only applicable in a subgroup of patients. Relative contraindications for a one-stage approach are summarized in Box 11.1.

In formulating the two-stage strategy, our policy is to limit the expected duration of the first stage to 8 h of anesthesia time. While arbitrary, similar time-based limits have been adopted by others as well.[3] We calculate expected operating room time at our institution by adding the expected operative times for the various component procedures, modified by the classification

Box 11.1 Relative contraindications for the lengthy one-stage option

- Patient priority for rapid return to work or activities.
- Patient priority to avoid blood transfusion.
- History of deep vein thrombosis, pulmonary embolus, or hypercoagulable state.
- Need for concomitant massive ventral hernia repair.
- BMI over 32 kg/m^2.
- Class 3 extreme skin excess.
- Lack of surgeon experience.
- Lack of adequate surgical assistance.
- Lack of adequate anesthesia or critical care backup.
- Need for large-volume liposuction.

Table 11.3 Advantages and disadvantages of combining versus staging body-contouring procedures in the massive weight loss patient

	Combining	Staging
Advantages	Patient convenience 'Get it all over with' concept Financial savings Less total time out of work or activities	Avoids lengthy operations Possibly lower morbidity and mortality Lower chance of blood transfusion More flexible 'touch up' options Less acute patient discomfort
Disadvantages	Lengthy operation Possibly higher morbidity and mortality Increased risk of blood transfusion Greater acute patient discomfort Longer one-time recovery	Multiple surgery and recovery periods Greater total cost Greater total time off work or activities

of skin excess in the individual patient (Table 11.2), and finally including the average anesthesia induction, wake-up, and preparation time.

An informed consent discussion then takes place outlining the various medically appropriate combining and staging strategies and their respective risks and benefits for the individual patient. The informed consent is carefully documented in the medical record. The signed consent form should also specifically include a statement that alternative staging and combining strategies were discussed. In the end, patients must come to their own conclusion about the best strategy for their individual case (Fig. 11.1).

In addition to operating room time, risk of transfusion, and risk of major medical complications, the surgeon must take into account several other issues when formulating the staging strategy. These include:

- patient comfort,
- postoperative skin relaxation and revision procedures, and
- potential technical interference between simultaneous procedures.

Hence there is no universal recommendation.

Patient comfort

A major truncal procedure (lower body lift or belt lipectomy), which generally constitutes the first stage in a multistage approach to body contouring, is a major undertaking in and of itself. If adequate tissue is resected, there is significant tension. The patient is quite limited in mobility and can experience significant postoperative pain. If additional areas, such as breast, upper extremities, or thighs, are treated simultaneously, it may immobilize the patient longer and make recovery somewhat onerous, especially if the patient has limited assistance at home. In our experience, some patients who have considered various staging options and have then elected a lower body lift as a first stage express relief that they did not opt for a larger one-stage procedure. By contrast, many of our patients who have undergone large, one-stage procedures are also happy with their strategy of enduring a one-time greater discomfort rather than multiple recovery periods.

Skin relaxation and revision considerations

Body-contouring specialists have uniformly noted that the stretched skin in the MWL patient is not normal in its elastic properties. In general, greater skin relaxation occurs postoperatively, and thus greater tension than in non-MWL patients must be employed during skin resection body-contouring procedures in the MWL patient. Nonetheless, the postoperative skin relaxation is variable, unpredictable, and frequently leads to the need for revision or additional resections due to the loss of skin elasticity and the apparent alterations in viscoelastic properties of skin in these patients. A multistage approach has the advantage of a built-in mechanism for addressing revisions from a prior stage. If a one-stage approach is selected, the patient must understand that some type of minor revision is almost inevitable. It should also be noted that, because of the damage within the skin, the quality of the scar may be better.

Technical considerations in combined procedures

The principles of body-contouring surgery are still evolving. All procedures, however, are designed to remove excess skin and redirect the remaining skin to reconstruct the ideal

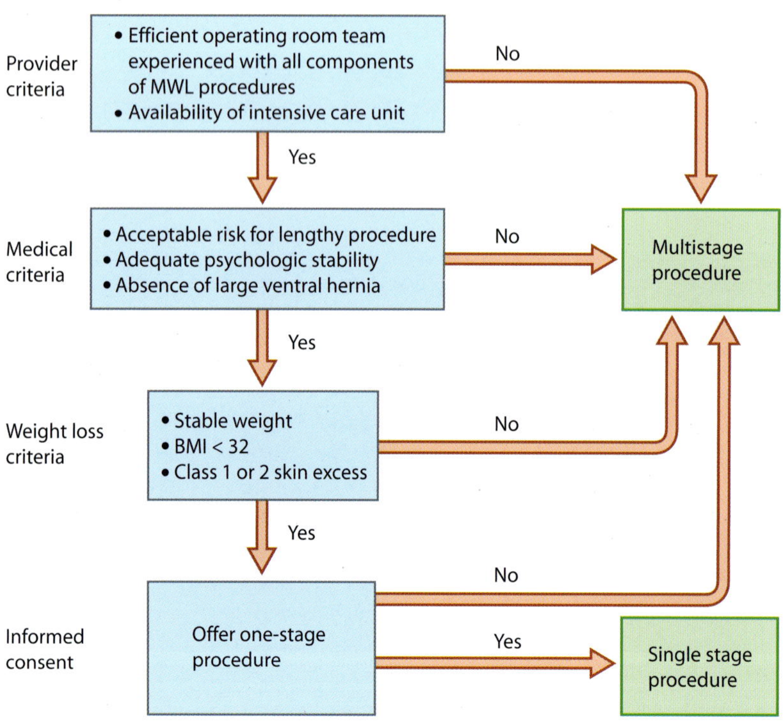

Figure 11.1 Staging algorithm.

anatomical form. Because of skin relaxation concerns, the vectors of pull in many of these procedures are substantial. In certain permutations and combinations of procedures, the surgeon may find that vectors of pull in various operative fields are counterbalancing, influencing, or complicating each other. In a lower body lift or belt lipectomy, for example, the abdominoplasty flap in the upper abdomen and flank is pulled inferiorly and laterally with great tension to meet the lower flap from the groin and hips. This may place some downward tension on the inframammary fold area and create some inferior displacement of the fold. If an upper body lift is performed simultaneously, the key principle of restoring the inframammary fold and its lateral extension to the correct position results in an opposite, superiorly directed vector on the very same upper abdominal and flank tissue. At a minimum, this may lead to increased technical difficulty during an already complex procedure.

It is possible that conflicting vectors of pull from simultaneous procedures may also lead to suboptimal results, asymmetries, or wound dehiscence. The surgeon must individually consider the vectors of pull of proposed combined procedures to ensure that the combination will not create technical problems or confounding conditions.

SURGICAL TECHNIQUE AND OUTCOMES

Detailed descriptions of techniques and outcomes for the various procedures are outlined elsewhere in this text. If multiple procedures are performed at one sitting, the usual precautions for lengthy procedures must be taken. These include:

- placement of a urinary catheter,
- sequential compression devices, and
- appropriate padding and checking of pressure points.

We do not routinely use prophylactic anticoagulants.

Procedures that involve multiple position changes, such as lower body lift or belt lipectomy, should be performed first. Currently, the most common positioning strategies are prone–supine and supine–lateral–lateral, although supine–lateral–lateral is also used by some surgeons. Our preferred sequence is to begin prone, performing the posterior body lift, the buttock autoaugmentation, the posterior thigh resection, and/or the posterior upper body lift resection. The legs are abducted and adducted at appropriate points in the procedure. Because the abdominal closure is the tightest, it is performed last, so that additional position changes are not required after completion of that component of the surgery.

Following the prone phase of the procedure, the patient is placed in the supine position for the remaining elements. We have found it useful to roll the patient to the supine position on an adjacent stretcher, and then move directly back to the operating room table. The remaining procedure is then completed, such as the anterior portion of the body lift, the anterior element of the thigh lift, brachioplasty, and/or breast surgery.

COMPLICATIONS AND THEIR MANAGEMENT

Most complications of combined procedures relate to an individual component procedure and are discussed in the appropriate section of the text. There is no evidence that seromas, wound dehiscence, and other common complications of individual procedures are increased in incidence when procedures are combined. In this chapter, discussion will be limited to those complications that are of particular concern in combined procedures. As outlined above, the major concerns about combining multiple procedures are complications that are associated with lengthy operative time. The most important and life-threatening of these is venous thromboembolism.

Death from pulmonary embolus is fortunately an extremely rare complication of body-contouring surgery. When it occurs, especially in the setting of aesthetic surgery, it is a devastating complication. In their recent review of thromboembolism in plastic surgery, Most et al. described a death from pulmonary embolus in an MWL patient following hernia repair, abdominoplasty, and thigh lift, despite the use of all appropriate perioperative precautions.[3] Abdominoplasty alone carries a reported incidence of 0.8% for pulmonary embolus.[4] When combined with other intraabdominal or aesthetic procedures, the incidence is higher, from 1.1% to 6.6%.[5,6] In other cosmetic procedures, such as rhytidectomy, deep vein thrombosis and pulmonary embolus were more likely if the procedure was performed under general anesthesia, according to results of a survey by Reinisch et al.[7]

A task force from the American Society of Plastic Surgeons stratified risk in office-based procedures.[8] Because all body-contouring procedures in the MWL patient require over 30 min of general anesthesia, all such patients fall into the 'moderate' or 'high' risk category established by the task force. Moderate-risk patients require comfortable positioning and sequential compression stockings. High-risk patients, including those with malignancy, obesity, or hypercoagulable state, are advised to use the same precautions as those for the moderate-risk patients, plus a hematology consultation and possible use of low-molecular-weight heparin before the procedure and daily in the postoperative period until ambulatory.

Several preparations of low-molecular-weight heparin exist. A common regimen for use of one of these agents is to administer dalteparin 2500 IU 1–2 h before surgery and then 2500 IU every day for 5–10 days after surgery. But to date there is no clear-cut evidence that low-molecular-weight heparin offers a distinct advantage over intermittent pneumatic compression stockings in this patient population, nor is there evidence that the marginal addition of low-molecular-weight heparin in addition to intermittent pneumatic compression stockings provides a distinct benefit in body-contouring surgery.

When deep vein thrombosis is suspected, it should be promptly and aggressively evaluated, initially with Doppler examination of the venous system. If a deep vein thrombosis is confirmed, treatment should begin immediately, and further evaluation for pulmonary embolus should be performed, including spiral computerized tomography scan.

Many reports involving combined body-contouring procedures appropriately focused on description of the techniques, and lack sufficient numbers to determine the incidence of low-probability events such as pulmonary embolus.[9] The term *belt lipectomy* was used originally by Gonzalez-Ulloa,[10] and was modified by Baroudi.[11] Currently, this term is generally applied to circumferential resections centered above the hips and along the waistline. Most early discussions of combined procedures were prior to the popularization of bariatric surgery.[12–15] Lockwood's seminal work involved description of the superficial fascial system and the pioneering design of many combined procedures in the MWL patient.[16–18]

In one of the first large series of body contouring in post–weight loss patients, presented by Dardour in 1986,[19] the single reported mortality in 300 patients was due to a pulmonary embolus. In 30 patients who underwent circumferential torsoplasty by Van Geertruyden,[20] one pulmonary embolus was noted. In Hamra's report of a series of 40 body lift patients,[21] no major complications were reported. Da Costa recently published the results for a series of 48 patients who underwent modified abdominoplasty after MWL.[22] These were limited procedures, averaging 180 min of total operative time, and there were no instances of pulmonary embolus.

Recent reports on combined body-contouring procedures in the MWL patient, performed by recognized experts at renowned centers of excellence, show a high incidence of pulmonary embolus. In a series of 32 patients who underwent belt lipectomy, which combines abdominoplasty with a circumferential trunk excision, Aly reported a 9.3% pulmonary embolus rate.[23] This series included some patients who were still overweight, but contained a group of 21 patients with MWL (average 187-lb [85 kg] preoperative weight loss). Their average operative time was 5.75 h, ranging from 4.86 to 6.93 h, and the average tissue resection was 10 lbs (4.5 kg). There was no mortality, and all patients recovered fully.

In Ellabban's series of 14 MWL patients who underwent abdominoplasty combined with medial thigh lift, all patients were given perioperative low-molecular-weight heparin as well as intraoperative sequential compression devices.[24] Operative times were remarkably low, with a mean time of 2 h, and the average mass of removed tissue was 70 oz (1995 g). No pulmonary embolus was noted. It is important to note that these combined procedures did not include circumferential resection.

Pascal described a series of 40 lower body lifts that combine high lateral tension abdominoplasty with circumferential skin resection and buttock lift. The incisions for the lower body lift are generally lower than for the related procedure of belt lipectomy. His group used low-molecular-weight heparin and sequential compression devices. There was no mention of average operative time or mass of resected tissue. No pulmonary embolus was noted.

Hurwitz reported eight cases of what may be considered the ultimate in combined body-contouring procedure: the total body lift.[25] This includes:

- circumferential abdominoplasty,
- lower body lift, and
- medial thighplasty.

It may also include brachioplasty and/or mastopexy and augmentation. Operative time ranged from 7–12 h, and transfusions ranged from 0 to 4 units. No pulmonary embolus occurred in these eight patients. One patient suffered from generalized edema and required readmission. These results are possible only with a very experienced team, and occasional use of the two-team approach with simultaneous surgery in two areas was noted. Even so, Hurwitz states that 'only the smaller and healthy weight loss patients should be offered these 1-stage procedures'.

CONCLUSION

The explosive popularity of bariatric surgery has created demand for a new genre of body-contouring surgery. Plastic surgeons performing these procedures on the MWL patient need to constantly examine their own practice and experience, as well as the needs and priorities of the individual patient, to make sound recommendations about how multiple procedures should be combined or staged.

- In the healthy MWL patient who is a candidate for treatment of numerous body areas, one-stage and two-stage approaches are medically appropriate options, with informed consent about the risks.
- Multiprocedure one-stage combinations should be performed only in appropriate patients by experienced surgical teams. Two-stage approaches are currently more common in most centers.

When undertaking lengthy combined procedures, careful medical evaluation and perioperative prophylaxis against deep venous thrombosis and other risks are essential.

REFERENCES

1. Steinbrook R. Surgery for severe obesity. N Engl J Med 2004; 350(11):1075–1079.
2. Mosteller RD. Simplified calculation of body surface area. N Engl J Med 1987; 317(17):1098.
3. Most D, Kozlow J, Heller J, et al. Thromboembolism in plastic surgery. Plast Reconstr Surg 2004; 115(2):20e–30e.
4. Grazer FM, Goldwyn RM. Abdominoplasty assessed by survey, with emphasis on complications. Plast Reconstr Surg 1977; 59(4):513–517.
5. Voss SC, Sharp HC, Scott JR. Abdominoplasty combined with gynecologic surgical procedures. Obstet Gynecol 1986; 67(2):181–185.
6. Hester RT Jr, Baird W, Bostwick J III, et al. Abdominoplasty combined with other surgical procedures: safe or sorry? Plast Reconstr Surg 1989; 83(6):997–1004.
7. Reinisch JF, Bresnick SD, Walker JWT, et al. Deep venous thrombosis and pulmonary embolus after face lift: a study of incidence and prophylaxis. Plast Reconstr Surg 2001; 107(6):1570–1575.
8. Iverson RE, ASPS Task Force on Patient Safety in Office-based Surgery Facilities. Patient safety in office-based surgery facilities: I.

Procedures in the office-based surgery setting. Plast Reconstr Surg 2002; 110(5):1337–1342.
9. Gonzalez M, Guerrero-Santos J. Deep planed torso-abdominoplasty combined with buttocks pexy. Aesthetic Plast Surg 1997; 21(4):245–253.
10. Gonzalez-Ulloa M. Belt lipectomy. Br J Plast Surg 1961; 13:179.
11. Baroudi R. Body contouring surgery in the 90s. In: Advances in Plastic and Reconstructive Surgery, vol 9. St. Louis: Mosby Year-Book; 1992:1–37.
12. Barrett BM, Kelly MV. Combined abdominoplasty and augmentation mammaplasty through a transverse suprapubic incision. Ann Plast Surg 1980; 4(4):286–291.
13. Pitanguy I, Ceravolo MP. Our experience with combined procedures in aesthetic plastic surgery. Plast Reconstr Surg 1983; 71(1):56–65.
14. Hallock GG, Altobelli JA. Simultaneous brachioplasty, thoracoplasty, and mammaplasty. Aesthetic Plast Surg 1985; 9(3):233–235.
15. Hauben DJ, Benmeir P, Charuzi I. One-stage body contouring. Ann Plast Surg 1988; 21(5):472–479.
16. Lockwood TE. Superficial fascial system (SFS) of the trunk and extremities: a new concept. Plast Reconstr Surg 1991; 87(6):1009–1018.
17. Lockwood TE. Lower body lift with superficial fascial system suspension. Plast Reconstr Surg 1993; 92(6):1112–1122.
18. Lockwood TE. Lower-body lift. Aesthetic Surg J 2001; 21:355.
19. Dardour JC, Vilain R. Alternatives to the classic abdominoplasty. Ann Plast Surg 1986; 17(3):247–258.
20. Van Geertruyden J, Vandeweyer E, de Fontaine S, et al. Circumferential torsoplasty. Br J Plast Surg 1999; 52(8):623–628.
21. Hamra ST. Circumferential body lift. Aesthetic Surg J 1999; 19:244.
22. Da Costa LF, Landecker A, Manta, AM. Optimizing body contour in massive weight loss patients: the modified vertical abdominoplasty. Plast Reconstr Surg 2004; 114(7):1917–1923.
23. Aly A, Cram A, Chao M, et al. Belt lipectomy for circumferential truncal excess: the University of Iowa experience. Plast Reconstr Surg 2003; 111(1):398–413.
24. Ellabban MG, Hart NB. Body contouring by combined abdominoplasty and medial vertical thigh reduction: experience of 14 cases. Br J Plast Surg 2004; 57(3):222–227.
25. Hurwitz DJ. Single stage total body lift after massive weight loss. Ann Plast Surg 2004; 52(5):435–441.

FURTHER READING

Matarasso A. Discussion. Is it safe to combine abdominoplasty with elective breast surgery? A review of ISI consecutive cases. Plast Reconstr Surg 2006; 118(1):213–4.

THE ROLE OF LARGE-VOLUME LIPOSUCTION AND OTHER ADJUNCTIVE PROCEDURES

12

V. Leory Young and Robert F. Centeno

Key Points

Liposuction

- If the patient needs debulking of subcutaneous fat in several areas, including the trunk, large-volume liposuction (LVL) may be an appropriate first stage of body contouring, especially if LVL will improve the aesthetic outcome of later staged excisions. This most often applies to patients with a BMI higher than 30 kg/m^2.
- If the patient chooses a major excisional procedure first, such as a circumferential body lift (CBL), identify remote areas (e.g. upper back, arms, thighs, or neck) that will benefit most from liposuction during the same surgery.
- Liposuction is useful for refining contour or removing residual subcutaneous fat several months after excisional procedure wounds have healed.
- Know your vascular anatomy, and be extremely cautious if performing liposuction near an area that will be excised in the same surgery to prevent disruption of a flap's vascular supply.
- If lipoplasty and an excisional procedure are performed during a single surgery, patient safety issues become more complex. Surgeons must be mindful of potential complications arising from both excision and liposuction and treat patients accordingly.

Mons reduction

- Improving the mons and genital area will improve function, hygiene, appearance, and patient satisfaction.
- Mons reduction can be safely combined with a CBL.
- Keep mons undermining to a minimum.
- Inform patients about temporarily decreased skin sensation, clitoral hypersensitivity in female patients, and prolonged edema and hyperemia following mons reduction.

Intergluteal reduction

- The skin length discrepancy and deforming effect of the posterior portion of a CBL can create a secondary deformity of the buttock. Intergluteal reduction or a V-shaped inverted dart incision in the intergluteal cleft helps minimize this deformity.
- The traditional posterior portion of a CBL incision is higher than is aesthetically ideal.
- To improve gluteal aesthetics, preserve the sacral triangle by lowering the central portion of the posterior body lift incision. Keep the incision at or below the level of the posterior iliac crest.
- Consult with patients about preferred underwear and bathing suit styles when designing incisions, but remind patients that fashion trends change. The goal of incision design should be the optimal aesthetic in the nude.

Autologous gluteal augmentation

- Thoracic spine/postural changes and anterior-inferior pelvic rotation associated with morbid obesity persist after massive weight loss and contribute to severe platypygia.
- The posterior component of a CBL causes flattening of the buttock.
- Autologous tissue of the lower back that would normally be discarded can be safely used to preserve or enhance projection in the gluteal region.
- Paucity of tissue overlying the coccyx and sacrum can be symptomatic, so preserving tissue in this area is important.

Axilloplasty

- Reducing the skin excess of the lateral chest wall/axilla can be safely combined with a brachioplasty, mastopexy or autologous breast augmentation, upper body lift, or CBL.
- Addressing this skin excess and recreating the lateral inframammary crease enhances the aesthetic results of breast procedures.
- Tissue that is normally discarded can be used for breast autoaugmentation as a well-perfused, well-described flap with known circulation.
- Preservation of critical axillary structures—including the brachial plexus, intercostobrachial nerve, lymphatics, and axillary fascia—will decrease morbidity.

Autologous breast augmentation

- The use of autologous axillary or lateral chest wall tissue to increase breast volume represents a good option for patients who do not want augmentation with an implant.
- Adding autologous tissue to the breast area provides increased volume and/or padding to prevent implant wrinkling and palpability if augmentation mammaplasty and/or mastopexy are planned.
- The normally discarded axillary tissue forms a lateral thoracoepigastric flap that is characterized by reliable perfusion and known anatomy.
- The use of the lateral thoracoepigastric flap is flexible enough to accommodate virtually all pedicle, skin excision, and breast pocket designs.

Liposuction plays an important role in body contouring of massive weight loss (MWL) patients and can be used to contour any body area that has excess fat. Suction-assisted (SAL), ultrasound-assisted (UAL), and power-assisted lipoplasty (PAL)—or their combination—are useful in the following contexts.

- Patients who need debulking of widespread subcutaneous fat prior to a staged excisional procedure.
- Patients who want or need additional contouring or removal of residual excess subcutaneous fat following an excisional procedure.
- Patients who have lipodystrophy in areas such as the upper back, thighs, or arms that may be improved with liposuction rather than excision.

Regardless of whether a patient has lost weight following gastric bypass surgery or through rigorous diet and exercise, weight loss will not be evenly distributed throughout all anatomical regions. Most patients lose visceral fat, which correlates with the reduction of their medical comorbidities, but significant subcutaneous fat may remain even after weight loss has stabilized. In most cases, areas of localized lipodystrophy are produced.

The volume of subcutaneous tissue plays an important role in the decision-making process when considering which procedures to undertake and in what order. As an example, loss of subcutaneous fat in the lower abdomen may be greater than in the upper abdomen. If a circumferential body lift (CBL) or panniculectomy is performed, patients may still have a large excess of subcutaneous fat in the epigastric region. Debulking this area with liposuction can simplify excisional procedures and produce a better aesthetic outcome. Liposuction is especially effective for removing excess fat in the back that is difficult to treat with a CBL. Another area that benefits from debulking prior to excision is the arms, which may retain significant excess fat even after patients have plateaued in their weight loss. If the arms are debulked with liposuction first, an excisional brachioplasty performed 3–6 months later—after the tissues have softened and vascularity has improved—will produce much better results. The thighs also benefit from debulking liposuction, as long as drains are used to prevent chronic seroma formation and infection.

For patients with significant subcutaneous volume, staged debulking liposuction can be safely performed before or after excisional procedures. For some patients, large-volume liposuction (LVL) as the first stage of body contouring may permit use of less extensive excisions or fewer staged procedures, as illustrated by the patient shown in Figure 12.1. The improvement in this patient's body contour would not have been possible without LVL, which prompted her weight loss. Limited liposuction combined with excisional procedures has been performed for years. Established combinations include:

- lower flank liposuction with abdominoplasty,
- submental liposuction with facialplasty,
- reduction mammaplasty with axillary lipoplasty, and
- CBL with thigh liposuction (Figure 12.2).

All these combinations share a focused use of liposuction based on known vascular anatomy and accumulated experience.

As the natural tendency toward innovation continues in plastic surgery, the literature increasingly reports on excisional procedures—such as abdominoplasty, thighplasty, and brachioplasty—combined in a single surgery with lipoplasty in areas that share a vascular supply.[1–7] Proponents believe that liposuction performed on or adjacent to flaps allows smaller excisions and improves aesthetic outcomes. Reports published thus far are interesting and suggest that less flap undermining is required if liposuction and excision are combined. However, more safety data are needed before we know whether the risk associated with these combinations is acceptable, and Matarasso advises that extensive liposuction with a full abdominoplasty is ill advised.[8] Patients must be properly informed about the potentially increased risks of delayed wound healing, infection, flap necrosis, or unfavorable scarring if excision and lipoplasty are combined. Above all, know your vascular anatomy before attempting to perform liposuction in or near an excision site. When in doubt, take a conservative approach rather than risk serious complications such as flap necrosis or delayed healing.

Issues of patient selection and informed consent have been covered elsewhere in this book. If liposuction is to be included in the body-contouring process, additional patient assessment must be done and consent obtained. By its nature, liposuction induces what may be considered blunt trauma injury. In addition, LVL may be associated with large fluid shifts that are dangerous—even fatal—if not handled appropriately. Patients should understand that they will have some excess skin and contour irregularities such as lumps, depressions, and wrinkles after LVL. The duration of recovery for LVL patients is approximately 3 weeks, but persistent swelling may last up to 6 months. Impressive skin retraction often occurs, especially after LVL, but final results will not be known for 3–6 months. Excision may be performed then if excessive skin laxity or contour irregularities remain.

PREOPERATIVE PREPARATION

The length of surgery and health history of MWL patients demand that multiple factors be addressed during the month or so prior to surgery, regardless of whether the planned surgery is LVL alone or excision plus liposuction. Some guidelines follow.

- Obtain clearance from MWL patients' internists or primary care physicians to ensure that they can safely undergo a large and lengthy operation. If patients do not have a physician, refer them to an internist.
- Pay special attention to cardiac health in patients undergoing LVL, because high-dose adrenaline (epinephrine) increases the risk for arrhythmias, fatal asystole, and myocardial infarction during surgery. Therefore hyperthyroidism, severe hypertension, cardiac

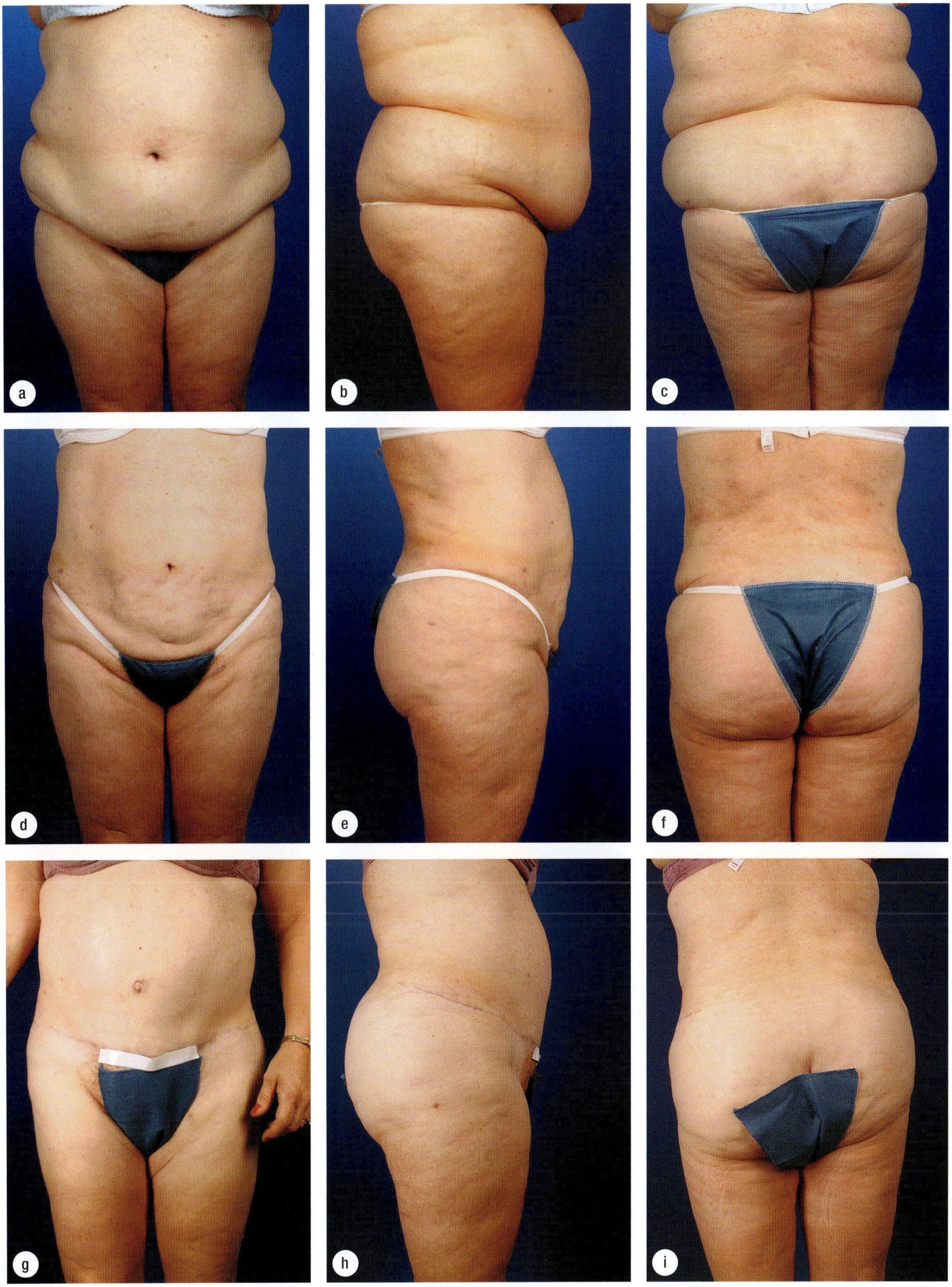

Figure 12.1 (**a–c**) This obese patient (BMI of 39 kg/m^2) underwent large-volume debulking liposuction (LVL; 18 000 cc aspirate), which enabled her to begin a rigorous walking program of 3 miles six times a week. (**d–f**) Ten months after LVL, the degrees of skin retraction and back improvement are impressive. For this patient, LVL became an impetus to massive weight loss by reducing her large amount of subcutaneous fat. (**g–i**) Five months after abdominoplasty. The patient originally thought about having a circumferential body lift, but her posterior contour was so dramatically improved that she opted for an abdominoplasty instead.

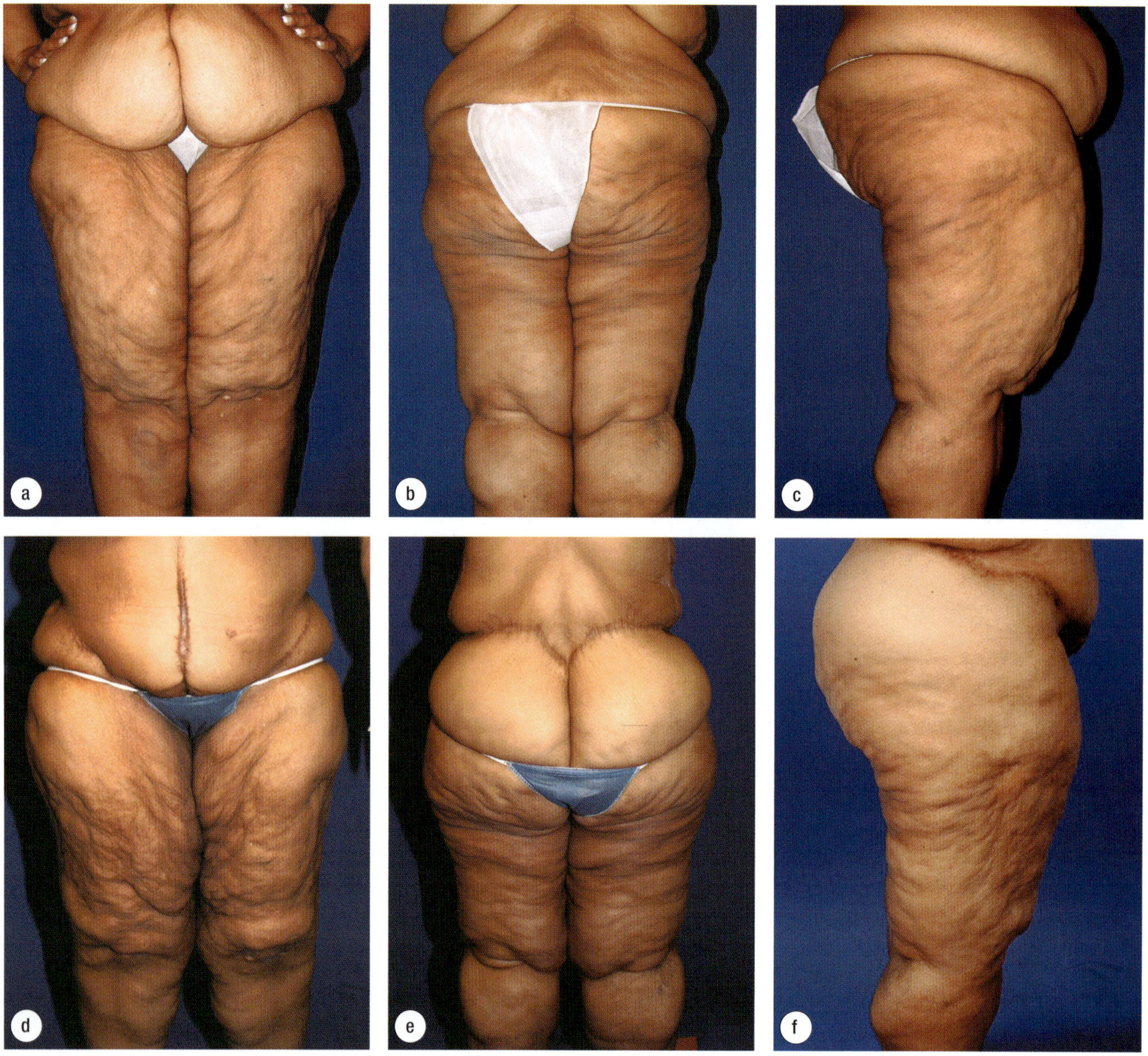

Figure 12.2 This 47-year-old patient had lost 130 lbs (59 kg) following gastric bypass surgery when she first came to us, and her BMI had gone from 69 to 46 kg/m^2. Multiple stages of body contouring were planned because of her high BMI. **(a–c)** Her first surgery consisted of a CBL, brachioplasty, and lliposuction of the thighs, with 7.5 L aspirated from each thigh (total 15 L). Her second surgery included reduction mammoplasty and arm liposuction (total 7.7 L). **(d–f)** Postoperative views taken 6 months after the patient's third surgery, which involved torsoplasty and secondary brachioplasty to further reduce skin excess and UAL of the lower back (5.3 L). The patient has continued to lose weight and her BMI is now 40. Her next planned procedure is additional liposuction of the thighs and an extended thighplasty. Although she has significant scars, the patient is pleased with her results.

disease, peripheral vascular disease, or pheochromocytoma are contraindications to lipoplasty.[9]

- Obtain a thorough health history, surgical history that includes all perioperative complications or problems, and complete list of current and recent medications plus herbal supplements. Ask specifically about birth control pills or hormone replacement therapy, because they increase the risk of thromboembolitic events. Request medical records rather than rely solely on what patients say.
- Assess patients for scars from prior surgeries (gastric bypass, cholecystectomy, caesarean section, etc.) that predispose to skin necrosis following liposuction, especially if superficial liposuction is performed in a diabetic patient. If a patient is at risk, modify the procedure to be less aggressive adjacent to scars.
- Check for the wide range of electrolyte, vitamin, and nutritional problems that affect MWL patients,[10] and optimize deficiencies at least 2 weeks prior to surgery. This

may involve intensive vitamin supplementation, protein supplementation, and nutritional counseling for at least a month before surgery.

- Carefully evaluate hematologic parameters, because low hemoglobin levels are frequent among MWL patients. Some may require recombinant erythropoietin to raise the hematocrit before surgery,[11] but this therapy carries an increased risk of hypercoagulability, requires intravenous iron therapy, and is costly.
- Type and cross-match patients in anticipation of the need for transfusion, a possibility that must be explained. Autologous blood donation should be discouraged, but directed donorship by family members can be arranged.
- Arrange for smoking cessation counseling to prevent wound-healing problems in smokers. To measure compliance with smoking cessation, perform continine testing 2 weeks prior to surgery, on the morning of surgery, and 2 weeks after surgery. A positive test before surgery should result in delaying the procedure until the patient stops smoking.

Marking

Patients undergoing liposuction alone should be marked in the standing position before receiving any sedative medications. They may be marked in the preoperative area, but we prefer to mark patients who will have excisional procedures (with or without liposuction) a day or two before surgery. Marking with indelible markers is best done in an unhurried and private environment to enhance accuracy and improve the patient experience. Preoperative marking takes time if done properly, because it demands careful measurements and double-checking.

- Make bilateral markings as symmetric as possible, and note any preexisting asymmetries.
- Delineate prominent areas such as folds or bulges to be liposuctioned, because they will be less apparent when the patient lies down.
- Border areas where liposculpture feathering is anticipated should also be identified.

Using differently colored markers facilitates color coding and indicates areas to be treated differently.

Prophylactic measures 30–60 min before surgery

Hypothermia prophylaxis

Because procedures are lengthy and large body areas are exposed, body-contouring patients are highly susceptible to inadvertent hypothermia, which is defined as a core body temperature below 36°C. Hypothermia has been found to increase the incidence of postoperative wound infections and inhibit tissue oxygen delivery and coagulation functions, thereby raising the risk of bleeding-related complications.[12] Begin warming the patient in the preoperative area with either heated cotton blankets or forced air blankets (such as a Bear Hugger) at least 30 min prior to surgery. Cotton blankets quickly lose their heat so must be continuously renewed. The objective of prewarming is to increase the heat content of the extremities so that heat will not be transferred out of the core during surgery.

Raise the operating room temperature to 73°F (23°C), which is the upper limit recommended by health-related government agencies.[13] Infection risk increases when temperature rises above 73°F and humidity is outside the range of 30–60%. Intravenous fluids, as well as liposuction infiltration fluids, should be warmed between 37 and 42°C with a fluid warmer to help maintain normothermia.[12] This includes the fluids begun in the preoperative area to replace deficits caused by overnight fasting. All fluids administered throughout the surgery and recovery room should be warmed. Do not heat fluids to temperatures higher than 42°C or burns may result. Warming the infiltration fluids is probably not necessary in UAL because the ultrasonic energy raises the temperature of tissues and fluids.

Thromboembolism prophylaxis

In 2004, the American College of Chest Physicians identified the following to be among the major risk factors for venous thromboembolitic events (VTEs) such as deep vein thrombosis (DVT) and pulmonary embolism (PE):[14]

- prolonged surgical time (more than 1 h),
- general anesthesia,
- patient age of 40 or more, and
- obesity.

By these criteria, essentially all MWL patients undergoing body contouring have a moderate to high risk for VTEs. PE usually arises from DVT in the legs at or proximal to the popliteal veins, with above-knee DVTs most often being the culprit. The frequency of DVT is between 15 and 40% of general surgery patients if no prophylaxis is given,[14] and 30–50% of patients with undiagnosed and untreated DVT progress to PE.[15] Even when prophylactic measures are taken, the risk of DVT lasts for at least 4 weeks after surgery.[14] Consequently, attention to VTE prevention must be a priority long after patients have gone home.

Mechanical prophylactic methods include compression stockings and intermittent pneumatic compression devices or venous foot pumps. Intermittent pneumatic compression devices or venous foot pumps are recommended for any plastic surgery procedure that lasts more than 1 h and for all patients undergoing general anesthesia.[16] The use of intermittent pneumatic compression devices or venous foot pumps should begin approximately 30–60 min prior to surgery.

Anticoagulant therapy is the most effective method of DVT/PE prevention and the only real option for patients with a prior history of DVT/PE or a hypercoagulability disorder. Anticoagulant choices include:

- low-molecular-weight heparin (LMWH);
- low-dose unfractionated heparin; and
- the recently approved drug called fondaparinux (Arixtra), which specifically inhibits the activation of coagulation factor X.

Clinical trials suggest that fondaparinux may be twice as effective as LMWH in preventing postoperative DVT, and its use requires no routine coagulation monitoring.[17] Adequate prophylaxis can be achieved by administering either LMWH or fondaparinux the morning after surgery, or at least 12 h following surgery completion. VTE prophylaxis should be continued until patients are fully ambulatory. For high- and very high-risk patients, continue chemoprophylaxis at home for 2 weeks, or longer if warranted by risk factors.

None of these anticoagulants has been found to increase clinically significant bleeding, and although postoperative hematomas are possible, they are uncommon. To help put bleeding risks in context, remember that acute adverse events occur in less than 1% of patients receiving transfusion[18] versus the 15–40% of general surgery patients who develop DVT. Concerns about bleeding during liposuction are probably justified because sites of bleeding cannot be visualized and addressed, as is the case with excision. However, we have not had adverse bleeding in LVL patients given postoperative chemoprophylaxis.

Antibiotic prophylaxis

- For patients not allergic to penicillin, begin administration of 1 g of cefazolin (Ancef) 30 min before surgery.
- Patients with a penicillin allergy are given 500 mg of clindamycin intravenously infused over 1 h immediately prior to surgery.
- Diflucan should be given to patients with yeast infections.
- In cases that take longer than 6 h, repeat antibiotics during surgery.

Draping

Place forced warm air blankets beneath the patient on the operating table and also cover patient areas outside the operating field, such as the head and extremities. The key to draping is to allow easy access for infusion and aspiration of the wetting solution. Areas wider than those to be suctioned are exposed so that the area being contoured can be blended into the non-contoured area. Drapes should not distort the body contours with their weight. After completing work on an area (or two symmetric areas), redrape the patient to retain heat.

SURGICAL TECHNIQUE

Anesthesia

Large-volume liposuction (5000 cc of aspirate or greater) and other body-contouring procedures in MWL patients are best performed using general anesthesia with endotracheal intubation. Because these patients typically must be repositioned during surgery, intubation assures maintenance of the airway. In addition, patients are more comfortable, oxygenation is ensured, and monitoring can be done to detect any problems. When anesthesia is induced, a Foley catheter is inserted to aid with fluid monitoring. We advise a distal esophageal probe or tympanic membrane device for constant monitoring of core body temperature.

Oxygenation

Most anesthesiologists administer oxygen at an F_iO_2 of 30–50% during general anesthesia. However, a large randomized and blinded study of intraabdominal surgery patients found that an F_iO_2 of 80% during surgery and for 2 h afterward reduced the incidence of wound infections by more than half when compared with the use of 30% F_iO_2 (5.2% versus 11.2%).[12] The use of 80% F_iO_2 may be especially important in lipoplasty patients who have received intentional vasoconstriction by adrenaline (epinephrine). Another benefit of using 80% F_iO_2 is that the incidence of postoperative nausea and vomiting is markedly reduced (approximately 50%) when compared with 30% for F_iO_2.[12]

Positioning

Position is dictated by the areas being treated with liposuction and same-surgery excisional procedures. The arms, flanks, back, hips, and outer thighs are most accessible to liposuction in the lateral decubitus position. The outer thigh offers a good example of the effect that supine or prone versus lateral position can have. In the supine or prone position, the weight of the body distorts the area and access is limited, in contrast to the lateral position that offers easy access and minimizes distortion. It is also much easier to evaluate results with inspection and palpation. The symmetry of areas can be assessed and refined in supine or prone positions. The abdomen, breasts, submental area, mons pubis, anterior and inner thigh, and knees are best treated in the supine position. When the patient is in a supine position, place a pillow under the knees to promote venous return flow through the popliteal area and thereby help prevent DVT.

Whatever position is chosen, it should allow easy access to the areas being treated and minimize the risk of distortion caused by position or pressure. A roll (folded/rolled linen) under the patient's chest or pelvis as indicated when in the supine position is used to prevent pressure or allow thoracic excision. Padding pressure points (i.e. joints) is important. The legs can be widely abducted to allow access, and in order to do so the ankles are positioned on padded arm shields.

Fluid management

Fluid management is always a challenge in LVL because of the risks of hypovolemia or fluid overload. Consequently, patients undergoing LVL require a rigorous fluid management regimen. The superwet technique is recommended to keep fluid infiltration and aspiration as close as possible to a 1:1 ratio (1 mL in and 1 mL out). The tumescent technique relies on larger amounts of infiltrate, with ratios as high as 3:1 to 7:1, and is therefore more likely to cause fluid overload. When managing fluids, remember that approximately 70% of the infiltrated wetting solution is not aspirated but remains in the subcutaneous tissues until slowly absorbed into the intravascular space.[19,20] Thus the majority of material in the aspirate is fat, not wetting solution.[21]

Use a data sheet to record the actual measurements of the amounts of fluid going in and coming out. The 'in' half of the 1:1 ratio includes the subcutaneous infiltrate plus any supplemental fluids given intravenously. The 'out' consists of 30%

of the suctioned aspirate (the other 70% of infused fluid is not aspirated), blood loss, urine output, and drainage through drains. Subcutaneous infiltration solutions are usually mixed in 1- or 3-L plastic bags with graduated markers of volume. However, measuring by volume markers is very inaccurate. Instead, measure the weight (in grams) dispersed from the bag. When using the 1:1 ratio of infiltration and aspiration, the volume of replacement fluids should be reduced to avoid the danger of fluid overload. The suggested amount for LVL is 0.25 cc of crystalloid for each cc aspirated over 5000 cc.[16,19] This is in addition to crystalloid intravenous maintenance fluid administered at a rate of 1.5–2.0 cc/kg per h. The amount of maintenance and replacement fluids should be monitored and adjusted to vital signs and urine output.

Along with keeping meticulous records of fluid amounts going in and coming out, a patient's heart rate, blood pressure, and urine output give important clues to the fluid status. The patient is hemodynamically stable if:

- the systolic blood pressure is over 100 mmHg,
- the heart rate is under 100 bpm, and
- the urine output is 0.5–1.0 cc/kg per h or greater.

Urine output is perhaps the best indicator of the need for supplemental fluids. The first sign of hypovolemia is usually tachycardia or a heart rate greater than 100 bpm. Young, healthy patients can often compensate by maintaining their blood pressure, but they tend to become tachycardic eventually.

Blood loss

During lipoplasty, the infiltrated wetting solution contains 1 cc of adrenaline (epinephrine) 1:1000 per liter of lactated Ringer's solution (for a final concentration of 1:1 000 000 per liter) to achieve vasoconstriction. Before adrenaline became part of the liposuction wetting solution, the estimated blood loss was as high as 45%. Some studies have determined that blood loss represents about 1% of the aspirate when adrenaline is added.[3,21] Karmo et al. compared hemoglobin levels before and 7 days after surgery, and found a mean decrease in hemoglobin (g/dL) of 0.93 ± 0.92 in SAL and 1 ± 0.64 in UAL for aspirate volumes up to 6000 mL. However, Cárdenas-Camarena and colleagues also evaluated the aspirate of patients undergoing LVL (5–22.3 L) and determined blood loss to be more in the range of 10% of the aspirate and higher after the seventh or eighth liter was aspirated.[22] The mean reduction of hemoglobin 1 week after surgery was 3.8 g compared to presurgical levels.

Transfusion is always a possibility with LVL or liposuction combined with excision. The guidelines for blood transfusion are a hematocrit below 23% or symptoms such as orthostatic hypotension and tachycardia. Patients with coronary or central nervous system atherosclerosis should be treated more aggressively. Hematocrit can be easily checked during surgery to assess patient blood loss, but results may not be entirely reliable for several days, until hematocrit equilibrium is achieved following final resolution of fluid shifts.[9,21] Healthy young individuals with normal preoperative hematocrits of approximately 40% can tolerate larger volumes of liposuction. Even though we have aspirated up to 34 L without giving transfusion to a morbidly obese patient, it is not uncommon to transfuse 2 units of packed red blood cells for aspirates over 20 L. Safety should be the first concern, and either the volume aspirated should be limited to an amount that maintains hemodynamic stability or transfusion should be available based on hematocrit and symptoms.

Fluid infusion

Surgeons should use the technologies and materials with which they are most comfortable. Neither LVL nor liposuction combined with excisional procedures should be attempted by the inexperienced because of the complex fluid management issues. Some general guidelines follow.

- Consider not including lidocaine when liposuction is performed under general anesthesia (as it usually is in MWL patients).
- Add 1 cc of adrenaline (epinephrine) (1:1000) for hemostasis per liter of Ringer's lactate (for a final solution of 1:1 000 000).
- Warm infused fluids to a temperature between 37 and 42°C for SAL.
- Keep in mind the 1:1 infiltration to aspiration ratio when infiltrating wetting solution.
- Infuse wetting solution with a blunt needle that connects the wetting solution tubing and pump. Klein needles are available in numerous lengths and diameters to address a wide variety of areas treated.
- Use small puncture wounds for infusion to minimize fluid loss through the incision.
- Place incisions in locations that can be used for aspiration.
- Infiltrate the wetting solution in all fat layers until the area to be aspirated and the tissues at its periphery are uniformly turgid or firm to palpation.
- Use a pump and tubing capable of very high flow rates.
- Wait 12–15 min following infiltration before aspiration. Vasoconstriction from adrenaline (epinephrine) is sufficient when the skin appears blanched.
- Perform sequential infiltrations and aspirations rather than infusing wetting solution in all areas to be treated before aspiration begins. If multiple areas will be suctioned, you can usually start aspirating the first infused area as soon as the next area to be treated is infiltrated.
- Limit epinephrine dosing to 10 mg/3 hr period. This dose may be repeated after 3 hrs.[23]

Application of ultrasound

Ultrasound-assisted lipoplasty is especially effective for treating fibrous or dense areas such as the back, flanks, and upper abdomen, as well as areas that received previous liposuction. UAL is less appropriate for superficial sculpting and refinements. We avoid using it in curved body areas because the cannula or probe lacks the flexibility needed to follow curves. UAL is applied as an intermediate step between infiltration and aspiration, with the ultrasonic probe being turned on for a minute or two after infiltration to emulsify fat, which is then aspirated in the standard suction-assisted manner. The length of ultrasound application varies by body area and patient, but ultrasonic energy sufficient to achieve fat emulsification has specific end points after which evacuation can be performed: a loss of tissue resistance to the probe and blood-tinged aspirate. When inserting the probe, place a skin protector and dry towel folded four times around the incision. Then keep the probe always moving to avoid dermal end hits and prevent thermal injury.

Because UAL emulsifies adipocytes—rather than destroying them with the mechanical avulsion of SAL—some believe that UAL is less likely to damage blood vessels and disrupt skin perfusion than SAL is, but this issue is far from settled. For example, some studies determined that skin perfusion is significantly better with UAL than with SAL,[24] and wound healing is reportedly faster with UAL.[25] Another analysis found no statistically significant difference in perforator vessel damage when comparing UAL and SAL.[26]

Surgeons should use the liposuction technique with which they are most comfortable, including combined technologies. Fortunately, reports of skin burns and necrosis have decreased as surgical proficiency and UAL technology have improved. Nonetheless, the potential for catastrophic complications arising from a combination of UAL, PAL, or SAL with an excisional procedure still exists.[27]

Aspiration

Large-volume liposuction is usually a debulking procedure, and relatively large cannulas (4–10 mm) can be employed. However, if cosmetic contouring in limited areas is being performed, smaller (2- to 4-mm cannulas) should be used. When large volumes are aspirated, speed is important. Studies have determined that the rate of aspiration is directly proportionate to cannula diameter, tubing diameter, and vacuum generated, and the rate of removal is inversely proportionate to cannula diameter and tubing length.[28] Therefore, using a cannula and tubing with the largest diameter and shortest length produces the fastest aspiration. However, in fibrous areas, it may be easier to pass small-diameter cannulas. The cannula design and size depend on the areas treated, the type of liposuction, and physician preference. The tip configuration of the cannula has minimal effect on the rate of aspiration.

Leaving a layer of superficial fat to minimize the risk of contour deformities (such as wrinkles, dents, or lumps) is recommended by many, and this superficial layer may facilitate skin flap mobility at subsequent excisional procedures. However, the goal of LVL is to debulk the area. We have found that superficial SAL, carried all the way to the dermis, provides more complete debulking and better skin retraction in the abdomen, flanks, and back. In fact, some patients with a panniculus have sufficient skin retraction to make a subsequent excisional procedure unnecessary. Others who planned a CBL after liposuction had an abdominoplasty instead, because the large-volume debulking removed so much fat that the need for the larger incision and more difficult recovery of a body lift was obviated (Fig. 12.1).

For debulking aspiration, we begin with a 6-mm cannula and finish the superficial layer using a 6-mm beveled tip cannula with a single large opening that behaves like a curette even though its edges are not sharp. This cannula essentially vacuums off any fat globules attached to the skin or fascia, which minimizes contour irregularities and produces better skin retraction. Smaller cannulas (3–4 mm) are more appropriate for refinement in the arms, submental area, thighs, and hips, where a superficial layer of fat should be left to minimize contour deformities.

Drains

Seromas are common after LVL in the abdomen, flanks, back, arms, and thighs, especially when large-diameter cannulas are used. When treating these areas, insert #19 hubless Blake drains to minimize seroma formation and speed recovery. The drains are removed when output reaches 30–50 mL or less per 24 h.

Wound closure

Would closure can be done with any absorbable or nonabsorbable suture and sealed with Dermabond dressings. We do not apply foam or compressive garments to the abdomen or thighs in the operating room because of concern about pressure injury and production of creases. When creases develop at the site of garment folds, they become relatively fixed and very difficult to eliminate. We apply TopiFoam to the submental area and cover it with an elastic head dressing. Arms also receive TopiFoam and are wrapped in Kerlix and Coban. Compression garments for comfort can optionally be used after drain removal.

OTHER ADJUNCTIVE SURGICAL PROCEDURES

In addition to body image disturbances, many MWL patients suffer from functional and hygienic issues caused by significant amounts of excess skin in the mons and genital area, buttock and anal region, and breasts and lateral thoracic wall. Along with skin excess, loss of tissue volume in some areas (face, breast, and buttock) produces significant contour deformities. During the past several years, we have noted increasing complaints regarding skin laxity in the facial region, upper abdomen, axilla, back, arms, and legs. Consequently, the adjunctive procedures described here have become more important for enhancing outcomes.

Deformities in these areas are not fully addressed by major body-contouring procedures. However, mons reduction, intergluteal reduction, autologous gluteal augmentation, axilloplasty, and autologous breast augmentation can make a huge difference in the final contour appearance, as well as in hygiene and clothing fit, of MWL patients. These adjunctive techniques are ideally combined with other body-contouring surgery. The lower body procedures are well suited for combining with the CBL as the core rehabilitative procedure, and add 1–1½ h to the operative time for all three surgeries.

An axilloplasty (~1 h) and breast autoaugmentation (2–3 h) work well when combined with upper body procedures. Alternatively, adjunctive surgery can be performed in separate stages of rehabilitation if combined procedures are not feasible. These smaller procedures are not metabolically demanding or lengthy, and may be done on an outpatient basis. When adjunctive procedures are combined together or performed in conjunction with a larger surgery such as a CBL or LVL, admission to the hospital for postoperative observation is advised.

Mons reduction

The suprapubic and genital regions are typically involved to a similar extent in MWL patients. Failure to contour these regions results in a suboptimal aesthetic outcome to the CBL, such as that seen in Figure 12.3, and decreased patient satisfaction, partly because problems with genital hygiene and function are not solved.

- In mild cases of suprapubic skin excess and lipodystrophy, standard liposuction of the mons will suffice.[29]
- In moderate cases of skin excess and lipodystrophy, excise an inverted triangular wedge of skin and tissue without undermining. Secure the superficial fascial system (SFS) of the mons to the anterior rectus fascia with '1' Ethibond or Vicryl Plus to prevent excess superior displacement. Then close in layers with 3-0 Monocryl (Fig. 12.4).
- A deep tacking suture at the lateral aspects of the mons "triangle" helps to restore a more normal contour after mons reduction.

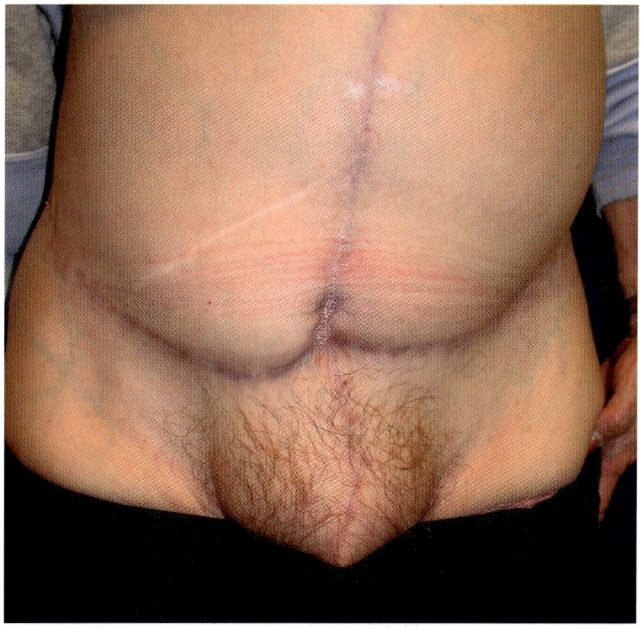

Figure 12.3 Early in our experience with circumferential body lift, we did not understand the importance of mons reduction. This patient illustrates the deformity that can result if mons reduction is not performed in conjunction with a lower body lift.

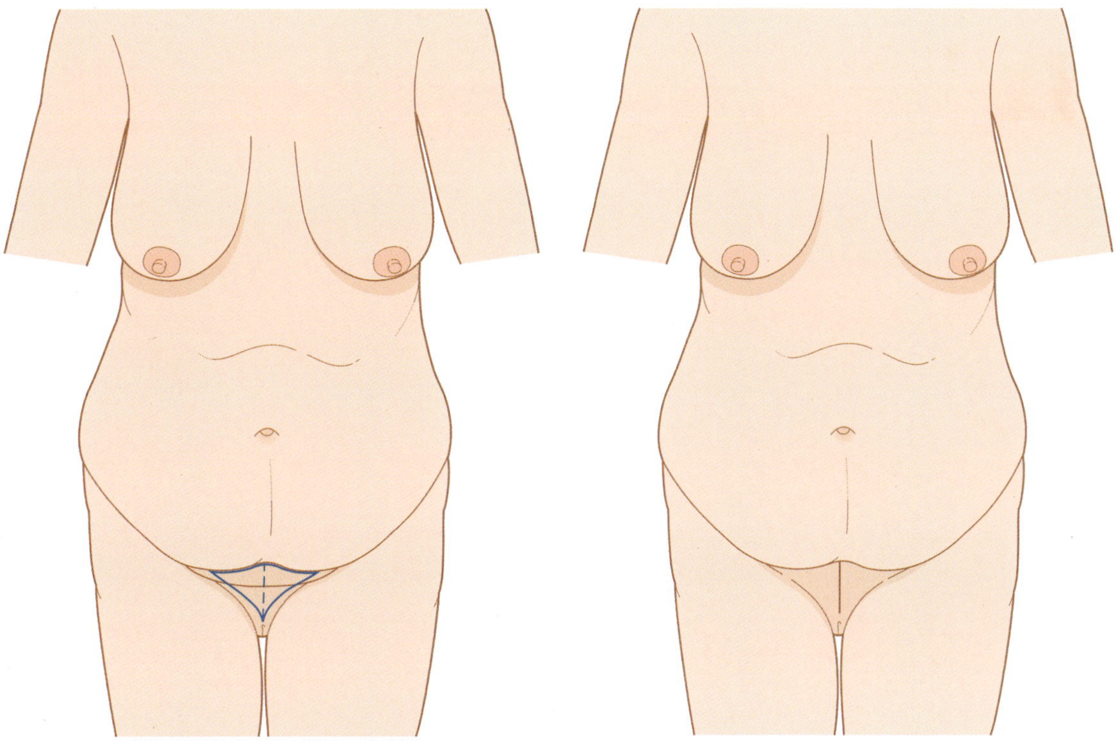

Figure 12.4 Perform mons reduction before closing circumferential body lift incisions.

The most severe cases of skin and tissue excess involve both the suprapubic region and the labia in women (Fig. 12.5), while men tend to have invagination of the penis (Fig. 12.6). With severe deformities in women, the triangular wedge excision is extended to include labioplasty of the labia majora (Fig. 12.7). Although men benefit from the triangular excision, a repeat excision or further debulking liposuction at a secondary stage is usually necessary to correct the most severe male deformities. Patients should be counseled that prolonged edema and reactive hyperemia is typical for procedures in the genital region.

Differences of opinion remain regarding undermining of the mons. An alternative approach is to manually de-fat the deeper tissue layers of the superior mons when it is significantly thicker than the abdominal flap.

Intergluteal reduction

An aggressive CBL can produce several buttock deformities, including a flattened appearance, an accentuated length discrepancy between the superior and inferior skin flaps, and bunching of tissue at the intergluteal cleft (Fig. 12.8). An intergluteal reduction will resolve these problems (Figs 12.9 & 12.10).

1. Resect the skin and subcutaneous tissue to the presacral fascia and secure the SFS with #1 Vicryl Plus.
2. Close in layers with 3-0 Monocryl.
3. Seal the incision with Dermabond to reduce fecal contamination.

An alternative approach is to design the CBL incision with a V-shaped dart at the center of the back to prevent the intergluteal deformity. However, published descriptions of this incision tend to produce a scar that is too high to be aesthetically pleasing. A significant component of gluteal aesthetics is the presence of the sacral triangle,[30] which disappears when a standard CBL incision with inverted dart is placed too high.

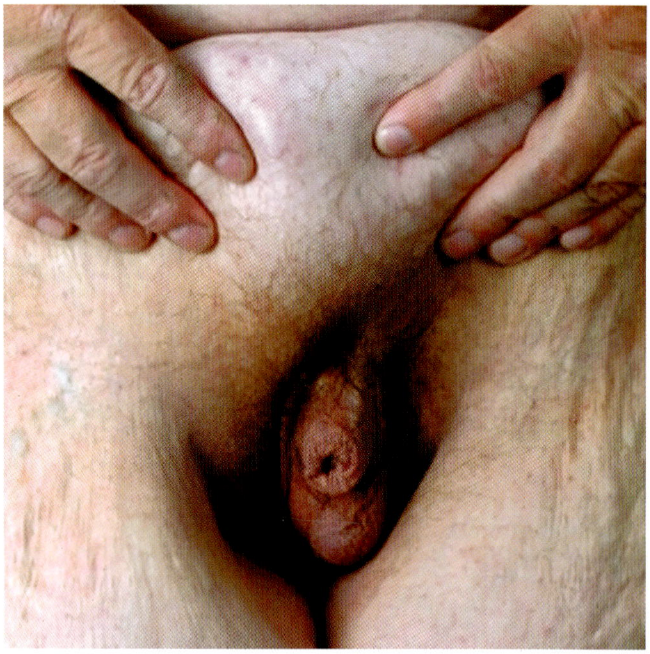

Figure 12.6 Excess skin and subcutaneous tissue can cause the penis to invaginate. The patient is holding up his extremely large panniculus.

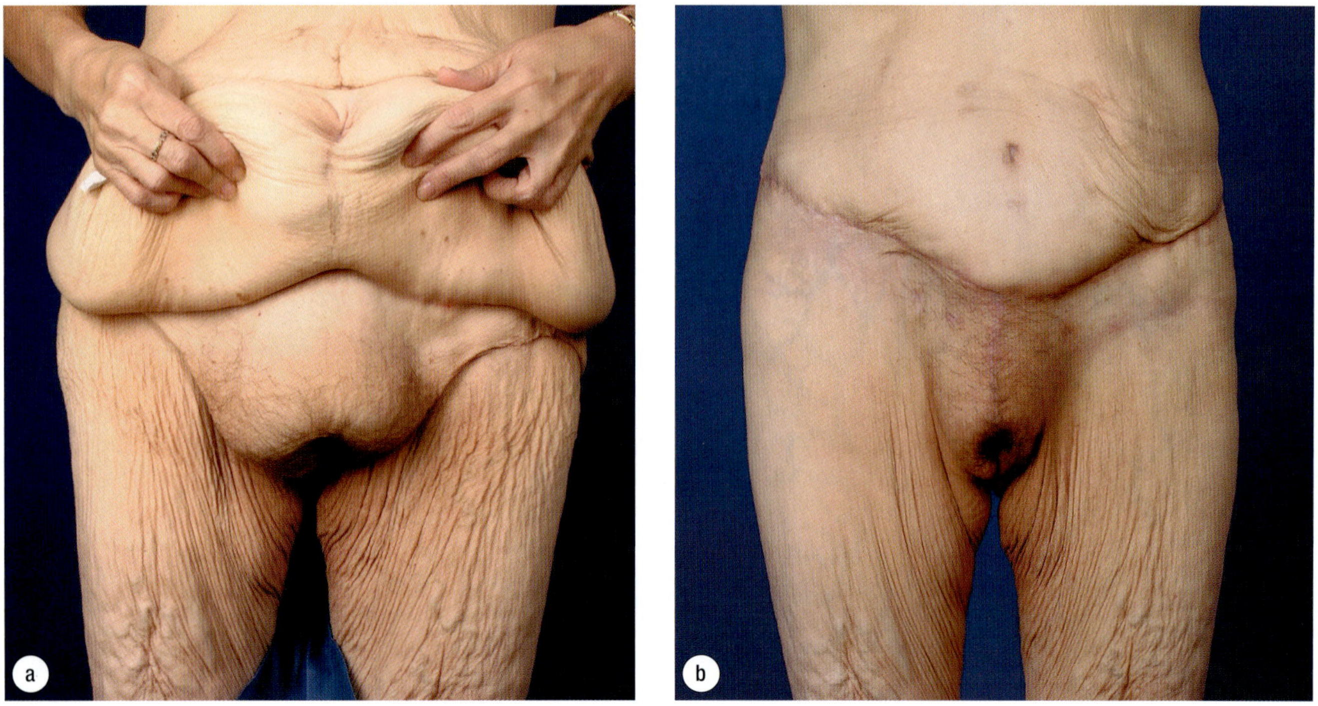

Figure 12.5 This 56-year-old woman lost 150 lbs (68 kg) over 18 months after gastric bypass. (**a**) Extreme skin excess of the mons pubis created persistent hygiene difficulties and discomfort. (**b**) Edema can be slow to resolve after mons reduction and labioplasty.

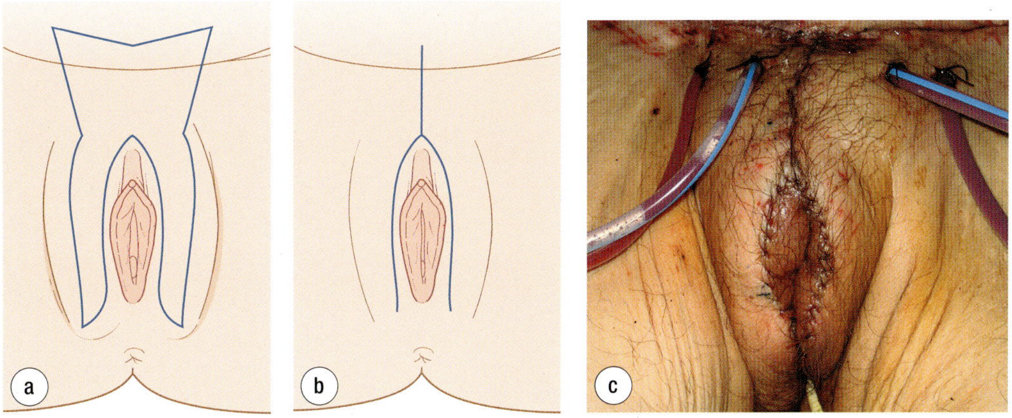

Figure 12.7 (**a** and **b**) For women, a labioplasty combined with mons reduction is often required. The superior vertical blue line (**b**) meets the mons reduction excision. (**c**) The patient shown in Figure 12.5 after labioplasty closure.

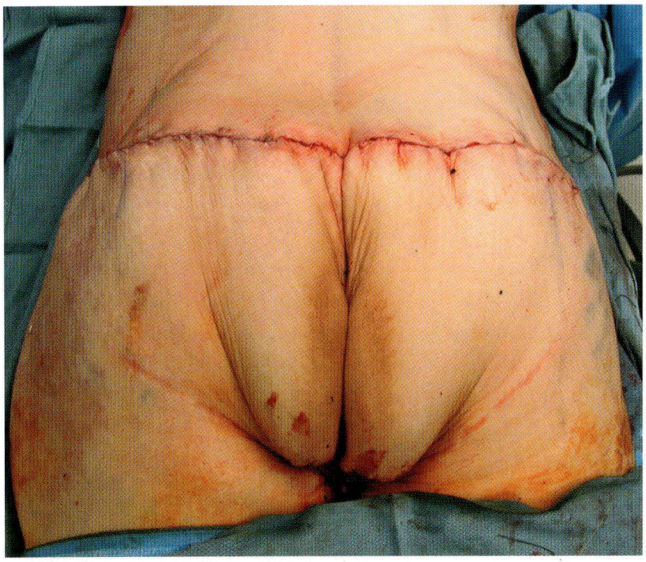

Figure 12.8 This patient displays the common buttock deformities often seen with circumferential body lift unless adjunctive procedures are performed.

Not only is the sacral triangle disrupted, but the buttock appears longer. By lowering the incision into the gluteal cleft, the sacral and gluteal aesthetic units are preserved.[31]

1. Preoperatively mark this portion of the body lift incision with the patient standing but bent forward.
2. After the patient is anesthetized and in the prone position, lower both the superior and inferior extent of the marked incision an additional 1–2 cm. This keeps the amount of skin resection unchanged, so that postoperative skin tension is not increased but the aesthetic results are improved.

Autologous gluteal augmentation

We now typically combine autologous gluteal augmentation and an inverted dart incision with the CBL. This approach solves the problem with buttock deformities that result from a body lift, and the inverted dart incision preserves gluteal aesthetic units (Fig. 12.11). Markings for gluteal autoaugmentation and the CBL are done at the same time, unless this adjunctive procedure is performed separately.

1. With the patient standing, mark the level of the mons pubis on to each buttock to identify the point of maximum projection.
2. When the patient is placed on the operating room table in the prone position, outline one of the flaps shown in Figure 12.12, making sure the flap is centered over the points of maximum projection.
3. The superior and inferior markings for the posterior portion of the lower body lift can then be adjusted to accommodate the autologous tissue. This usually requires moving the CBL markings inferiorly by a few centimeters.
4. The safety and adequacy of the skin resection must be reconfirmed. If the flap cannot be positioned appropriately or the size is inadequate to achieve good projection, gluteal augmentation should be abandoned so as to not compromise the safety of the body lift.
5. Perfusion of the autologous flap can be confirmed with a Wood's lamp and fluorescein dye.

Figure 12.13 shows deepithelialized island and moustache flaps. All three flaps have technique commonalities. The inferior skin and subcutaneous tissue are elevated to accommodate the flap volume, and flaps are anchored to the gluteal fascia at the desired level with #1 Vicryl Plus. The SFS is closed with #1 Vicryl Plus and the dermis with two layers of 3-0 Monocryl. Staples are added for reinforcement. Although the propellor and moustache flaps are similar, we no longer use the propellor flap because the moustache flap provides significantly more autologous tissue for augmentation. With both flaps, the superior half of each side is imbricated, and the postsacral tissue is left in place to provide padding. Fat grafting may be performed secondarily to refine results, but should not be necessary when a moustache flap is used.

Axilloplasty

Many patients who seek upper body contouring complain about excess skin and adipose tissue in the axillary and chest

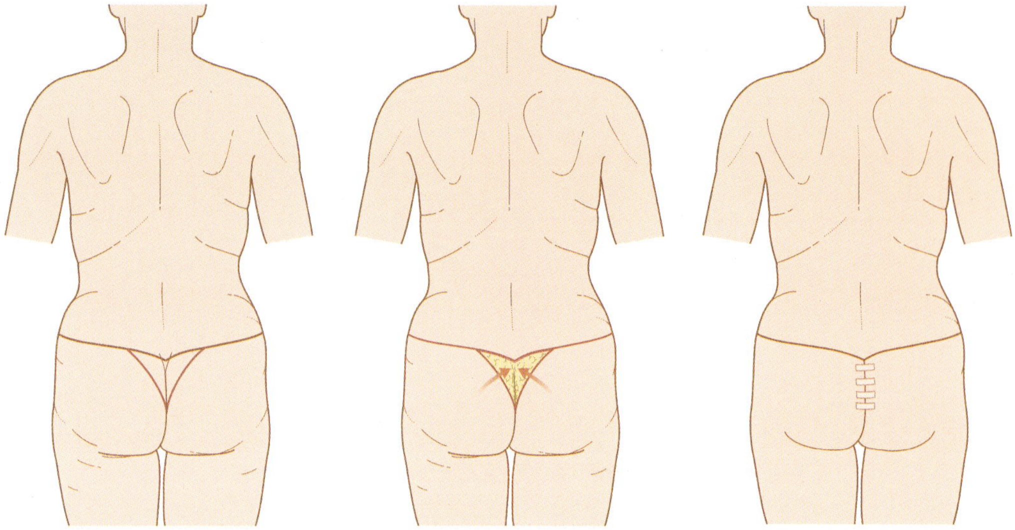

Figure 12.9 Intergluteal reduction involves excision of a triangular wedge of skin and tissue included as part of the body lift.

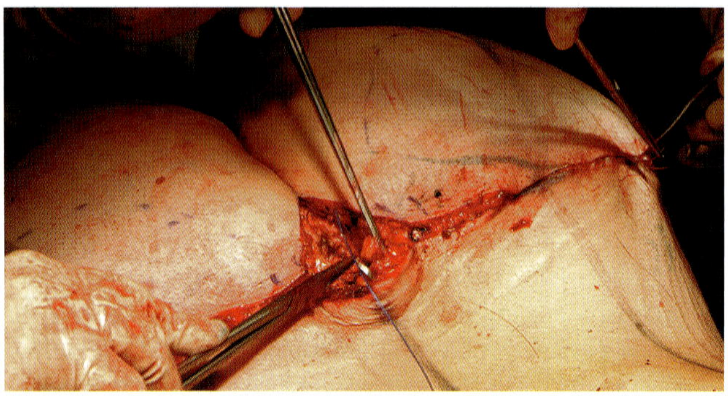

Figure 12.10 Intergluteal reduction may also be performed by incorporating a V-shaped dart of excised tissue into the body lift incision.

wall area lateral to the breast. For patients with mild skin and adipose excess in the axillary region, the best treatment is axilloplasty, which can be combined with other procedures, including mastopexy, autologous breast augmentation, brachioplasty, torsoplasty, and even CBL.

1. For marking, have the patient stand with arms fully abducted, then grasp the axillary skin excess and manually advance it in a superior-medial direction.
2. Mark the inferior point of greatest advancement (Fig. 12.14).
3. The superior marking is usually placed immediately posterior to the anterior axillary line or pectoralis border.
4. The inferior incision begins horizontally and abruptly curves superiorly to end in the axilla.
5. Preserve the axillary fascia and underlying neurovascular structures when the skin and subcutaneous tissues are resected.
6. Carefully secure the SFS to the axillary fascia prior to skin closure.

Autologous breast augmentation

The use of autologous tissue for breast augmentation can play an important role in body contouring for MWL patients because of their pronounced loss of breast tissue volume and moderate to severe skin excess. Breast recontouring typically involves restoring volume and reducing the skin envelope. The skin laxity and lack of tissue make augmentation with an implant especially challenging. Autologous augmentation represents a safe alternative that can be accomplished in one stage while simultaneously addressing surrounding deformities, as shown in Figure 12.15.

A variety of flap configurations are possible for breast autoaugmentation.

1. Mark the patient for a Passot "no vertical scar" mastopexy[32] with the superior-lateral limb extended more vertically to reach immediately behind the anterior axillary fold (Fig. 12.16).
2. The inferior-lateral limb is extended into the axilla as it would be for an axilloplasty. This allows the lateral chest wall and axillary subcutaneous tissues to be utilized as a perforator flap. The flap can be based inferiomedially and left attached to the inferior pedicle or to the chest wall if a superior-medial pedicle is preferred.[33–35]
3. Pinch and manually advance the axillary skin to determine how much tissue is available for the flap.
4. After the markings are confirmed on the operating room table, deepithelialize the axillary skin and mark the flap with methylene blue.
5. Begin dissection distally and progress medially while preserving the superficial fascia of the lateral chest wall to protect the underlying neurovascular structures.
6. Rotate the flap superior-medially and inset with absorbable sutures to create a breast mound.
7. Secure the superficial fascia of the axillary skin to the superficial fascia of the chest wall.
8. Redrape the breast skin flaps and close in the usual fashion.

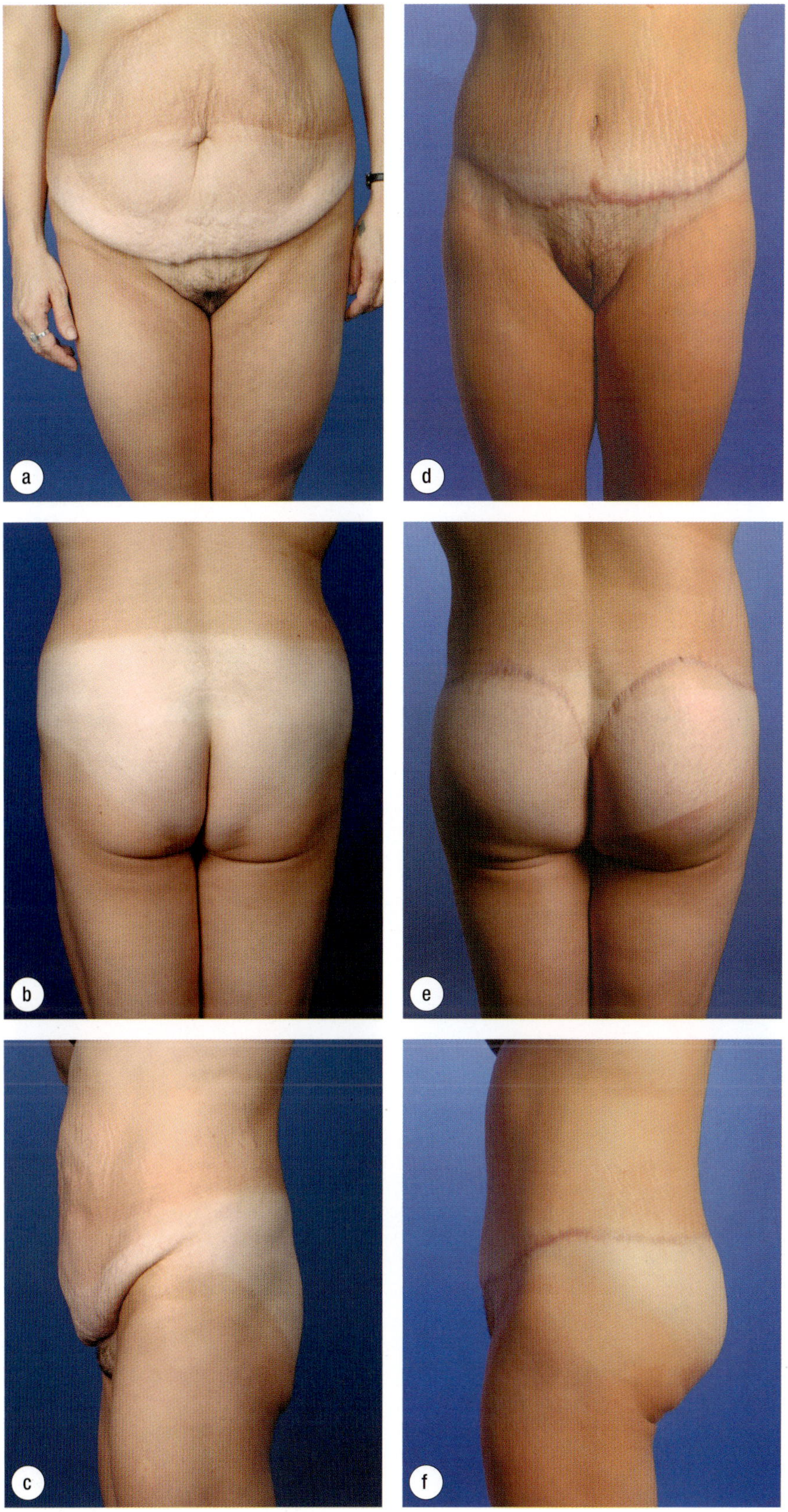

Figure 12.11 (**a–c**) This 28-year-old woman lost approximately 50 lbs (23 kg) through dieting, and her BMI went from 32 to 25 kg/m^2. (**e–f**) Five months following CBL and gluteal autoaugmentation with a moustache flap. The existing flatness of her buttocks would have been made worse with CBL alone, but the addition of the moustache flap produced good projection of the buttocks at the same level as the mons pubis, which is considered the ideal position. The inverted dart incision along with the autoaugmentation have greatly enhanced the gluteal aesthetic units.

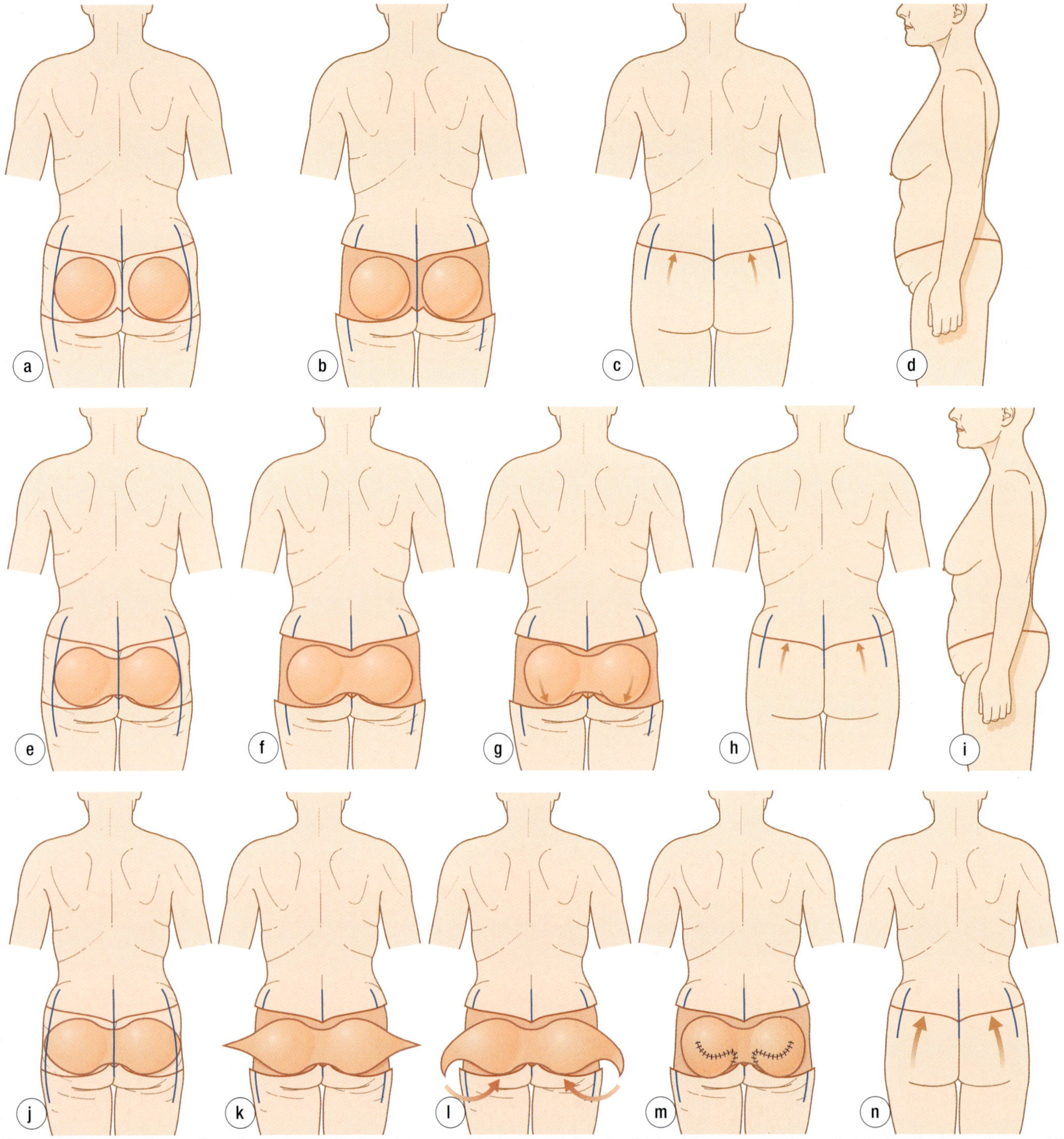

Figure 12.12 Three flap configurations are possible for autologous gluteal augmentation. (**a–d**) Island flaps produce 'normal' gluteal projection and are useful when the amount of presacral tissue is adequate. (**e–i**) A peanut flap is larger and produces mild augmentation. (**j–n**) The moustache flap provides the most tissue for gluteal augmentation.

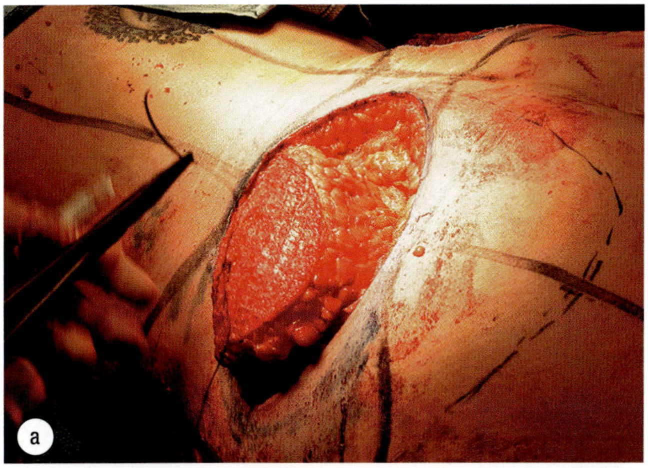

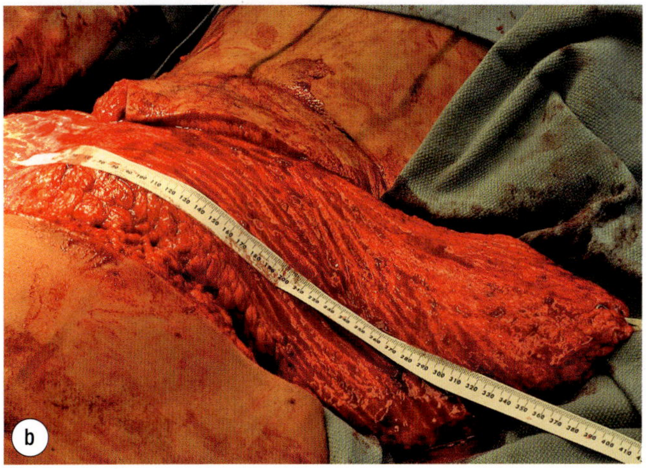

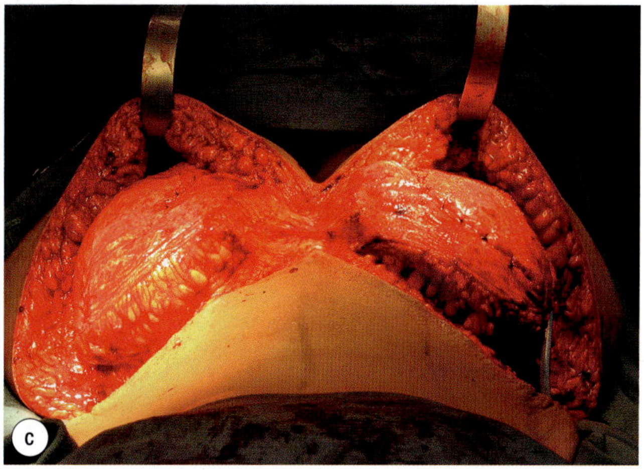

Figure 12.13 Dissection of island or moustache flap. (**a**) After island flap dissection, the dermal islands are beveled away through the fascia, and the superior half of the flap is imbricated. (**b**) For a moustache flap, the lateral extensions are dissected to accommodate the size of flap appropriate for the patient. (**c**) The "handlebars" of the moustache flap have been rotated medially and imbricated to create an anatomical mound of gluteal tissue. After creating either gluteal flap, the posterior portion of the circumferential body lift is then dissected and the inferior flap pulled superiorly to cover the new gluteal mounds.

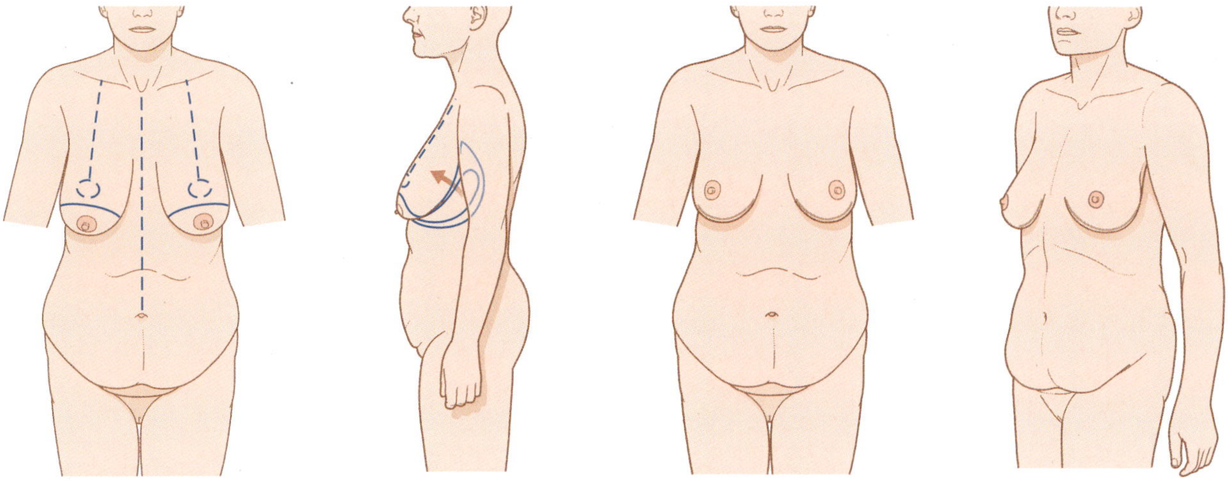

Figure 12.14 Markings for axilloplasty show rotation of the flap used for autologous breast augmentation.

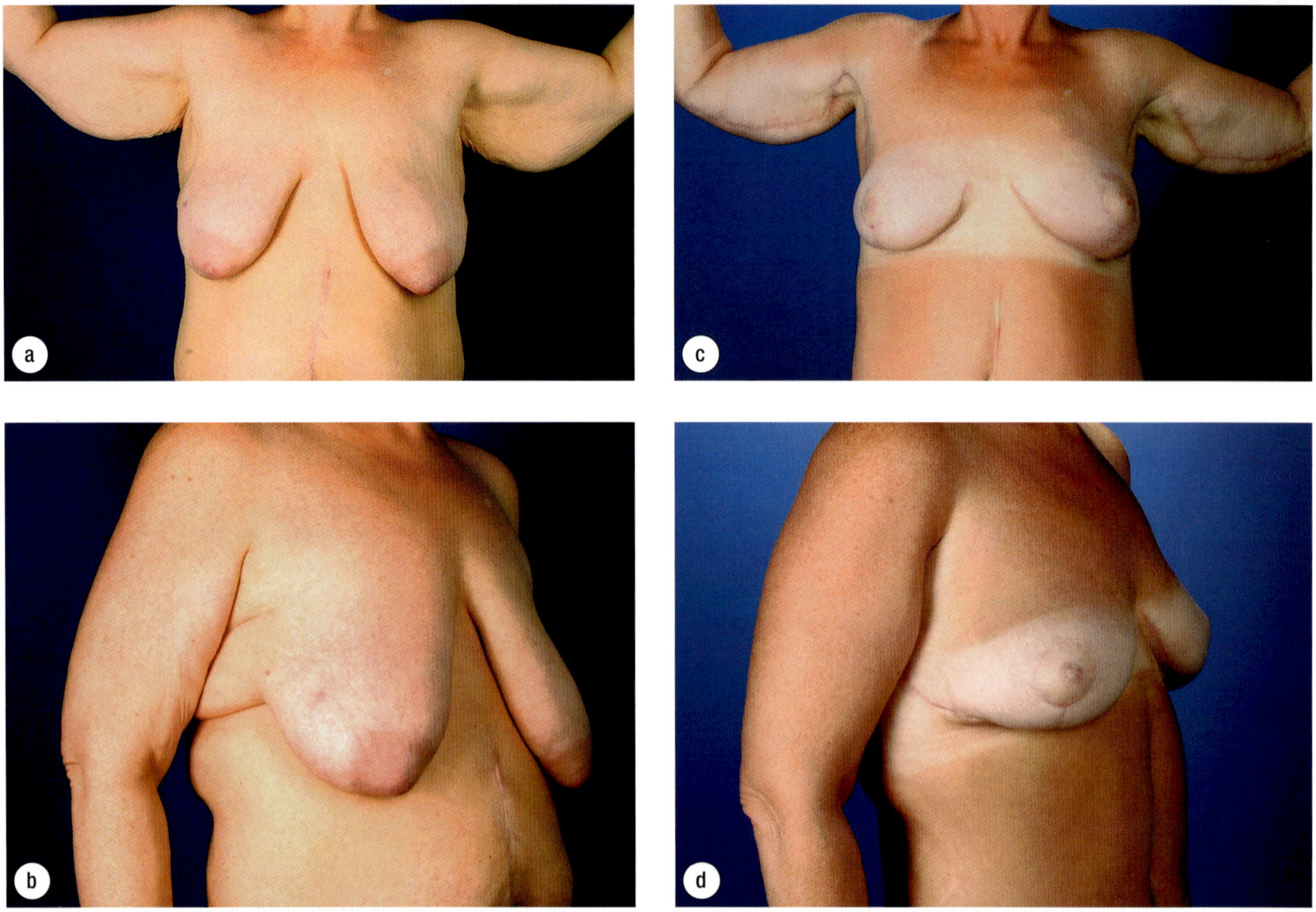

Figure 12.15 (**a** and **b**) Preoperative views of an MWL patient with a loss of breast volume and excess skin of the breasts, arms, and axilla. (**c** and **d**) Six months after autologous breast augmentation combined with axilloplasty and brachioplasty. Since this patient's surgery with a Wise pattern mastopexy incision, we have adopted the Passot "no vertical scar" mastopexy technique. The Passot technique solves the problem of lateral displacement of the nipple-areolar complex seen in this patient.

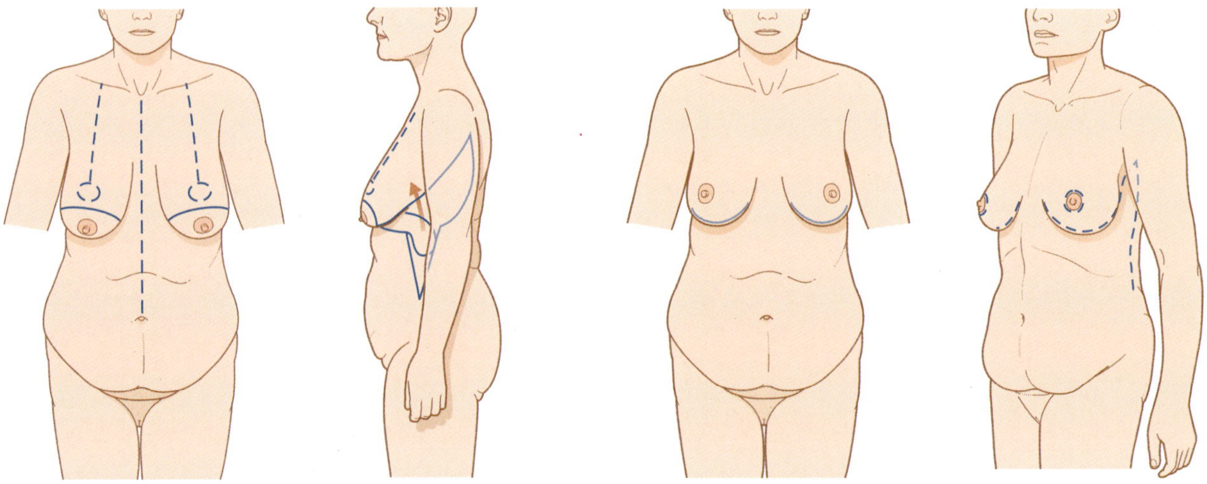

Figure 12.16 Autologous breast augmentation simultaneously enhances volume of the breast while reducing excess skin of the axilla and lateral chest wall. This illustration shows incorporation of a lateral thoracoepigastric flap for breast augmentation as well as torsoplasty. If torsoplasty is not performed, the vertical incision on the side of the torso will be much shorter.

Wound dressings

We no longer routinely use dressings on long incisions for several reasons. They impede the ability to monitor skin flaps and intervene in a timely manner should problems arise. Additionally, as edema increases over the first 1–3 days, a taped dressing becomes constrictive and can produce shearing forces that cause blistering. These blistered areas are then subject to postinflammatory hyperpigmentation, which is bothersome and long-lasting. To prevent this complication, we now use Dermabond in lieu of dressings. Dermabond 'seals' incisions and prevents bacterial contamination, permits observation of healing, and accommodates edema.

The posterior incision of a CBL, as well as intergluteal reduction and gluteal augmentation incisions, are vulnerable to another vexing problem: minor wound dehiscence. Flexed posture when the bed is in a semi-Fowler's position and early postoperative edema seem to contribute to a higher rate of minor superficial posterior wound separations. This problem has been significantly reduced by adding a scant row of reinforcing staples to the posterior aspect of the incision after Dermabond has dried. These staples are removed at the first postoperative visit to reduce permanent 'track' marks on the skin.

OPTIMIZING OUTCOMES

Lipoplasty is an essential component of body contouring in MWL patients and can play a variety of roles, especially for debulking before excision and for refinement of results in a staged procedure following excision. In many instances, liposuction reduces the need for excision or minimizes excision size.

Aesthetic outcomes in MWL body contouring are in large part significantly related to BMI. Because better results are achievable in patients with a lower BMI, surgeons are wise to begin incorporating adjunctive techniques with lower BMI patients. As experience grows, adjunctive procedures can be added for patients with higher BMIs and more complex deformities.

The types of adjunctive procedures described here can dramatically improve the aesthetic results of body contouring and produce high levels of patient satisfaction.

Perioperative management is critical in body contouring. Proper fluid management must be carefully addressed in LVL. In addition to stressing the maintenance of normothermia, we have adopted more aggressive VTE prophylaxis because MWL patients are at increased risk for this dangerous and potentially fatal complication.

Counsel patients and family members about expected difficulty with routine daily living tasks after surgery, especially if combined procedures are performed. Patients may initially need assistance for transferring in and out of bed, taking care of hygiene, and following early ambulation guidelines. Equipment to help with such tasks can be rented at surgical supply stores. Disposable supplies such as adult diapers, moist wipes, anesthetic or antibiotic creams/ointment, and peroxide are also useful during the first days after discharge.

POSTOPERATIVE CARE

Massive weight loss patients, including those undergoing LVL, demand close postoperative scrutiny. They should be kept in a medical facility for at least one night to make sure that they have fluids carefully managed, are hemodynamically stable, and do not require transfusion. On average, our multiprocedure patients prefer 2–3 days of hospitalization. Guidelines for the immediate postoperative period follow.

- Continue forced air and fluid warming in the recovery room. Once on the floor, extra warming should not be necessary.
- Continue fluid resuscitation until oral intake is sufficient. The goal is to ensure adequate urine output, a systolic blood pressure greater than 100 mmHg, and a pulse rate below 100 per minute. This generally means 125–150 mL of crystalloid per hour. If hypovolemia is evident, treat with a crystalloid fluid challenge of 500 mL/h. Use diuretics to treat fluid overload, which is characterized by hypertension, jugular vein distension, full bounding pulse, cough, shortness of breath, or moist crackles on auscultation of the lungs. If not addressed, fluid overload may progress to pulmonary edema and congestive heart failure.
- Apply topical 70% dimethyl sulfoxide (DMSO) to improve tissue perfusion if ischemia is noted near incisions in the intraoperative or early postoperative period.[36] DMSO should be reapplied every 4 h until circulation in the area improves. (This is an off-label use.)
- Start the diet with clear liquids and advance as tolerated, keeping in mind that many gastric bypass patients cannot tolerate high-sugar diets. Pay particular attention to protein intake in a suitable form. Close communication with the patient's bariatric surgeon facilitates consultation if a general surgical issue should present.
- Check hematocrit and hemoglobin immediately postoperatively and at 12 and 24 h later to assess red blood cell loss. Many LVL and MWL patients will manifest an anemia with a hematocrit below 30%. In these cases, a fluid challenge of 500 mL/h may lower the pulse rate and raise blood pressure. Increasing the amount of crystalloid might produce further hemodilution. If a patient becomes tachycardic or develops orthostatic hypotension, transfusion may be necessary. Two units of packed red blood cells are required when the hematocrit is below 23%.
- Maintain patients on an F_iO_2 of 80% through a 'non-rebreather' mask for the first 2 h after surgery to decrease the risk of infection, minimize nausea, and ensure optimal tissue oxygenation. Then switch to standard oxygen through a nasal cannula for 24 h.
- Continue prophylactic antibiotics for 24 h after the preoperative dose. No studies have determined that prophylactic antibiotics administrated for more than 24 h after surgery are of any benefit, but they should be continued if infection is present.

- Continue DVT prophylaxis with intermittent pneumatic compression devices and stress early mobilization. Intermittent pneumatic compression devices should be removed and replaced after walking until the patient is discharged. Encourage patients to begin ambulation the day after surgery. If appropriate, continue anticoagulation prophylaxis with LMWH or fondaparinux for 1–4 weeks after surgery or until fully ambulatory.
- Manage pain with morphine or meperidine (Demerol) patient-controlled analgesia and/or oral narcotics as needed. Gradually wean patients to non-narcotic pain relievers. Some body-contouring patients report chronic pain after surgery that may result from nerve injury. Gabapentin (Neurontin) and/or amitriptyline (Elavil) are sometimes effective for treating the type of burning pain patients describe.
- Discontinue the Foley catheter early on the first postoperative day to encourage ambulation.
- Order a complete blood count and basic metabolic panel for the morning after surgery. Glucose monitoring may also be warranted. Common electrolyte abnormalities that follow LVL include lowered sodium, potassium, and blood urea nitrogen levels in the early postoperative period.[34] Liver enzyme testing has revealed significantly lowered levels of albumin and protein that are consistent with hemodilution and lowered blood viscosity. In addition, levels of plasma aminotransferases significantly increased in LVL patients, a possible indication of injury to adipocytes or skeletal muscles or hepatocellular damage.[37] Creatine kinase levels also may be elevated.
- Leave drains in place until output is in the range of 30–50 cc in 24 h. If drainage is prolonged, perform sclerosis with a high-concentration doxycycline solution (100 mg per 10 cc of 0.9% saline solution) infused through the drain. Prior to sclerosis, infuse with 0.5% marcaine for anesthesia. Clamp the drain for 15 min and then return to suction. Because the doxycycline concentration is higher than recommended for infusion, it must be specially ordered for off-label use. Infusion can sometimes be painful, and analgesics are recommended. Injection into a seroma cavity can be performed, but it must not be into the subcutaneous tissue because doxycycline can cause fat and skin necrosis.
- Occasional massage therapy is often useful to help speed the resolution of edema following liposuction.
- Compressive binders and garments should not be used routinely in the immediate postoperative period, because they may interfere with already-challenged perfusion of skin and/or flaps and impair the ability to monitor blood flow. Drains inadvertently placed beneath a binder can cause pressure necrosis. Later in the postoperative course, it may be prudent to add a compression garment to reduce swelling, dead space, and discomfort associated with ambulation.

COMPLICATIONS AND THEIR MANAGEMENT

Liposuction

Recent statistics place the rate of significant complications secondary to lipoplasty in the range of 0.3%[16] to 1.8%.[38,39] Major complications include:

- hemorrhage (usually resulting from visceral perforation),
- hematoma (particularly in the retroperitoneal space if the fascia is penetrated),
- skin or fat necrosis (major) or skin slough,
- infection,
- necrotizing fasciitis,
- pulmonary edema (resulting from fluid overload),
- lidocaine toxicity,
- DVT,
- PE,
- fat embolus,
- cardiac arrhythmia, and
- death.

Minor complications are:

- contour irregularities,
- scarring,
- prolonged edema,
- paresthesias,
- anemia,
- hypovolemia,
- hemodilution that requires blood transfusion, and
- thermal injury from ultrasonic energy.

Seroma is perhaps the most common complication of liposuction, but its frequency can be greatly reduced with drains. There is no evidence of increased complication rates when aspirate volumes of ≥5000 cc are compared with volumes <5000 cc.[16,40]

Massive weight loss patients who undergo debulking liposuction with or without excisional procedures have the potential to develop the typical complications of liposuction plus some additional risks. Contour irregularities such as wrinkles, lumps, or dents occur in almost all MWL patients, but they are generally tolerant of such irregularities if the possibility has been discussed preoperatively. If excessive skin laxity remains after liposuction—and it usually does—staged excisional procedures are the only option for correction. Some patients, however, accept the skin excess if the fat debulking is sufficient to make them more physically comfortable.

The risk of lidocaine toxicity becomes real if the total delivered dose exceeds 35 mg/kg. Lidocaine toxicity can be completely avoided by omitting it from the infusion solution. Kenkel and colleagues determined that only about 10% of infiltrated lidocaine is aspirated, and lidocaine toxicity may not manifest for 8–16 h after surgery.[41,42] The time to peak for the lidocaine metabolite monoethylglycinexylidide may be even longer, up to 28 h. (Because lidocaine is metabolized in the liver, it should not be used in patients with liver dysfunction.) Therefore the period of potential lidocaine toxicity lasts longer than is commonly believed. However, the analgesic effect of lidocaine is not long-lasting. Kenkel et al. found that even though lidocaine is present in blood for up to 18 h, it does not remain at a therapeutic dose in local tissues for more than 4–8 h. Most surgeries performed in MWL patients require general anesthesia because procedures are lengthy and rigorous monitoring is essential. Patients receiving LVL or liposuction plus excision are going to require opiate analgesia postoperatively, as well as hospitalization. Therefore the need for lidocaine is non-existent in these patients.

Fat embolism has been reported with liposuction, although its frequency is unknown. Estimates place this complication in the range of 1:100 000 to 1:300 000.[43] Fat embolization occurs when small globules of fat migrate through the venous circulation to the lungs. It usually does not produce significant symptoms unless there is a large amount of embolization, but symptoms may include tachycardia, tachypnea, elevated temperature, hypoxemia, hypocapnia, or thrombocytopenia. In contrast, fat embolism syndrome is an inflammatory and biochemical condition associated with free fatty acids released into the blood that produce a syndrome of petechial rash, respiratory distress, and cerebral dysfunction approximately 24–72 h after surgery. A suggestion for preventing fat accumulation and emboli is continuation of intravenous fluids for 24 h after surgery to flush fatty material through the circulatory system.[40]

Blindness has been recently reported in patients undergoing liposuction who develop a significant anemia and decreased retinal circulation.[44] This makes it very important to monitor the hematocrit in these patients and keep them well hydrated and volume expanded to avoid hypotension.

Skin necrosis is uncommon in liposuction, except in diabetic patients and people who have scars from previous procedures. Because many MWL patients meet these criteria, they should be warned in advance of the necrosis risk.

Mons reduction

If undermining can be avoided, postoperative complications such as skin necrosis and delayed wound healing are uncommon because tissues in this area are very well vascularized. However, lymphatic drainage is compromised when mons reduction is combined with a CBL or thigh lift. This results in prolonged postoperative lymphedema and hyperemia that can resemble cellulitis. Empiric antibiotic therapy can be used but is often unnecessary. Sensation is temporarily altered but usually resolves. Hypersensitivity of the clitoris in women can be a problem if aggressive lifting and reduction of the mons are performed. It may improve over time but can lead to permanent discomfort. Should this be a problem, desensitization creams can be helpful.

Intergluteal reduction

The most significant complication associated with intergluteal reduction is delayed wound healing. This region is a 'watershed' of blood supply that may become compromised by overresection and undue tension on the closure. Having the patient bend over when marking the central posterior incision adds an additional safety margin. Closure of 'dead space' with a layered closure helps prevent seromas that could lead to wound separation. Covering the anal region with a povidone–iodine (Betadine)-soaked towel prevents contamination of the sutures during closure, and sealing the incision with Dermabond reduces fecal contamination. Careful attention to cutting the deep SFS sutures close to the knot helps lessen suture burden, extrusion (spitting), and potential infection. This procedure can be eliminated by incorporating an inverted dart incision into the CBL and/or gluteal augmentation.

Autologous gluteal augmentation

Complications directly related to autologous gluteal augmentation are relatively uncommon in our practice. The robustness of vascularization in the area produces good flap viability, which can be confirmed with a Wood's lamp and fluorescein dye. Small areas of fat necrosis are typically allowed to resorb on their own. Seromas due to large dead spaces can be avoided by putting drains in the most dependent portion of the gluteal pocket. If seroma does occur, management is important because it can precipitate wound dehiscence. (Sclerosis with doxycycline was described earlier.) We do not routinely use quilting sutures in this area, but they may be helpful.

Delayed wound-healing rates for our CBL patients with and without gluteal augmentation do not appear to be significantly different. Nonetheless, inferior flap undermining and tension on the closure increases when gluteal augmentation is added, and this can lead to wound-healing problems plus anorectal hypersensitivity and maceration due to overexposure of the anus. Maceration is usually self-limited and can be managed by topical anesthetics such as hydrocortisone (Anusol), a 'doughnut' cushion for sitting, frequent positional changes, high-fiber diet, sitz baths, or baby wipes for cleansing.

Until gaining experience with gluteal autoaugmentation, we advise careful preoperative planning and conservatively sized island flaps to avoid overresection that may lead to wound-healing problems, skin necrosis, and dehiscence. Although this may limit the quality of initial results, aesthetic outcomes will significantly improve with experience. Secondary excisional touch-up procedures such as adjunctive flank liposuction and infragluteal fold excisions can further refine aesthetic outcomes.

Axilloplasty

The critical neurovascular structures of the axilla are less likely to be injured if surgical dissection remains above the axillary fascia. Inevitably, the fascia will be violated from time to time. The structures most likely to be injured are the intercostobrachial nerve, the lower roots of the brachial plexus, and the axillary lymphatics. Injury to the intercostobrachial nerve can be treated by neurorrhaphy or proximal transposition. Because brachial plexus injury is more problematic, it is best avoided; if injury does occur, prompt consultation with a peripheral nerve specialist is recommended.

Inadvertent excision or transection of lymphatics results in lymphorrhea and lymphoceles, but these can be prevented by tying off the afferent channels if nodes are involved in the tissue to be resected. If problems occur, distally inject lymphazurin blue and surgically localize the involved afferent channels with ligation.[45] Sclerosis of a lymphocele with high-dose doxycycline (100 mg per 10 cc of 0.9% normal saline) is sometimes helpful. Wound dehiscence in the axilla results from undue tension caused by overexcision. Anchoring the SFS to the axillary fascia with #1 Vicryl Plus should help reduce tension on the skin closure.

Autologous breast augmentation

Complications from autologous breast augmentation utilizing a lateral thoracoepigastric flap in conjunction with axilloplasty and mastopexy can largely be avoided with careful preoperative planning. Skin excision with a Passot "no vertical scar" technique makes redistribution of the axillary skin and lateral breast flap easier than when a Wise pattern excision is used. It also reduces the problem of lateral displacement of the nipple-areolar complex. It is often helpful to mark the lateral breast flap immediately posterior to the anterior axillary line or the pectoralis major muscle border. Doing so leaves a small margin of extra lateral breast flap skin that helps prevent overresection. In addition, careful dissection and leaving a layer of adipose tissue over the lateral chest wall prevents injury to the fourth and fifth intercostal nerves. Once the autologous tissue is added to the breast mound, tension on the breast skin can be significant. Meticulous pedicle dissection avoids compromising the circulation of the nipple areolar complex.

CONCLUSION

Almost all MWL patients will benefit greatly from liposuction added as part of the staged procedures often required to achieve optimal aesthetic results. Circumferential debulking liposuction is especially useful for patients who have excess subcutaneous fat, particularly if it is distributed throughout the body, as is typical in patients with a BMI of 30 kg/m^2 or higher. In this context, LVL can have a major impact on final body contour if performed as the first stage. Other patients have localized lipodystrophies that are easily treated with liposuction. For patients who prefer not to undergo multiple staged excisional surgeries, liposuction offers an alternative with few risks and quick recovery time. If too much excess skin remains after liposuction, an excisional procedure can be scheduled.

The complexity of deformities after MWL is unprecedented in plastic surgery. Body contouring in this population challenges our ingenuity, creativity, and surgical skills on a regular basis. The adjunctive techniques described here have enabled us to improve clinical outcomes and enhance satisfaction among our patients.

REFERENCES

1. Brauman D. Liposuction abdominoplasty: an evolving concept. Plast Reconstr Surg 2003; 112:288–301.
2. Cárdenas-Camarena L, González LE. Large-volume liposuction and extensive abdominoplasty: a feasible alternative for improving body shape. Plast Reconstr Surg 1998; 102:1698–1707.
3. Hunstad JP. Body contouring in the obese patient. Clin Plast Surg 1996; 23:647–670.
4. Vogt PA. Brachial suction-assisted lipoplasty and brachioplasty. Aesthetic Surg J 2001; 21:164–167.
5. Abramson DL. Ultrasound-assisted abdominoplasty: combining modalities in a safe and effective technique. Plast Reconstr Surg 2003; 112:898–902.
6. Avelar JM. Abdominoplasty without panniculus undermining and resection: analysis and 3-year follow-up of 97 consecutive cases. Aesthetic Surg J 2002; 22:16–25.
7. Saldanha OR, de Souza Pinto EB, Matos WN, et al. Lipoabdominoplasty without undermining. Aesthetic Surg J 2001; 21:518–526.
8. Matarasso A. Liposuction as an adjunct to a full abdominoplasty revisited. Plast Reconstr Surg 2000; 106:1197–1202.
9. Iverson RE, Lynch DJ, ASPS Committee on Patient Safety. Practice advisory on liposuction. Plast Reconstr Surg 2004; 113:1478–1490.
10. Alvarez-Leite JI. Nutrient deficiencies secondary to bariatric surgery. Curr Opin Clin Nutr Metab Care 2004; 7:569–575.
11. Goldberg MA. Perioperative epoetin alfa increases red blood cell mass and reduces exposure to transfusions: results of randomized clinical trials. Semin Hematol 1997; 34:41–47.
12. Sessler DI, Akça O. Nonpharmacological prevention of surgical wound infections. Healthc Epidemiol 2002: 35:1397–1404.
13. Mangram AJ, Horan TC, Pearson ML, et al. Guideline for prevention of surgical site infection, 1999. Hospital Infection Control Practices Advisory Committee. Infect Control Hosp Epidemiol 1999; 20(4):250–278.
14. Geerts WH, Pineo GF, Heit JA, et al. Prevention of venous thromboembolism: the Seventh ACCP Conference on Antithrombotic and Thrombolytic Therapy. Chest 2004; 126:338S–400S.
15. Young VL, Watson ME. The need for venous thromboembolism (VTE) prophylaxis in plastic surgery. Aesthetic Surg J 2006; 26:157–175.
16. Rohrich RJ, Beran SJ. Is liposuction safe? Plast Reconstr Surg 1999; 104:819–822.
17. Nijkeuter M, Huisman MV. Pentasaccharides in the prophylaxis and treatment of venous thromboembolism: a systematic review. Curr Opin Pulm Med 2004; 10:338–344.
18. Sazama K, DeChristopher PJ, Dodd R, et al. Practice parameter for the recognition, management, and prevention of adverse consequences of blood transfusion. Arch Pathol Lab Med 2000; 124:61–70.
19. Matarasso A. Superwet anesthesia redefines large volume liposuction. Aesthetic Surg J 1997; 17(6):358–364.
20. Trott SA, Beran SJ, Rohrich R, et al. Safety considerations and fluid resuscitation in liposuction: an analysis of 53 consecutive patients. Plast Reconstr Surg 1998; 102:2220–2229.
21. Karmo FR, Milan MF, Silbergleit A. Blood loss in major liposuction procedures: a comparison study using suction-assisted versus ultrasonically-assisted lipoplasty. Plast Reconstr Surg 2001; 108:241–247.
22. Cárdenas-Camarena L, Tobar-Losada A, Lacouture AM. Large-volume circumferential liposuction with tumescent technique: a sure and viable procedure. Plast Reconstr Surg 1999; 104:1887–1899.
23. Brown SA, Lipschitz AH, Kenkel JM, et al. Pharmacokinetics and safety of epinephrine use in liposuction. Plast Reconstr Surg 2004; 114:756–763.
24. Gupta SC, Khiabani KT, Stephenson LL, et al. Effect of liposuction on skin perfusion. Plast Reconstr Surg 2002; 110:1748–1751.
25. Hasen KV, Greve S, Casas LA. Differences in wound healing between ultrasound-assisted lipoplasty and suction-assisted lipoplasty in in-

verted T-pattern breast reduction surgery and chest wall contouring. Aesthetic Surg J 2001; 21:27–31.

26. Blondeel PN, Derks D, Roche N, et al. The effect of ultrasound-assisted liposuction and conventional liposuction on the perforator vessels in the lower abdominal wall. Br J Plast Surg 2003; 56:266–271.
27. Cedidi CC, Berger A. Severe abdominal wall necrosis after ultrasound-assisted liposuction. Aesthetic Plast Surg 2002; 26:20–22.
28. Young VL, Brandon HJ. The physics of suction-assisted lipoplasty. Aesthetic Surg J 2004; 24:206–210.
29. Matarasso A, Wallach S. Abdominal contour surgery: treating all aesthetic units, including the mons pubis. Aesthetic Surg J 2001; 21(2):111–119.
30. Cuenca-Guerra R, Quezada J. What makes buttocks beautiful? A review and classification of the determinants of gluteal beauty and the surgical techniques to achieve them. Aesthetic Plast Surg 2004; 28:340–347.
31. Centeno RF. Gluteal aesthetic unit classification: a tool to improve outcomes in body contouring. Aesthetic Surg J 2006; 26:200–208.
32. Lalonde DH, Lalonde J, French R. The no vertical scar breast reduction: a minor variation that allows you to remove vertical scar portion of the inferior pedicle Wise pattern T scar. Aesth Plast Surg 2003; 27:335–344.
33. Hurwitz DJ, Golla D. Breast reshaping after massive weight loss. Semin Plast Surg 2004; 18:179–187.
34. Van Landuyt K, Hamdi M, Blondeel P, et al. Autologous breast augmentation by pedicled perforator flaps. Ann Plast Surg 2004; 53:322–327.
35. Lossing C, Elander A, Gewalli F, et al. The lateral thoracodorsal flap in breast reconstruction: a long term follow up study. Scand J Plast Reconstr Surg 2001; 35:183–192.
36. Young VL, Boswell CB, Centeno RF, et al. DMSO: applications in plastic surgery. Aesthetic Surg J 2005; 25:201–209.
37. Lipschitz AH, Kenkel JM, Luby M, et al. Electrolyte and plasma enzyme analyses during large-volume liposuction. Plast Reconstr Surg 2004; 114:766–775.
38. Gilliland MD, Commons GW, Halperin B. Safety issues in ultrasound-assisted large-volume lipoplasty. Clin Plast Surg 1999; 26:317–335.
39. Matarasso A, Hutchinson O. Liposuction. JAMA 2001; 285(3):266–268.
40. Cárdenas-Camarena L. Lipoaspiration and its complications: a safe operation. Plast Reconstr Surg 2003; 112:1435–1441.
41. Kenkel JM, Lipschitz AH, Shepherd G, et al. Pharmacokinetics and safety of lidocaine and monoethylglycinexylidide in liposuction: a microdialysis study. Plast Reconstr Surg 2004; 114:516–524.
42. Matarasso A. Lidocaine in ultrasonic-assisted lipoplasty. Clin Plast Surg 1999; 26(3):431–439.
43. Grazer FM, de Jong RH. Fatal outcomes from liposuction: census survey of cosmetic surgeons. Plast Reconstr Surg 2000; 105:436–446.
44. Foroozan R, Varon J. Bilateral anterior ischemic optic neuropathy after liposuction. J Neuroophthalmol 2004; 24:211–213.
45. Stadelmann WK. Intraoperative lymphatic mapping to treat groin lymphorrhea complicating an elective medial thigh lift. Ann Plast Surg 2002; 48:205–208.

INDEX

F

G

H

I

J

L

M

N